Citizenship and Mental Health

Citizenship and Mental Health

Michael Rowe

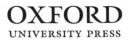

OXFORD
UNIVERSITY PRESS

OXFORD
UNIVERSITY PRESS

Oxford University Press is a department of the University of
Oxford. It furthers the University's objective of excellence in research,
scholarship, and education by publishing worldwide.

Oxford   New York
Auckland   Cape Town   Dar es Salaam   Hong Kong   Karachi
Kuala Lumpur   Madrid   Melbourne   Mexico City   Nairobi
New Delhi   Shanghai   Taipei   Toronto

With offices in
Argentina   Austria   Brazil   Chile   Czech Republic   France   Greece
Guatemala   Hungary   Italy   Japan   Poland   Portugal   Singapore
South Korea   Switzerland   Thailand   Turkey   Ukraine   Vietnam

Oxford is a registered trademark of Oxford University Press
in the UK and certain other countries.

Published in the United States of America by
Oxford University Press
198 Madison Avenue, New York, NY 10016

© Oxford University Press 2015

Library of Congress Cataloging-in-Publication Data
Rowe, Michael
Citizenship and mental health / Michael Rowe.
   pages cm.
Includes bibliographical references.
ISBN 978–0–19–935538–9
1. Homeless persons—Mental health.   2. Homeless persons—Mental health services.
3. Community mental health services.   4. Citizenship.   I. Title.
RC451.4.H64R69 2015
362.196890086'942–dc23
2014028624

9 8 7 6 5 4 3 2 1
Printed in the United States of America
on acid-free paper

to Kai Erikson, friend and mentor

CONTENTS

Acknowledgments   ix

Preface   xiii

1. Introduction: Citizenship Roots in Outreach Work   1

2. Citizenship and Community Organizing: *Citizens*   10

3. Citizenship and Individuals: The *Citizens Project*, Early   35

4. Citizenship and Individuals: The *Citizens Project*, Ongoing   63

5. Going to the Source: Citizenship Measure Development and Validation   94

6. Taking Citizenship to Scale: The *Citizens Collaborative* I   114

7. Taking Citizenship to Scale: The *Citizens Collaborative* II   134

8. Taking Citizenship to Scale: The *Citizens Collaborative* III   160

9. A Model of Citizenship and Mental Health   189

10. Conclusion   200

Notes   205

Bibliography   221

Index   233

ACKNOWLEDGMENTS

An author of a book on citizenship rooted in practice ought to have some friends to thank. I have many.

The encounters of people who were homeless and mental health outreach workers pointed the way to citizenship and mental health. Therefore, I owe thanks to all the staff and clients of the New Haven outreach team during my tenure as project director from 1994 to 2000. Later, hundreds of participants in citizenship interventions and studies contributed to the learning that persuaded me this book would be worth writing.

Patty Benedict and Lezley TwoBears, who have run two major citizenship projects from 1997 to the present, delved into their back pages for stories of people and events otherwise lost to our official records. Madelon Baranoski showed me how the limitations of diverting people from criminal justice to mental health systems of care, a good thing in itself that failed to address clients' aspirations to become valued community members, paralleled the limitations of outreach work that inspired the citizenship approach in the first place, thus giving the work its second start.

Larry Davidson, Michael Sernyak, Robert Cole, Ezra Griffith, Michael Hoge, and Kyle Pedersen, like Patty and Madelon colleagues in the Yale Department of Psychiatry, have encouraged and supported me and offered wise counsel. Alison Cunningham generously gave a home and her own participation to several citizenship projects at Columbus House. Margaret Bailey is an invaluable partner in our current efforts to develop citizenship-oriented care at the Connecticut Mental Health Center in New Haven.

Former Commissioner Thomas Kirk, Commissioner Patricia Rehmer, and Chief Operating Officer Paul DiLeo of the Connecticut Department of Mental Health and Addiction Services have funded many of our citizenship programs and gone well beyond that with their ideas and enthusiasm. Jean-François Pelletier of the University of Montreal and Yale has been stalwart in expanding the scope of citizenship and mental health to Montreal and internationally. Then-State Senator, now Mayor of New Haven Toni Harp and State Representative Toni Walker have also championed this work.

Research team members and investigators, administrative and program staff, volunteers, student film makers and committee members for citizenship projects have enriched the citizenship efforts that I report on here. They are Nathan Aguilar, Kimberly Antunes, Margaret Bailey, Chyrell Bellamy, Patty Benedict, Lily Berneker, Robert Bessard, William Bromage, Stacy Brown, Lucile Bruce, Josephine Buchanan, Matthew Chinman, Ashley Clayton, Mark Costa,

Mary Dansinghani, Elizabeth Flanagan, Matthew Gambino, Donald Gildersleeve, Kevin Johnson, Larry Davidson, Kimberly Guy, Annie Harper, Yolanda Herring, Jeffrey Johnson, Bret Kloos, Nancy Leisa, Alice Mattison, Rebecca Miller, Paul Mitchell, Victoria Molta, Christina Decker Morris, Lorraine Myers, Luz Ocasio, Maria O'Connell, Patty Osborn, Rachel Payne, Kyle Pedersen, Jean-François Pelletier, Michelle Piczko, Allison N. Ponce, Raymond Raw, Tomas Reyes, Hilary Rogers, Johnny Santos, Lesley Schwab, Jordan Sloshower, Mary Snyder, Erica Stern, Dawn Stewart, Thomas Styron, Lezley TwoBears, Timothy Walsh, Barbara Wells, Devone Williams, Bridgett Williamson, and Summer Willoughby. I apologize to those whom faulty memory has caused me to leave out or who joined us after this book went to press.

My co-authors on citizenship papers and reports are well represented in the text and references for this book, which would be poorer and thinner without their ideas, analysis, and writing. They are Neil Aggarwal, Kimberly Antunes, Madelon Baranoski, Chyrell Bellamy, Patty Benedict, Ryun Black, Josephine Buchanan, Matthew Chinman, Ashley Clayton, Anne Boyle Cross, Larry Davidson, Paul Falzer, Charles Garvin, Vincent Girard, Annie Harper, Bret Kloos, Christopher Jewell, Rebecca Miller, Jenny Noia, Maria O'Connell, Jean-François Pelletier, Allison N. Ponce, Lesley Schwab, David Sells, Michael Sernyak, Erica Stern, Lezley TwoBears, and Melissa Wieland.

Christ Church and Father David Cobb have provided free program space for the *Citizens Project* for the past 14 years. David O'Sullivan of the Community Soup Kitchen has shared his storage space there with us, left meals for students, and freely given of his and his staff's time for special citizenship events. What good works they've done. Daniel Rowe carefully proofread and edited the manuscript before I sent it off to Dana Bliss, my editor at Oxford University Press, who guided and cheered me on, gave me an extension when it was clear I wouldn't meet my first deadline, and supported the writing of this book and the basic premises behind it.

In addition to the Connecticut Department of Mental Health and Addiction Services, I am grateful to a number of organizations and institutes that have funded citizenship projects since the late 1990s. They are the National Institute of Mental Health, the Yale Institution for Social and Policy Studies, the Melville Charitable Trust, the Carolynn Foundation, the CMHC Foundation, Columbus House, the Connecticut Mental Health Center, the Haymarket Foundation, Citizens Bank, and the United Way.

I came to sociology after working in human services and the arts for years. I was happy to be accepted into the program at Yale, with little knowledge of the faculty in sociology but with the conviction that I'd been given a chance to combine my work and intellectual-creative lives. Early on during my first semester, a fellow student, Paul, and I walked across town to the School of Epidemiology and Public Health on a tip that we could find an easier introduction to statistics course there than was being offered on our side of town. We didn't find one, but weaving our way through the building we chanced on the school's library, and a book sale. Paul picked up a book, said "Kai Erikson's book," and showed it to me. The book was *Everything in its Path*, and Kai Erikson was Chairman of the Department of Sociology at the time. I bought it. By the end of the day I knew I'd come to the right place and that I had to become a student of the man who wrote it. Recently rereading *A New Species of Trouble*, another Erikson masterwork, I treated myself to another object lesson in Professor Erikson's ability to communicate the incommunicable in collective disasters through his superb prose, his imagination and probing mind, and through making room for the testimony of people who experienced those disasters at a moment in time but continue to experience them across it. I've been fortunate to keep in touch with him over the years through our periodic lunches at Caffé Bravo on Orange Street. And one other thing—when you read his books you've met the man, and when you meet the man you've been introduced to his books. I'm honored to dedicate mine to him.

My son Jesse died in 1995 after the signal events in the development of the New Haven outreach team that led me to my citizenship work had occurred. My and my family's experience with Jesse during his three-month hospitalization conferred citizenship on us in a country no one would choose to visit but that settles deep inside you, as has our memory of him and his whole life. I'm indebted to them, too—my wife Gail, my son Daniel, and my daughter Cassandra. A citizen needs a home. They give me a good one.

Thank you all.

PREFACE

Citizenship is a way of thinking about membership in society. My work as a medical sociologist on the topic began, before I recognized it, with mental health outreach to people who are homeless. Recognition came late for me because our iterative learning process—how to find people who were homeless with mental illnesses outside the confines of mental health clinics and social service agencies, how to make contact and build trust with them, how to help them get disability entitlement income or dental care while slowly persuading them that mental health care or housing were worth considering as well—suggested that, masters of one task after another, our prospects, and those of our clients, were boundless. It was only when we learned that helping people move into their own apartments did not automatically make them neighbors and community members that citizenship came into our ken, or we into its.

Since then we've undertaken four main stages of practice and evaluation—a community intervention, an individual and group intervention, empirical measurement, and in-progress work to develop "citizenship-oriented care" for the Connecticut Mental Health Center, the public mental health center for the New Haven area, as a pilot project for "taking citizenship to scale" for the Connecticut Department of Mental Health and Addiction Services. Each of these stages followed roughly the same pattern as that of our outreach work apprenticeship, with achievement of mastery at one stage announcing the need to move on to another. During this time, study of political and social philosophy and sociology has informed my thinking about citizenship's range, from participation in the warp and woof of life in the city-states of ancient Greece, to individual rights and freedoms from the Age of Enlightenment, to a recent shift in focus from the mainstream to the margins of social life, where citizenship claims are increasingly being made by and for excluded groups.

An occasional critique of our work has been that citizenship is too much about its legalities to be a useful framework for thinking about the community membership of people with mental illnesses. Participants in our intervention and measure development studies have given the best answer to this critique. Their citizenship ideas and goals, it turns out, range as wide as does the literature on the topic. Then, too, the poverty and discrimination and stigma they experience that pushes them to the social, psychological, and economic margins of society seem to me to call for a broad citizenship perspective.

A more specific instance of the legal critique is that citizenship's meaning and uses in mental health care will be limited by the distractions of the public focus on whether or not its rights, protections, and obligations will be extended to undocumented immigrants. This aspect of citizenship hit home for me in talking to staff of a clinic that provides care to undocumented Latino immigrants. If you can't check "Yes" by the "Legal Citizen" box, their comments made clear, it's unlikely you'll be able to check "Yes" by the "Participation" and "Valued Roles" and "Sense of Belonging" boxes. But the fact that citizenship is and has been denied to some does not negate its practical and symbolic importance. In fact, its inclusionary and exclusionary elements and the way these play out for individuals, communities, and countries lie at the core of its meaning and significance in the "lives" of all three.

Over time, after making the case for what citizenship can bring to the mental health field, I took to giving another response to these caveats. "Yes," I would say in so many words, "let's talk about citizenship—what it is, for whom, and under what conditions. Who gets to define and have it? Who is squeezed or liberated by it? And what do the answers to these questions say about its value and uses in general and in relation to mental health care?" These are conversations worth having, with the excluded as well as the included having an equal say in public settings.

Another factor that puts in question the idea of linking citizenship and mental health is the larger direction of public mental health care in the United States. If effective treatment and a life in the community constitute a dual goal, we need to test the dual hypothesis that effective clinical treatment, narrowly defined as addressing mental health symptoms, can have a positive impact on people's community lives and that a "life in the community" can have a positive impact on people's clinical symptoms. With such needed evaluation, though, mental health care should attend to what people with mental illness hope for—a life lived with others, love, a chance to achieve their dreams, the kinds of things that pretty much everyone wants.

Yet health care is changing in the United States, with the Affordable Care Act (ACA) being the biggest driver of change. The ACA has already increased the availability of primary health care for millions of Americans and should increase the availability of mental health care as well, both by disallowing pre-existing conditions as a rationale for denying coverage and mandating parity between physical and mental health coverage. Increased access to mental health care is not guaranteed, since laws against denial of and for parity in coverage are undercut if psychiatrists and other mental health clinicians accept my private insurance but don't accept your Medicaid. Even bracketing this problem, the ACA's eventual impact on social aspects of mental health care is unknown, as the act focuses on medical care as traditionally defined. Thus the place and impact of citizenship and other "social recovery" approaches are not assured. At the same time, though, the ACA does advance the notion of engagement in one's own care, including reviewing one's own chart, along with preventive care, and these are citizenship-friendly, if not specifically citizenship-oriented, values and practices.

Our current research-to-practice group of clinicians, peer staff, administrators, and researchers began with the idea that we would develop and evaluate a citizenship intervention to be linked to clinical care at a mental health center. If successful, the intervention might provide a means for grafting a stronger social approach to mental health care, with robust links to community opportunities and resources, onto a medical one with psychosocial elements. The more we've talked about the notion of citizenship-oriented care, though, the more we've come to see that it won't put down deep roots without the rich soil of a home institution that supports citizenship efforts and aspirations.[1] This means that citizenship-oriented care won't work unless patients, or clients, and staff share and reflect in their inter-actions a common understanding of citizenship. And we're in agreement that such a shared understanding of citizenship implies the center's participation in its home community and society at large.

Following from what I've said about the iterative quality of outreach work that led me to citizenship, this book on citizenship and mental health can't truly be finished, or not now. We are in the midst of our work and research on developing citizenship-oriented care for mental health centers and clinics, including ways to make more community resources available to them and their clients. But coming up on 20 years of research and practice, it's time to sum up what we've learned and make the case for the wider application of the citizenship framework in mental health care.

Let me give one note and make three points before moving on. The note is that I refer to the Connecticut Mental Health Center, the setting of our current citizenship-oriented care efforts and home base for most of our previous citizenship research, as "the mental health center," "the center," or the like for the remainder of this book, to give a little narrative distance for readers, and for me.

The first point is that a portion of the research my colleagues and I have con-ducted involves the use of statistical methods and analytical procedures that would leave many readers cold. Thus I limit such details here to what's essential for under-standing what we did and found, and refer interested readers to the published arti-cles, referenced in the text, for more detail.

Second, on language and terminology, I use the term "client" instead of "patient" for people receiving outpatient mental health services. A full explana-tion of the reasons for this could fill a book chapter, but suffice it to say here that both terms are used by mental health professionals and persons receiving services in different settings. "Client," I think, is the more common term when writing in the area of social and community inclusion for people with mental illnesses and for people receiving outpatient mental health treatment. I also use the terms "case manager" and "case management" instead of the newer current terms, "care manager" and "care management," the latter based on the notion that "I'm not a case and you're not my manager." I do so in part because the former terms will be more familiar to most readers. More importantly, though, I want to maintain the tension between the person-to-person connection that mental health care often strives for *and* bureaucratic distinctions of "helper" and "the one helped" suggested by "case manager" and "client." Neither set of terms—client versus patient or case manager versus care manager—is perfect, and both elide the medical and social tensions of public mental care, although I'll revisit this tension.

Third, on the relevance of a citizenship framework for mental health care in the United States and perhaps beyond, this book takes up the topic of what such an approach to the community and social inclusion of people with mental illnesses is and might be. Yet citizenship as an applied theory emerged from mental health care in Connecticut, and that mainly in New Haven, with much of its funding coming from the Connecticut Department of Mental Health and Addiction Services. This means that our citizenship work has occurred in the Northeast and in a liberal city in one of the most liberal states with, arguably, the most progressive state mental health authority, in the country. And it has been developed and practiced by a particular set of researchers, staff, and participants working under certain social, institutional, and professional conditions.

Still, application of a theoretical framework of citizenship should reach far if it's worth taking up at all. One qualification to the caveats I've just given about the "generalizability" of this work is that the research design for one of our studies— development of a survey instrument to measure individual achievement of citizenship—can be reproduced in other settings both nationally and internationally. The reproduction of that process, or variations of it, in other settings, will no doubt yield a set of citizenship items that show commonalities with, and differences from, the citizenship measure developed in a small corner of the world called New Haven, Connecticut. In fact it has already, in Quebec.

Yet this book deals with more than measurement. It involves community-level interventions—*Citizens*, up first—a group intervention aimed at helping individuals "make it" as citizens; the *Citizens Project*, next up; and an attempt to take citizenship to scale in a large mental health center as a pilot project for the state of Connecticut—the *Citizens Collaborative*, last up before outlining a model of a citizenship-oriented system of mental health care that, indeed, hopes to be relevant beyond the site of its preceding interventions. The very qualifications of theory, practice, and measurement that comprise the citizenship work I take up here beg to be challenged, validated, or modified beyond their original borders. I will try to set that next stage of citizenship work on the road in this book, after telling the story of the road it's been on since the mid-1990s.

Citizenship and Mental Health

1

Introduction

CITIZENSHIP ROOTS IN OUTREACH WORK

Jim? I couldn't see him young. He seemed gray. Not his hair, that was more sandy than gray. No, gray like the survivors of collective disaster in a Kai Erikson book who lift off the page before you real as your hand but separate, too, like with dirt under their fingernails.

Of course Jim was young once. It was a failure of imagination on my part that painted him gray. Or the triumph of a different sort of imagination as our team psychiatrist might have suggested. There is an otherness to the experience of homelessness, he told us. We need to acknowledge it, then reach across its chasm. Not too swiftly or easily, though, and keeping watch for an influx of imagination that isn't tethered to observation but is, instead, a projection of our own fears or fascination or both.[1] I agree, and would only add that a pause before such "other" experience is a form that respect can take, as long as you don't wallow in it.

Jim was living on the streets of New Haven in 1994 when outreach workers found him one cold fall morning asleep on a ledge under the Water Street highway bridge for Interstate 95. Or found a pair of neon yellow sneakers sticking out from one end of half a dozen blankets encasing what they took to be a body, and that of a man since few women slept under highway bridges at the time.[2] Not wanting to wake this person at 5:30 in the morning, they came back at the end of their early morning outreach run. The man with the neon yellow sneakers was gone, along with others who slept up there that the outreach workers already knew. They asked around at the soup kitchens and drop-in centers about a man who wore neon yellow sneakers. Finally someone said, "That's Jim. Try the library." They went to the main branch facing the New Haven Green where people who were homeless were allowed to sleep with a book propped open in front of them and walked around half bent over looking at feet under tables. They found the sneakers, and Jim.

I met Jim later that fall at the Downtown Evening Soup Kitchen on rounds with an outreach worker named Julie. He sat on a low wall by the driveway of the church parish house where dinner was being served in the basement. For some

1

reason we never learned, he wouldn't go in there. Someone brought him up a plate of food. Julie introduced me. She had business to conduct with Jim, so I drifted off a few paces.

"How are you doing?" she asked.

"Not well," he said.

"I'm sorry to hear that…So, have you thought about applying for SSI [Supplemental Security Income, a federal disability entitlement program] since we talked the other day?"

"What's the use?"

"It could help you…to have some money. You really should think about it."

John gave Julie a man of the world look.

"How old are you?"

"I'm in my 20s."

"Well, I'm 55 and I've made too many mistakes in my life," said Jim, and walked away from her.

Jim could turn an outreach worker's questions back on her with aplomb. He did it to me, too, that winter at a Catholic church on a desolate stretch of Grand Avenue a few blocks from the New Haven Green. I got coffee up at the front of the basement community room, thinking I shouldn't be eating food that was meant for others. This was the bonehead move of a novice ethnographer, one that set me apart from the people I wanted to talk to even more than my unruffled streetless appearance did. The room was dim and dully lit, with seven or eight long rows constructed of fold-up tables pushed together end-on-end to butt up against the far wall. Picture yourself spotting a friend who is sitting, like you, at the end of a row but one over and on the far side of his table from you. To talk to him privately you have to get up, walk all the way to the front of the room and over to his side of the next table, then down the length of the room again to where he's sitting.

I saw Jim at the far end of a row. I walked down the aisle and sat down cata-corner to him. This was from Making Contact 101—don't sit straight across from the person you want to talk to. He might take it to be challenging. I could have asked Jim's permission, too, but thought that might come across as too formal. I tried to make eye contact, having got a sideways glance from him on my way down. He ignored me.

"Hi, Jim. Do you remember me?"

He scowled and gave me another sideways look.

"Yes I do."

There was a long pause. I cursed myself for not taking some food.

"How are you doing?"

He didn't look at me this time.

"You asked the question, you already know the answer," he said.

Another long pause. I sipped my coffee.

"How's the food here?"

"You asked the question, you already know the answer."

More coffee. Jim picked at his food, critically.

"Have the outreach workers been able to help you with things?"

Another sideways look.

"You asked the question, you already know the answer."[3]

Jim stood up, picked up his plate, and walked away.

He had me dead to rights. Did he remember me? I asked him. Yes, he was polite enough to say, but I already knew this from the glance he gave me as I walked down the aisle, and he knew that I knew it. How was he doing? I asked. He was homeless and eating in a soup kitchen. How well could he be doing? Still I pressed on. And how was the food here? It was soup kitchen food, and he had noticed I wasn't eating it. Unable to admit defeat or with Poe's imp of the perverse in my heart,[4,5] I asked if the outreach workers were helping him. But I was the director of the outreach team, wasn't I? So I knew the answer to that question, too.

Jim was not looking to be found, or not by us. He didn't deserve any help, he told us, and he wasn't buying what we had to sell in any case. Set apart as he seemed, though, Jim knew people on the street. He managed to share a ledge with others under the Water Street highway bridge. And somebody had to carry his dinner up to him at the Downtown Evening Soup Kitchen, since he wouldn't go in to fetch it himself.

It was different with Ed, one of the outreach workers, though. It wasn't just his persistence when Jim kept walking away from him. Outreach workers are persistent, period. But Ed, a "peer" outreach worker, that is, one with personal experience of a mental health or addiction problems or both, found a way to connect with Jim. We didn't know then what we'd learn a few years later from our research, that peer workers have a knack for making contact with and persuading people who are "unengaged" in care to accept it.[5,6] This is not to say that non-peers have no such knack, but that peer workers have a step on them at the outset.

Assertive mental health outreach, or homeless outreach, took its imperative from the "new homelessness" of the late 1970s and early 1980s when mostly single folk, poorer and more likely to have a mental illness than homeless persons from the Skid Row days that preceded them, started showing up in the downtowns of cities across the United States.[7] Few mental health centers were making deliberate efforts to reach out to people on the street at the time, and people on the streets returned the favor by avoiding them in droves because of previous negative experiences such as having been hospitalized against their will or having to offer up personal information that such places are obliged to collect or the exigencies of homeless life—choosing lunch at the soup kitchen over an appointment with a clinician, for example— that impinged on their ability to keep appointments with clinicians, or other reasons.[8]

Outreach workers leave their offices for the streets, soup kitchens, shelters, and drop-in centers where people who are homeless congregate. They meet people "where they are" both geographically and existentially and have high respect for their strengths as survivors of homelessness.[9] Workers start small with their prospective clients, bringing food, clothing, and other basic goods with them on their rounds. With rare exceptions such as an imminent mental health crisis or cold weather that could kill you, they don't insist that people accept help. Instead, they offer an array of services including access to primary medical care, housing, help getting a job or applying for disability income support, referral to substance abuse treatment, and other services. They try to provide these things based on their clients' stated preferences, hoping eventually to persuade them to accept mental health treatment as well.[10–15]

The New Haven outreach team was part of a federal project called ACCESS, for Access to Community Care and Effective Services and Supports. ACCESS was a nine-state, eighteen-site, six-year study of care for people who were homeless with mental illnesses run by the Substance Abuse and Mental Health Services Administration, better known as SAMHSA, pronounced SAM-SUH.[16,17] New Haven ACCESS was one of those 18 sites. The heart of each of the 18 programs was a mental health outreach team lodged in a local mental health "system" of care. The national research involved the largest-ever test of the theory of systems integration in human services

Systems integration theory first became popular during the 1960s and 1970s, when the rapid growth of human service programs, coupled with factors such as deinstitutionalization—the massive discharge of chronic mentally ill persons from state hospitals—led to increasing complexity and "fragmentation" of programs that often rendered services inaccessible to people who needed them.[18] Systems integration was proposed as a way to coordinate services by creating policy and program linkages within and across different systems of care such as mental health, housing, and disability entitlements.[19] From a public financing perspective, systems integration held out the promise of increasing the efficiency and economy of existing services while undercutting the need to expand them.[18,20,21]

Systems integration has been an elusive goal for planners and policy makers, with little empirical evidence to show that, when it is achieved, it leads to better client outcomes.[22] Coordination, as Janet Weiss has written, is often done around trivial issues by organizations that systematically exclude others with controversial agendas.[23] Roland Warren and colleagues found that 1960s Model Cities programs designed to increase coordination and innovation among urban social service agencies accomplished neither because gatekeeping organizations defined a narrow range of objectives for social reform and resisted change. Then, too, service integration work tends to disregard the fact that many issues, such as federal economic policy and its effect on unemployment, are beyond the scope of local or regional efforts.[24] Finally, Warren argues, defining the solution to poverty as a social service challenge leaves its causes unexamined and shifts attention to clients' personal deficiencies.[25]

All this said, the national ACCESS project and its application of systems integration theory have a different story to tell than the one I'm telling here. The New Haven outreach team was a project of the local public mental health center, which provided leadership, clinical care, and case management. Several private nonprofit social services agency partners brought shelter, housing, job training, and additional case management expertise and services to the team. After receiving outreach team services, clients generally were transferred to ongoing office-based care at the mental health center.

As project director I ran the team with a clinical coordinator from the mental health center and the program director of a local emergency shelter. As a sociologist I studied homeless outreach, observing workers on their rounds, going out on the streets and into soup kitchens, drop-in centers, and emergency shelters on my own or with a guide who'd been homeless himself. I also interviewed people who were homeless and outreach workers. Over time I came to see the meetings taking place between the two parties as social, rather than clinical, encounters. This made sense, my being a sociologist not a clinician, and this view of things would eventually lead me to citizenship, but the term and concept were far from my mind in the early days of building the program.

The social encounters of outreach workers and people who were homeless were not casual ones from the outreach worker's perspective, and were anything but accidental. They included the elements of material or well-defined goods such as housing and mental health treatment and of symbolic or intangible goods such as a sense of belonging where you were or where you hoped to get to. They also included mutual perceptions and negotiated understandings, spoken or unspoken, about the price that people would have to pay for goods and services they accepted. These encounters took place at the physical borders of New Haven—in shelters, soup kitchens, and drop-in centers, the places where people who were homeless were allowed to operate and the people they served were tolerated. The borders of such sites could be marked by their out-of-the-mainstream location in poor sections of town or by their own contained, set-off space and function in mainstream public spaces such as the Downtown Evening Soup Kitchen behind the First and Summerfield Methodist Church that overlooked the historical and social heart of the city, the New Haven Green. These encounters also took place at the social and economic borders of the New Haven community where marginalized folk received health and social services while the big business of the city took place a few stone throws away.

Homeless encounters involve instrumental elements such as the possibility of having one's own apartment, expressive elements such as the wish to belong, and combinations of them such as receiving mental health care and taking on the title of "mental patient." Ultimately, these encounters were negotiations and transactions over goods and identity and the price attached to each.[26] There was the price of a loss of privacy or, better said, of anonymity, since people who are homeless hardly have the privacy of those residing in apartments with doors they can lock behind them. Agreeing to become a client of the mental health center, to participate in research associated with the ACCESS project, and to apply for disability entitlement programs also meant having to answer many questions people could avoid on the street. Those questions and their inevitable repetition from one program to another were one reason that some people avoided such programs in the first place.

In accepting services from the outreach team there was the price, too, of being reminded of the very exclusion and marginalization for which the goods and services outreach workers had to offer their clients were to be the remedy. Not to overstate the case—it's not as though people who were homeless forgot about their exclusion and marginalization—but the act of accepting or applying for such goods and services could put their marginalization in a particular, and painful, light for them. The benefits of acceptance were evident in the forms of treatment or service received, income gained, housing, and more. These benefits were not associated with status-generating resources, though, but with being disabled persons entitled to public support. Thus the uses of the information people had to give up and the acts of giving of the information were ineluctably associated with the wounds of stigma, discrimination, and dependence on others for access to, and continuing enjoyment of, benefits received.

The identity of being a "housed person" had to be weighed against the reality of giving up the difficult but known life of homelessness. For some, homelessness at least gave the satisfaction of being able to survive it and the bitter conviction that those among the comfortably domiciled who looked down on them wouldn't last a week on the streets. By contrast, there were practical and emotional worries that came with housing, such as how to manage an apartment, the responsibilities of paying bills, cooking your own meals, and others. And there were the dignity violations[27] of having to accept SSI disability income or using food stamps in the days before you could swipe your debit card at the checkout counter like everyone else. "You feel like less of a man," one man told me, "like you shouldn't be getting these things . . . 'Feed me, clothe me, house me, I'm finished.'"[28]

Of course, people who were homeless were well aware of the stigma attached to it. Angela, a woman in her 40s who'd been living on the streets for years, developed a strong working relationship with one outreach worker, Don. Heading into the coldest weekend of a bad winter she finally agreed to come inside, but only after Don, having begged her for hours to take a room in a boarding house he'd found for her, took the risk of feigning disgust and started to walk away from her. Angela gave in. She didn't want to disappoint Don, or have him be angry with her.

We were uncertain about Angela's past. She probably had two children in Florida whom, we thought, the state had taken away from her. She definitely had a bum leg from being hit by a car. We thought she had cognitive deficits as well and, if so, that these may have come from a head injury caused by the probable accident that ruined her leg. I talked to Joe about my wanting to interview Angela, and he talked to her. She declined at first but then agreed, with Joe's assurance that I could be trusted. Unlike many of the interviews I conducted in the Burger King in the doomed mall across from the Green, this one took place at the outreach team's offices, perhaps to reassure Angela with others around, although at this late date I don't recall. The beginning of the interview went like this:

"When you were without a home, what do you think was the cause of it?"
"I never said I was without a home."
"You weren't?"
"No. I never said that to anybody."
"OK."
"Not me."
"How long have you been in New Haven?"
"I have never said I've been homeless."
"OK, OK."
"I have never said that."
"Alright. So you've been at your place on Howard Avenue for a year or so?"

What I remember—the abjectness of my apology—doesn't come across on the page. The dialogue also lacks the image of Angela jumping out of her seat across from me, ready to bolt. I include it here for its connection to an understanding of identity transactions on the way to citizenship that I gained by "stumbling into awareness," as Erving Goffman wrote of ethnographic research.[29] The most dangerous assumptions, I've come to think, are the ones you don't recognize as such. Why? Because you know they are facts, not assumptions, so there's nothing to question.

A clinical assessment of Angela's statement that she hadn't said she was homeless might suggest that delusional thoughts should, in clinical parlance, "be ruled out." After all, Angela had been sleeping in the basement level of the old Malley's abandoned parking garage. Sounds pretty homeless, doesn't it? Yet consider this. In 1995 several definitions of homelessness were in play in the United States. Some included "couch surfing" from one friend's apartment to another and some did not. Some included a guaranteed, or fixed "length-of-stay," bed in an emergency shelter and some did not. The definition of homelessness for the ACCESS project was "literal" homelessness—staying in an emergency shelter or sleeping on the streets or vehicles or abandoned buildings "not fit for human habitation."[30] The current SAMHSA definition of homelessness includes "transitional" housing, meaning housing with support services that serves as a sort of way station between homelessness and permanent housing, with the requirement that residents move on by a certain time determined by the agencies that run them, not by SAMHSA.[31] So what does homelessness mean?

Angela didn't truck with such definitions, in any case. She may have been thinking of one of the older meanings of home as "a land of origin, a native soil...the place to which one really belongs, even though quartered elsewhere; the place to which one dreams of returning,"[32] as Erikson describes it. Or she may have had in mind a more contemporary meaning of home that he describes as "the outer envelope of personhood."[33] And I suspect that Angela wasn't about to acknowledge to me, a total stranger but for word of mouth, that she'd been stripped of that part of her personhood and now belonged to one of the most stigmatized groups in our society, regardless of what I knew of her situation. That was not a happy identity to be pegged with. And note that Angela didn't tell me she *hadn't* been homeless. She said she had not *told* me she had been.

Ed, like almost everyone else on the team, was new to outreach work. It hadn't been that long since he'd been homeless himself. Now married and with a baby on the way, he and his wife had just bought a house. He was eager to do the work but unsure of himself. Tracy, the public health nurse and his outreach partner, was his mentor. But Ed was a quick study and managed to connect with Jim, different backgrounds or no, Jim having grown up in rural Pennsylvania and Ed in New Haven, Jim being a Veteran and Ed not, Jim being white and Ed African American, Jim in his mid-50s and Ed in his early 30s.

Ed had learned two things about Jim, he told me. The first was, "Don't try to talk to him before he eats. He'll just be grouchy." The second was that out on the street, people were always asking for things from him. "Got a dollar, Jim?" "Got a cigarette, Jim?" "Got an extra blanket, Jim?" So Ed decided he would always bring something to him—a cup of coffee, a sandwich, socks. And it worked. "I got my hook in him," he said.

Ed was a good listener, too, and Jim, after running through his list of "too old to be helped," "don't deserve help," and "leave me alones," began to dole out bits and pieces of his story. He came from a large, poor family. When he was 17 a younger female cousin told her parents of Jim's romantic interest in her. He was drummed out of the family, nuclear and extended. He joined the army. Given his age when we met him I calculated this must have been around the time of the Korean War. He earned an honorable discharge and drifted south. Eventually Jim came back north, roamed the eastern seaboard for years drinking himself out of one menial job after another, and wandered north to Connecticut, having renewed contact with at least one family member, his sister in Meriden twenty miles northeast of New Haven. She took him in, but a couple of months later asked him to leave because of his drinking.

Jim came to New Haven. He slept under highway bridges and other outdoor sites and ate in soup kitchens. It appeared that, like many others, he wasn't sleeping on the streets because of having been refused shelter because of his drinking or disruptive behavior but that he deliberately avoided them because of their noise, their rules, and the lack of security they offered for his few possessions. He continued to resist the services that Ed began to float in his company. The blankets and sandwiches were enough, he said. But Ed persisted. Eventually, Jim agreed to apply for SSI with Ed's help. He got it. Then Ed persuaded him to come to our office a mile away from the mental health center to see our psychiatrist, Dori Laub, whom he'd met a few months before in the soup kitchen. Finally, Jim went apartment hunting with Ed, found a place, and agreed to try it out.

Getting Jim off the streets was a tall marker point for the outreach team. We'd come of age, had proved ourselves, and proved wrong the naysayers at the mental health center who thought we'd never get this or that one who'd been "in the system" years before to accept mental health care or housing. A couple of weeks after this watershed moment, though, Ed came into our weekly team meeting looking troubled. When his turn came he said Jim had told him he wanted to move back to his spot under the Water Street highway bridge. There, he said, he had friends. He knew what to do. He didn't look and feel out of place. It would be better for him back there. Jim's mental health symptoms had flared up, too. He thought the people in the television shows were speaking directly to him, and continued to think so after turning off the television, and then after unplugging it. It's possible these symptoms were independent of Jim's new living arrangements, but recent research suggests that social isolation may be a trigger for psychosis rather than, or in addition to, being caused by it.[34]

As we talked in the team meeting we realized that two big changes had happened in Jim's life at precisely the same time. One was moving into his apartment. The other was that, with Jim safely ensconced in his new apartment, Ed headed back out to the streets and spent little time with Jim. Thus at the moment when Jim may have needed Ed's support the most, he and we had taken our foot off the gas. We agreed that Ed should spend more time with Jim, which he did, stopping by his apartment, showing him how to use his appliances, taking walks with him around the neighborhood, taking him to see Dr. Laub, and accompanying him to a social club for people with mental illnesses.

It worked. But for me, Ed's announcement at the team meeting reverberated after the blast of it. Outreach work was not the answer to the community inclusion of people like Jim. In pushing the work as far as it would take our clients and us we had simultaneously pulled back the curtain on it. The outreach team could do many things. We could leave our offices to look for people who didn't want to be found. We could make contact and build relationships with people who affirmed their human worth and right to be part of society rather than survivors at its margins. We could offer them tangible services including housing, which ends physical homelessness. What we couldn't do were three things. First of all, we couldn't turn them into neighbors of the areas they moved into. Housing alone didn't come with that status. Second, if we couldn't turn our clients into neighbors, then we couldn't offer them the status of community members, either. And third, we couldn't offer our clients full citizenship in our democratic society.

2

Citizenship and Community Organizing

CITIZENS

Outreach workers are practical folk, but they are passionate and idealistic, too. They will move heaven and earth to get people like Jim and Angela off the street, but none, I think, would accept the idea that a shriveled life in the domiciled community is good enough for their clients because at least they're not homeless anymore. This, in addition to the fact that talking about "community" and "community member," with the sentimental connotations that cling to them, begs the question of what communities and neighborhoods people who are homeless will end up living in and whether or not they will feel socially connected or safe in them, along with their fellow neighbors and community members. To say this is not to say that they won't or can't, but that these are open questions.

In practice, though, workers' ability to support a life in the community for their clients, once housed, is limited. They can help people manage the transition from homelessness into housing, but being domiciled falls well short of being a part "of" one's community rather than simply living "in" it.[1] In New Haven, a dual isolation from their peers in the homeless community and alienation from the domiciled community left many people nominally housed but with their anti-status as marginalized persons intact.[2] Only having access to the instrumental goods of social and economic resources and the expressive good of experiencing membership in society through building relationships and taking on valued roles could earn them the status of first-class citizenship.

Jim and others who managed to function on the streets for years without help from outreach workers found themselves dependent on them or other mental health staff for social contact once they entered housing. Sometimes, as for Jim, homelessness can look more like home than your own apartment. Lezley TwoBears, Assistant Director of the Community Soup Kitchen during the latter 1990s, helped us identify people who were eligible for our services and introduced us to them. Her recollections of this dilemma during a recent interview were similar to mine at the time:

*You guys had done a good job getting people into housing and now they were com-
ing back to the soup kitchen, homeless again. What happened? What did we do
wrong? What was it about being homeless and being housed that wasn't meshing?
What did we not understand about the street and housing? Why wasn't it as simple
as we thought it would be?*[3]

Later in the interview Lezley, who became the director of *Citizens,* the main topic
of this chapter, answered her own question:

*So we would get people into housing, in these tiny apartments mostly, people
who'd been more visual than linguistic out on the streets. They had to look for
clues constantly, who was doing what to whom and what it might have to do with
them, outdoors, on the street, all those things to see and figure out. And suddenly
they're in these apartments that are like a box, claustrophobic, like one of those
sensory deprivation chambers. How would any of us do that after being out on the
street? And then think about having a mental illness, or a criminal history, or a
drug addiction. We'd be done.*

Outreach workers argue, convincingly I think, that human contact and trust provide the foundation for persuading people to accept help. This was especially the
case in New Haven for those who had been homeless for long periods and had
mental illnesses of long standing. Once housed, peoples' relationships with their
outreach workers could help them remain in housing, a point we missed at first with
Jim. Those relationships, though, can be two-edged swords, helping people hang
on but delaying their acquisition of new social networks and social "moments"[4]
that may put them on a path to feeling like, and being recognized as, neighbors
and community members. Supportive housing programs offer people their own
leases and optional case management in an attempt to strike a balance between
encouraging their autonomy and giving them the support they need to achieve it,
but they have not been shown to increase people's social inclusion and community
participation.[5-7]

Nor has outreach work. But this fact might better be said to represent not
the limitations of the work so much as what lies outside its proper boundaries.
Still, outreach workers' growing awareness of the limits of their help puts them at
risk of bad faith in their homeless encounters, of making promises they can't keep,
especially considering the hopes and aspirations they may foster and then dash in
their clients. Outreach workers try to keep the focus on what they *can* do, but rarely
include a buyer beware clause in the contract they negotiate with their clients. So,
if being homeless confers a shadow citizenship on people and bounded citizenship
is a likely result of a simple move into housing, what does first-class citizenship in a
democratic society look like? Here, I went to the social science and social philosophy literature on citizenship, the first of many trips that would follow.

For Aristotle, "Man is a political and social animal and the state both represents and embodies the highest form of human association." To be a citizen, a

status that excluded women and slaves, was to adhere in values and action to civic duties and "virtues," known as the "civic republican" model of citizenship. The "liberal state" model of citizenship emerged from the Age of Enlightenment in Europe starting in the late seventeenth century. In it, the state exists for the purpose of protecting and ensuring the enjoyment of individual rights and freedoms.[8]

In the nineteenth century two Frenchmen, Alexis de Tocqueville surveying American democracy and Émile Durkheim surveying the breakneck passage from traditional to industrialized societies in Europe, wrote of the critical roles of secondary institutions such as churches, civic associations, businesses, and other institutions as buffers between the individual and the state during an era of upheavals in social and cultural life.[9,10] Thomas Marshall, writing in the aftermath of World War II, described three forms of citizenship rights—civil and legal rights including freedom of speech and property ownership, political rights including the right to vote and, most recent of the three in terms of recognition and government action, social and economic rights to health care, education, and welfare.[11]

Citizenship is an elastic concept in contemporary social and political theory. For Thomas Janoski, the heart of it is the relationship between the individual and the state. The state, he says, gives legal sanction to citizenship norms, while civil society provides structures, institutions, and the associational context that mediate between citizens and the state. Janoski writes of the theoretical traditions of Marshall's developmental model of legal, political, and social rights balanced with taxes, military, and other service obligations to the state, and of solidarity and social change associated with Tocqueville and Durkheim and expressed in part through civic participation and volunteerism. He distinguishes between substantive citizenship in which stigmatized groups gain rights and recognition as full citizens, and formal citizenship in which immigrants become naturalized citizens. He also distinguishes between passive legal and social rights and obligations that people have by virtue of being legal citizens, and active participation in exercising those rights and obligations through political action, civil disobedience, and other means. Janoski notes the simultaneous process of expanding citizenship rights through social movements to include previously excluded groups and barring access to those rights though legal entrance requirements. Finally, he describes four categories of citizenship rights—legal rights or liberties, political rights including voting, social rights that support economic subsistence, and participation rights such as decision making among individuals and groups. For each category, corresponding obligations to the state balance the rights that pertain to it.[12]

Robert Bellah and colleagues write about citizenship as political participation at three ascending levels—the politics of community in which people reach moral consensus in face-to-face interactions, the politics of interest involving conflicts between opposing interest groups, and the politics of the nation by which politics is raised to the level of statesmanship and local interests give way to national goals and ideals. The American culture of radical individualism, they argue, favors an autonomous middle-class form of individuality that excludes others from full membership in society while failing to come to terms with the power of large institutions. Effective citizenship can be enhanced by strengthening voluntary organizations and community associations, fostering democratic social movements to check the power of government and its bureaucracies, and linking people across localities in a national dialogue supported by religious and civic "communities of memory."[13]

For Pnina Werbner and Nira Yuval-Davis, democratic citizenship is a contested concept shaped by cultural and political elites between forces of normalization and forces of difference. Like Janoski, they note that citizenship both opens up new arenas of freedom for previously excluded groups and restricts freedom through legal and procedural limits. They argue for a shift in discourse toward social and cultural difference and the global dimensions of citizenship.[14] Citizenship, Ruth Lister observes, has historically been hostile to large segments of humanity and thus claims a false universalism. Still, she sees it as a powerful theoretical tool for laying bare the processes of social exclusion for the use of excluded groups as a political tool for gaining access to the full benefits of membership in society.[15]

Simon Duffy writes that social justice theory has paid little attention to the needs of people with disabilities. He proposes a citizenship theory of social justice based on the dignity of all persons and the value of diversity and difference. A foundational value and mechanism of the theory is "personalization," by which "users"—the preferred term for "consumers" or clients in the United Kingdom— are at the center of care, co-designing and producing the services they receive and maintaining control over their own support as a reflection of and means of achieving, social justice. Among the key principles of the theory are respect for all and a just organization of society so that all can achieve citizenship. The six *keys* to citizenship are authority over one's own life, purpose and meaning, resources, home, support, and contributions or "giving back" to others.[16]

Matthew Gambino, an historian and psychiatrist, studied the history of psychiatry and institutional care during the first six decades of the twentieth century through the lens of St. Elizabeth's Hospital in Washington, DC. St. Elizabeth's was also Erving Goffman's fieldwork site for his influential theory of "total institutions" in which people with mental illnesses receive intensive training in becoming mental patients and institutional citizens,[17] a master status that will characterize them and their relationships with others permanently, whether they remain incarcerated or eventually are discharged to their home communities. Gambino takes an historical and cultural view of psychiatry's role via mental institutions as both reflecting and helping to construct modern American ideals and realities, as they attempted to foster "the reconstitution of mentally-distressed men and women for proper citizenship," while at the same time promoting a "highly gendered and racialized vision of American life."[18]

Elizabeth Anderson writes that in a just society, citizens stand in relations of equality to each other and are guaranteed equal access to the social conditions in which they can flourish in freedom. Distribution of goods based on principles that show respect for all citizens is justified to assure this flourishing of free persons. The principles of justice identify the goods to which citizens should have access and to which they are entitled. That is, people should not have to debase themselves to demonstrate their worth to receive goods that should be available to all. Anderson writes that most of the things we do and want as individuals involve participation with others. Such participation, she notes, is impossible for people who are, in effect, excluded from society.[19]

Chantal Mouffe writes of an "explosion" of challenges to the Western individualistic, rational, and universalist view of citizenship that minimizes the role of conflict in public life. A new democratic order, she argues, will balance the need for consensus and shared values and the need for antagonisms in a pluralistic democracy with special attention to marginalized groups whose status as an "underclass" places them almost beyond the pale of the political system of society.[20] Axel Honneth argues that self-respect and self-esteem cannot be achieved in isolation. They must come, instead, from others' recognition of your equal and shared humanity and worth. This process occurs at the societal level through social conflict in which excluded groups assert their rights to full inclusion in the form of full social and political participation and a decent standard of living and economic security.[21]

Citizenship and Mental Health

In my study, two dialectical pairs of citizenship themes struck me as most relevant to the work of citizenship and mental health. The first pair involves individual rights and freedoms paired, and in tension with, civic-collective participation. The second involves mainstream status with citizenship rights and obligations that is paired, and in tension with, marginalized status and membership with restricted rights and obligations. With these in mind, the definition of citizenship I decided on, with modest changes over a decade and a half of research and colleagues' suggestions, is this:

> *Citizenship is a measure of the strength of the person's connection to the 5 Rs of rights, responsibilities, roles, resources, and relationships that society makes available to its members through public and social institutions and the associational life of neighborhoods and local communities.*[2,22,23]

To be citizens, people need material means, the opportunity to connect with others in common activity, and a sense of belonging and entitlement to exercise their rights and responsibilities that comes about through others' recognition of their worth.[21] Citizenship includes instrumental elements of practical knowledge and skills linked with opportunities and resources, and affective elements of participation and valued community membership, along with community recognition of the previously excluded group's legitimacy and full membership in society.[2] This framework of citizenship falls most neatly within what Janoski calls the Tocquevillian–Durkheimian tradition, which Bellah and others draw upon. Like Werbner and Yuval-Davis, it focuses on opening up citizenship opportunities for excluded and marginalized persons. Of Janoski's four types of citizenship rights, it has to date placed most emphasis on social and participation rights, yet efforts to secure these rights overlap with those to secure political and legal rights, and self- and other advocacy have been part of our citizenship-based interventions from the outset.

The citizenship framework resonates Norma Ware and colleagues' description of the process through which people with mental illnesses develop their capacities for connectedness and citizenship. Social connectedness involves building and maintaining reciprocal relationships, while citizenship involves the rights and privileges and corresponding responsibilities that members of democratic societies enjoy.[1] The framework also draws on social capital theory for its focus on developing personal networks as a means of increasing social opportunity and participation,[24-26] and on identity theory with its investigations of how roles and group membership shape people's social participation and enhance their mutual commitments,[27,28] determine their self-concepts and foster self-esteem,[29-31] and bolster their claims to social identities.[32]

Citizenship work also takes place in the context of other socially oriented theories and practices in mental health care, among them recovery, social inclusion, and capabilities. Each of these directly or indirectly responds to the fact that the deinstitutionalization and community mental health movements of the 1950s through the late 1970s never successfully came to grips with what the New Haven outreach team also found in the mid-1990s—that even the most innovative forms of mental health care do not provide their clients with an entrée to a full membership and participation in the community,[2] that is, "a life in the community,"[33] with "fullness," "participation," and "a life" not based on a quantitative comparison to a mean or range among individual citizens, but to the individual's capacities as supported by the elements of citizenship and Honneth's "recognition."

RECOVERY

Recovery is the dominant paradigm in contemporary US mental health care. William Anthony, a founding father of psychiatric rehabilitation, provided an early and influential definition of recovery as "a deeply personal, unique process of changing one's attitudes, values, feelings, goals, skills and roles...a way of living a satisfying, hopeful and contributing life, even with the limitations caused by illness...Recovery involves the development of new meaning and purpose in one's life as one grows beyond the catastrophic effects of mental illness."[34]

Larry Davidson and David Roe describe two forms of recovery. Research dating back to the early 1970s has demonstrated partial, episodic, and full clinical recovery *from* schizophrenia, previously thought to be an incurable disease with a progressive downward course.[35] Recovery *in* or *outside of* mental illness,[36] sometimes called "social recovery," involves building and "having a life" in spite of the debilitating social effects of mental illness and a message of hopelessness that many have experienced as coming packaged with clinical care.[37] The authors trace the roots of social recovery to the independent living, civil rights, and psychiatric survivor movements of the 1960s and 1970s, also noting that the concept of living a life "in" recovery from mental illness was borrowed from 12-step groups such as Alcoholics Anonymous.

In social recovery, people achieve self-determination and full membership in society *even if* they continue to experience symptoms of mental illness.[38,39] People need not return to, or achieve, a "normal" state of functioning, as mental illness is only one aspect of a person's life. Recovery involves coping with one's disability while also striving to overcome the socially and economically disabling impacts of poverty, inadequate housing, and lack of valued roles. People with mental illness can have friendships, intimate relationships, and hold down jobs. They can join others in worship or recreation, school, and work, and can build a life based on their goals, values, and desires[35] rather than a life of "avoiding stress." Recovery is also associated with a number of clinical and psychosocial practices, including supported housing, peers as staff in community mental health care, and "recovery-oriented practice" in clinical care.[38]

Social recovery, even with its social and political roots, has come under criticism for emphasizing the subjective status of being "in recovery" over social and structural inequities that work to the exclusion of people with mental illnesses.[39] Kim Hopper argues that recovery minimizes the roles of state, culture, and society in mental health reform.[40] Alison Edgley and colleagues draw on Noam Chomsky's work to advocate for a relative shift in the work of recovery from individual autonomy and responsibility toward creativity and interdependent mutuality in nurturing communities.[41] Another criticism of social recovery and of clinical recovery, both, is that some persons with mental illnesses are too severely impaired to have or achieve either.[42] An anti-recovery (AR) and pro-recovery (PR) debate starting from this point might contain some of these points:

> **AR:** *You're holding out hope to people who can't achieve recovery of any sort. And how does that leave them? Just as ill as before but with hopes dashed and probably blaming themselves for not recovering.*
>
> **PR:** *First of all, recovery at the individual level is a personal thing, a way of thinking about yourself and of coping with your illness. You can't define it for someone else and then say they can't achieve what they may not have been aiming for in the first place. Second, you don't know who "those people" are until you've seen them not recover according to your assessment of them and their situation. That's the definition of a stacked deck. How do you know if and when someone will "take up" the project of their own recovery? I don't.*
>
> **AR:** *But then you're defining recovery so loosely that it becomes meaningless. Or means anything and everything, which amounts to the same thing. And*

> *that's a kind of bad faith, in the promulgation of it. Recovery is bound to send some people—the most severely and chronically ill folk, that is—to the back of the bus.*[43]
>
> **PR:** *The back of the bus syndrome applies to any approach in mental health care—the possibility that that could happen and the need to guard against it. There's a tension there, for sure, but it doesn't apply only to recovery.*
>
> **AR:** *But recovery is RECOVERY. It screams "GETTING BETTER." It ups the ante too high. Wellness or inclusion, less so.*
>
> **PR:** *Only because recovery has been defined by others for people with mental illnesses. Now, recovery is for those same people to define for themselves.*

Of course this debate could go on, and it has no obvious winner. I think it's fair to say, though, that recovery advocates and practitioners can benefit from continuing "devil's advocacy" work in mapping out and defining its territory and, no more but no less than other socially oriented approaches to mental health and health care, from continuing to ask themselves the questions, "Who are we sending to the back of the bus?" and "What do we do about it?"

SOCIAL INCLUSION

In their ethnographic–qualitative research, Ware and colleagues found that six personal capacities—responsibility, accountability, imagination, empathy, judgment, and advocacy—are central to achievement of social inclusion for people with mental illnesses. These core capacities can be integrated into mental health care such that, with increased "occasions" to engage in choice making that attention to personal capacities makes room for, people will employ those capacities for achieving social inclusion outside mental health systems of care.[4]

Davidson and colleagues argue for adoption of a broad conceptual framework of inclusion based on a disability paradigm. Social inclusion, with elements of friendship, reciprocity, and hopefulness, not only supports social recovery, but being "in recovery" requires a foundation in social inclusion to support people's efforts to overcome marginalization, discrimination, and stigma. Social inclusion supports people's sense of belonging through opportunities for friendship, personally valued activities, and cultivation of hope. As these opportunities increase, people are more available for, and open to, spontaneous life-affirming "moments" that strengthen their sense of personhood and foster a more positive attitude toward their lives, even when the evanescent moment of grace has passed on.[44]

Social inclusion among European Union nations has a more structural–institutional bent than its American counterparts. Hilary Silver contrasts the US view of poverty as lack of income for purchasing necessities to the European view of poverty as social deprivation, lack of participation, and comparatively lower living standards. European policies to promote inclusion cross bureaucratic domains such as housing, health, and income support, and treat social inclusion as a long-term process passing through a number of transitional stages. Each stage in this process must include the participation of previously excluded persons in local and national policy making. Silver argues that attention to the European form of social inclusion could transform policy and public debates in the United States both by connecting individuals across excluded groups that are normally isolated from each other and by connecting social policy agencies across domains.[45] An example of the latter in the United States is the federal Interagency Council on Homelessness, which developed a plan leading to SAMHSA's 1993–2000 ACCESS project. This project, in turn, funded the New Haven outreach team and 17 other programs linked to local mental health and social support systems of care across the country.[46]

Difficulties with social inclusion include its multiple definitions, a lack of structured instruments to measure it, and lack of agreement on its primary domains.[45] Like recovery, the long reach of social inclusion could encourage its wider adoption in mental health policy and practice in the United States. Lack of attention to measurement of the concept and resistance to learning from European models, however, could slow its progress.

CAPABILITIES

Some mental health researchers have adapted capabilities theory from Amartya Sen's work on alleviating poverty and deprivation in developing countries. Sen, Hopper writes, argues that income and goods are not adequate measures of "well-being" because they don't take into account people's choices about their own goals. People's "functionings" are the practical choices they can make and the endeavors they can pursue, and poverty is not merely a lack of income but a deprivation of choice and social participation.[47] Well-being may come from benefits given by others, but dignity violations can come with them, too.[48] "Agency freedom," for Sen, is the capacity to pursue one's goals as a responsible agent. "Wellbeing freedom" involves the things that people can do without bringing their personal aims into play.[49] Capabilities, then, involves not only what people *do*, but what they *can do* if they want to and *about* the things that matter most to them.

Hopper points out that if well-being means having basic securities, and capabilities means the exercise of one's capacity as a moral agent, then capabilities can pose a risk to people's basic securities, since it urges recipients of care to become makers and doers of their own projects.[50] A well-known example of the recipient–doer dilemma in the mental health field is the reluctance of people who've been awarded federal Supplemental Security Income (SSI) to risk losing it by taking a part-time or full-time job. Taking the job, usually with no long-term security, will eventually trigger termination of the person's SSI benefits. Trial periods of work with resumption of SSI benefits if needed are an option, but not a widely known or trusted one for recipients. Capabilities theory challenges mental health systems to play or fold on "strengths-based" care and supports. Success in addressing disability, Hopper contends, depends upon supporting people's enhanced capacities and their conversion to empowered social roles and ventures.[50]

A strength of capabilities theory is its specificity. Of all major socially oriented theories in contemporary mental health care in the United States it is the least vulnerable to devolving, or being devolved into, vague generality. A possible weakness of the theory lies in the particulars of translating its elements rooted in economic reform in developing countries to mental health reform in the United States, although its principles seem to be well suited for the latter. A question I mull over with the theory as applied to people with serious and disabling psychiatric disorders is whether or not it risks excluding people whose capacities and capabilities, at a particular time or across time, make paid work too high a bar for them. Another way of putting this is, does capabilities have a critique of the hegemonic value of work in American society and, as a result, the narrowing of what constitutes a valued contribution to society?

Citizens

A citizenship agenda, my colleagues and I have argued, should not only support individual efforts to achieve full community membership, but push communities to welcome people in from its margins as well. Surveying the community in which we were trying to find housing for people like Jim, we thought about enlisting the help of community members and institutions. Jim and others might choose not to take advantage of some opportunities that open up for them as the result of such efforts, but saying no to an opportunity and not being able to vote on it at all are two different things. Perhaps Sen would say that the first situation involves the exercise of personal agency, while the second involves a "wellbeing deprivation." Yet few policy and programmatic responses to homelessness, at the time of the New Haven ACCESS Project's tenure, included systematic efforts to address the question of whether or not people who were homeless could become full members of their communities and society.

We decided to put our citizenship framework to its first test with a community-level approach through a project to be called, simply, *Citizens. Citizens* would have three broad aims—to increase neighborhood, community, and business support to people who were homeless and about to enter housing, raise public awareness of the needs and aspirations of people who were homeless, and foster cooperation among community organizations, homeless persons, and social service providers in New Haven. A "Community Council" made up of homeless or formerly homeless persons, providers of mental health and other services, and other community members would decide how to carry out these aims.

The Melville Charitable Trust funded the project. Columbus House, the largest agency serving people who are homeless in New Haven, agreed to administer it and

I supervised it. We hired Lezley TwoBears as the director. Lezley knew about people who were homeless and lived on little but their wits, their friends on the street, and their resilience. "I watched people not die because they simply refused to do so," she wrote.[51] She hired Patty Benedict, an activist in the American Indian community in Connecticut who, like Lezley, also had experience in mental health advocacy work.

Our next step was to recruit representatives from our three constituency groups for the Community Council. John and Ted had been homeless and had mental illnesses. They also had some organizing and advocacy experience though the People's Center, a longtime grass roots organization in New Haven. David, a client of the mental health center, was eager to do anything to help. Keeping him on task and on point with the message of citizens in his conversations with people at the mental health center was a challenge. Florence, a friend of David's who had earned a PhD and MPH before mental illness interrupted her academic trajectory, was an early recruit who stayed with the project through its second iteration, which I'll take up in the next chapter. Florence had not been homeless, but had been at risk of it.

Peggy, who had found an apartment and got reconnected with mental health treatment through the outreach team, was another early recruit. I had written about Peggy as an "essential client," one who took outreach workers and teams to their professional and emotional limits and exemplified the best of what they could do. Peggy was in her early forties when the outreach workers met her. She had a serious and disabling mental illness and had dropped out of treatment. She dressed in many layers of purple clothes and waved around a plastic Luke Skywalker sword when strangers came near her. Her price for talking to outreach workers was that they bring clothes and food to her friends.

Peggy had endured many tragedies. Two of her children had died in a house fire, one of her sisters was killed in a freak accident, and another was dying of cancer. Perhaps purple was her color of mourning, outreach workers surmised. Peggy refused the help they offered her because the team received federal funds, and she thought the government wanted to imprison her for her past work with Amnesty International. Her refusal, though, was also spiced with her anger toward family members for trying to get her into mental health treatment. One day, Peggy agreed to visit Columbus House to take a shower. Later, she washed her clothes there and took a peek at the sleeping quarters on her way out. A few weeks later, the police brought her to the Yale-New Haven Hospital emergency room after she threatened them for disrobing the statue of a Civil War hero dressed in her purple clothes. She accepted the outreach team's help now because she saw them as rescuing her from the hospital.[52] This is only the beginning of the story of Peggy and the outreach team, but workers helped her to find an apartment, renew her beautician's license, and make plans to get back to work. Her contribution to *Citizens* was slim, practically speaking, but her connection to it was a reminder of what we were about and of the inner resources that could come into play with help from others that come in the right place at the right time.

The homelessness and mental illness folk tended to come and go as council members because of instabilities in their lives or because the project didn't generate jobs for them as we, and they, had hoped. Other members of this group who occasionally sat in on council meetings had a connection to Lezley from her soup kitchen days. One was Jennie, a poet in her twenties who was in and out of prison, drug treatment programs, and homelessness. "So bright and so addicted," said Lezley. One day, at her wit's end, she took Jennie aside. "I've done everything I can for you," she said. "You can't get yourself into recovery because you're too clever for that. You have to outmaneuver yourself. When you kill yourself I will wail at your funeral. I will throw myself on your dirt. I will bawl over you in your grave like a mother for her child."

Lezley's intervention was a risky one, the taking of which requires that you know who you're talking to and what kind of connection you have with them. And even then it's risky. Such interventions do occur outside of professional clinical care, though, and modified versions of them occur in care as well, especially at its margins, as in homeless outreach work. An example of the latter is Joe's feigned anger at Angela in the last chapter, successful because it got Angela to come inside on a dangerously cold weekend. But what if she'd not responded to his feigned anger? Would he have had to come back and try to work out another solution with Angela for the cold weekend? How likely would success have been in that case, his status and influence with her diminished by his first failure and his tacit admission of it in coming back?

Jennie is married now and is a counselor at a drug treatment program and a minister. "She calls me every year and sings Happy Birthday to me," said Lezley. "She tells me, 'Without you I'd be dead.'"[3]

Richard Weingarten, director of peer services at the mental health center at the time, counted among the service provider group, but his lived experience and role also connected him to the "homelessness" sector of people who were likely to be, or have been, clients of the mental health center. Alison Cunningham, director of Columbus House, and Edward Mattison, director of a peer-based agency for people with behavioral health disorders, were council members along with others associated with the mental health care system. Sheila Masterson, director of a "special services district" in New Haven that advocated for and supported local businesses, and Ruth, owner of the building that housed the outreach team, were the most dependable community members.

The Community Council was to be a "community coalition"[53] that would address topics of homelessness and mental illness that were "rooted in a larger social, cultural, political and economic fabric"[53] by drawing on the perspectives and resources of diverse sectors of the New Haven community. Colleagues in the Yale Department of Psychiatry proposed an evaluation with participant observation, analysis of written material—minutes, planning documents, and other material— and weekly "process logs"[54] in order to measure organizational development over time. The process log form asked questions about recent internal and external contacts, type of activity conducted such as presentations to community partners, and planning for more substantial projects such as a hoped-for jobs program. Council members and staff showed a healthy reluctance to complete the logs, but most finally did so. The evaluators presented their findings periodically at council meetings to help the group make mid-course adjustments.[55]

We began with two working hypotheses. First, there would be a tendency for representatives of social service organizations to dominate the project development and governance and so, participants would need to make concerted efforts to shift the relative locus of power away from them. We knew that housing the program in a social service agency rather than a council of churches or voluntary association might delay the process of gaining community support and, perhaps, build in a tendency for the project to "act like" a social service agency. We decided, though, that the advantages of sponsorship from an agency that dealt with homelessness and mental illness would likely outweigh its disadvantages, especially since the Melville Charitable Trust was funding us on a year-to-year basis and wanted to see tangible returns on its investment.

Our second hypothesis was that there would be tension and conflict between the long-term goal of establishing a more welcoming social and economic environment for homeless persons in general, and the immediate goal of helping individuals who were homeless now. This tension, we thought, would reflect the interests of representatives of each of the three sectors represented on the Community Council.

We were frustrated at times in trying to recruit strong council members. Here's Lezley, looking back:

> *We were surprised that the grant came through. I wasn't an administrator. There was no real structure to the project and no one telling me what to do... [but] if I'd been with an agency that was more uptight, I wouldn't have been as free to make mistakes. I think we just decided that we'd explore how people who were homeless and people who were housed are different and similar, and what one would say to the other, to get to the point where we could figure out how to help people who were homeless come into housing. I think we knew more about what we weren't at the beginning than what we were. "Are you a...?" Fill in the blank. We didn't know. "Do you...?" Fill in the blank. We didn't know. We were who we weren't before we were who we were. So we said, Let's find our place in relation to homelessness and community and what community meant to each group—people who had homes and people who didn't.*

Our hope that the New Haven community, or a substantial sector of it, would adopt the project proved to be wildly unrealistic. In part because of this, regular membership on the council had dwindled to a core group of four near the end of the second year and day-to-day program operation and oversight resembled that of a traditional small social service program, with Lezley as the project director, Alison as the sponsoring agency's executive director, and me as the guy from the mental health center. The three of us made most decisions and gave progress reports to the council.

As I Sat on the Green

It was around this time that the idea of a book written by homeless people came to the fore. Lezley, Patty Benedict, and a nationally known writer of fiction, Alice Mattison, who had volunteered for years at the Community Soup Kitchen, took the lead. Lezley recalls it this way:

> *That's what crystallized into our purpose, to introduce these communities to each other. What were the commonalities among people that made them part of a community? What were the parts of being a community that people in housing didn't consider in people who had a community without homes? Because we knew there was a homeless community...but it was a hidden community.*

The book consists mainly of interviews with people who were homeless that Lezley, Patty, and Alice conducted. *As I Sat on the Green* only briefly discusses the citizenship concept, but it did address the objective of community education. It also speaks, in their own words, of how people who are homeless fight to create, shape, and protect a positive identity for themselves with a sense of their own dignity and self-worth.

Denise is described in the book as a 28-year-old widow, part white and part African American, and lesbian. At 18 she married a man who became a drug smuggler from Cuba to the United States and was killed during a drug raid. At the time when she became homeless she was, as she put it, "one of those close-minded people who thought that people who are homeless are all drug addicts that were gonna beat me up and take all my stuff."[56] Denise was interviewed in a women's shelter, having been refused entry in a drug rehabilitation program because she was clean at the time. Such are the ways, at times, of social service bureaucracies and their funding sources. Denise had been close to getting a job managing a convenience store when the owner called to speak with her and discovered she was living in a shelter. Like Angela in my interview with her, she did not endorse being homeless:

> *I'm just temporarily displaced. My home is where I am. I carry my home with me, I am my home.*[57]

And how did she find the strength to cope with all she'd been through, the interviewer asked her?

> *I think it's just a sheer mean streak. I think it's just a sheer desire to be alive. I think it's just curiosity. I want to know what happens after this.*[58]

Kelvin was born in North Carolina. He grew up there and in New Jersey and Connecticut. He did well in high school academically and was captain of the football team. Kelvin went to college, where he was a star again both academically and athletically. Shortly before graduation, though, he tried crack cocaine:

> *It was all immediately déjà vu. Even though I didn't realize I'd had it before, I recognized the feelings, the sensation immediately. Over time I began to put together the pieces, realizing just how much dope I had been exposed to as a child.*[59]

Kelvin had been homeless for six years at the time of his interview. He was cut off from his family. "I was never nothin' to my family," he said.[60] He'd had many jobs, as a mural painter, doing temporary work in construction, roofing, and plumbing, but hadn't fulfilled what his high school and most of his college career predicted for him:

> *Every time I get involved in something that seems to be leading to something big, something really significant, I get tremendously scared. Sometimes, I even duck out... I'll do something self-destructive, that's the story of my life. But I've been working on all that.*[61]

Several of the people who told their stories in the book gave well-attended readings in New Haven and around the state. The book's main contribution, in addition to giving people who were homeless the chance to speak for themselves, was to counteract the reification of these same people as overwhelmingly single, without children, and homeless for years beginning in some vague past that did not include a family of origin. Many of the book's speakers had grown up in or around New Haven, had family members in the area, and in various combinations had been married, had children, and had long employment histories, sometimes in professional or well-regarded trade positions. They had lived difficult lives, all of them, many with chaotic and early traumatizing experiences in their families of origin. But they planned to return to work or get better jobs, go to school, reunite with their children, and take back control of their lives. Few, interestingly, offered a social critique of their situations to match their critiques of themselves and the mistakes they'd made.

Representation of the Governed: the Leadership Project

Citizens never lacked for ideas and activities. Some important networking and planning was done for a jobs project, for example, that would focus on training and job placement for people who were homeless and training for employers on cultural aspects of worker–supervisor relationships. The idea for the project came from our learning that many of the people we were trying to help were motivated to work and, often, had specific job skills and experience. What they lacked or could use brushing up on were social skills and workplace savvy. During one meeting, Lezley gave me a lesson in "cultural competence" or, as Lezley put it, "How do you touch someone on the shoulder when you don't know if that will start a war?"[3] A few of us were talking about how a supervisor could mistake the shy or insecure behavior of an employee who doesn't make good eye contact for untrustworthiness.

"That's right," said Lezley. "For example," she said, looking at me, "I don't look you in the eye."

"What do you mean, you don't look me in the eye?"

"I don't look you in the eye."

"You're doing it right now!"

"No, I'm not. But you think I am. In my culture [American Indian], looking someone in the eye is a sign of disrespect. So I've learned how to *almost* look you in the eye."

Unfortunately, time on what, in the event, would be a three-year project, was running out. Our jobs project came too late in the game for us to get it off the ground.

Lezley, and Patty as well, sat in on many mental health system housing and jobs committees, and spread the word about *Citizens*. "No one knew quite what to do with us," Lezley said. "We weren't really part of the mental health system, so there was no reason to come to *our* meetings... ." One of those meetings, though, which Patty and I attended, sparked the creation of the *Leadership Project*, an undertaking less ambitious than the jobs project but that set the stage for the *Citizens Project* of the next chapter. A little background is in order.

In 1994, the Clinton Administration mandated a new funding approach for its Housing and Urban Development programs. Instead of a survival-of-the-fittest, or fittest grant writer, process, HUD now mandated local consensus for local housing and rental assistance programs for people who are homeless that it funded. Localities were to develop a "Continuum of Care" plan that listed its priority applications to be submitted under the imprimatur of a to-be-established Continuum of Care Committee. The plan would also have to be accepted for, and included in, the city or regional planning document in which the committee was located. Predictably, the New Haven Continuum of Care Committee became a service provider monopoly after a contentious beginning that included professional mediation. In fairness to the agencies, it was their job to fight for their clients and their own survival, and only an intervention by the New Haven City Administration or citizen lobbying would have been likely to create a more balanced public, nonprofit, client, and other private citizen involvement.

The Continuum of Care mandate was slow in the adoption, but by the late 1990s policy had become fact. HUD also wanted to see people who were homeless sitting on local Continuum of Care Committees. There was much discussion among New Haven committee members about how to do this. At the meeting Patty and I attended, a young African-American man who had been invited by an agency representative spoke angrily and nonstop for about 10 minutes about the lack of representation of homeless people on the Continuum of Care Committee, the self-interest of the social service agencies, and the hypocrisy of the whole process. He finished, got up, left, and never returned.

Patty and I talked afterward about the missed opportunity and what a citizenship approach might be able to offer. We knew some agency directors wanted to encourage client representation, and some had tried to do so, without success. We wanted to offer an program that would be empowering for people who were or had been homeless, would help social service organizations and action groups fulfill their promise of client representation, and would have an impact on improving services. A pilot board training and internship program seemed to be the way to go.[62]

We talked to some people who were homeless and some agency directors and city officials. Some who were homeless said the search for housing and work or the need to focus on their mental health or getting clean from drugs stood in the way of board membership for them. Others spoke of being undervalued on the rare occasions when they did have the chance to speak to agency administrators or of being intimidated by the prospect of doing so. A few denigrated their own perspectives and knowledge as survivors of homelessness. Agency directors and board members spoke of not knowing how to encourage client involvement and not having been able to identify many people they considered stable enough to participate on their boards and committees. A few spoke of previous negative experiences with clients as board members, including their inconsistent attendance or inappropriate behavior. We also found that the structure of services for clients works against their representation, as clients are encouraged to focus on their own recovery, find housing, and move beyond their experience of homelessness rather than advocate for changes in the programs that serve them.

It became apparent, then, that people who were homeless had no real say in the administration of programs that served them. There was, that is, no representation of the governed, and the governors lacked a forum for considering the insights and information the governed could offer. In addition, the governed were deprived of the opportunity for personal and group empowerment that membership on boards and committees could offer them.

A few private foundations gave us small grants. Patty, who would be director of the *Leadership Project*, drafted a curriculum and class schedule with help from people who were homeless and agency directors. Classes would meet twice a week for three hours each on interpersonal skills, public speaking, assertiveness training, negotiation and conflict resolution, board and committee training including Robert's Rules of Order, reading budget reports, the state legislative process, networking and advocacy, and homelessness. Students would be paid $10 for each class and $20 for each Board meeting during a six-month internship after class graduation. Classes would be held in the evening to accommodate students who worked during the day.

Students were recruited through agency contacts, flyers posted in shelters and soup kitchens, and group discussions at soup kitchens and shelters. Fifteen people applied and had an interview with Patty, who talked with them about the importance of having a support group in place for what might prove to be a challenging experience for them. Of the 15, almost all had an addictions history and about half had a mental illness. Although they weren't asked this question, one-third reported that they had AIDS or were HIV positive. All had been homeless, but only two were at the time of their interviews. Most had attended college or a technical school, most had a support system, and a few had some previous board or action group experience. Only three were employed.

Patty accepted 10 applicants, six men and four women, as students. She contacted directors of almost two dozen local and statewide agencies and a City of New Haven's human services administrator about sponsoring internships, telling them they would have to appoint a board member to serve as a mentor to the intern and a liaison to her. Four agencies—a statewide anti-homelessness coalition that agreed to take two interns, Columbus House, the New Haven Mayor's Select Committee on Homelessness, and a small nonprofit organization that distributes food vouchers to people who are homeless—made the cut.

Class instructors included a peer outreach worker, a community mental health care manager, an attorney, a United Way administrator, social service administrators, a lobbyist, a legislator, and Patty. Each class, held in the conference room of a supportive housing agency, began with an update on how students were doing, in general and with the course. Patty found that she needed to schedule individual time with students before most classes to talk with them about personal crises or their anxiety about the course and a looming internship.

Initial classes, on leadership itself, went well. During a class on interpersonal skills, though, a few students were rude to the instructor, a peer outreach worker. Patty confronted them at the beginning of the next class. Not only was their behavior unacceptable, she said, but it was self-defeating at the level of advocacy for the homeless community. And not having been one of the rude ones didn't excuse anyone, she added. Students had to take individual and collective ownership of the class. She asked them to develop a set of class rules. To her surprise, the ones they adopted were stricter than the ones she would have imposed. And they worked. During the final class sessions, for example, participants challenged instructors who spoke on homelessness, but did so on point, not ad hominem.

Early on it became clear that the students were developing a sense of community, even of being "a family." Here are some post-graduation comments from students:

The fellowship that was created was really good. I liked the way the class worked together and how we developed our own rules for the class. I met a lot of good people that I still keep in touch with.

I learned how individual ideas can apply to the group and how to be part of a group and work within it ... What happened to one of us happened to all of us. Who would have thought that we would all chip in and put on a cookout together?

This training helped me to build my self-confidence and gave me a reason to get back involved in advocating for the homeless community. It was beneficial to my sobriety and gave me an added incentive to be sober. I liked feeling like the project belonged to us and how we got to create our own rules for the classes. People from the classes still see each other on a regular basis, even those that didn't graduate.

Of the 10 students, one man left to enter a residential drug treatment program. A woman, selected as an alternate, took his place. Another woman left because the classes conflicted with her work schedule. A man left when his housing program pulled him out the class because of his drug use. A woman, thought to be using drugs, dropped out of sight. Another woman who stayed almost to the end of the class period began drinking and dropped out.

Five people graduated from the program. Education distinguished them from their colleagues who left—all five had attended college or trade school. Also, the nature and quality of participants' writing in the class surveys pointed to the importance of education in students' understanding of the training material. In their written evaluations of public speaking, for example, comments of community college or trade school graduates were descriptive and directly related to content, as in, "We had the opportunity among ourselves to express ourselves' throughout the speeches," and "I enjoyed us just communicating as a group." Two of the non-graduates by contrast, wrote comments such as, "The class and TV man," and "When we got up to speak."

Students saw the course as being successful. Even some of those who dropped out stayed in touch with Patty and spoke highly of it and of their fellow students. Students thought future courses should be longer to allow for more role playing on board membership, more assertiveness training, and more time spent on developing interpersonal skills.

There were no differences between school graduates and non-graduates on knowledge of class subjects prior to the class or their assessment of whether or not the class helped them prepare for board membership. Most students gave the public speaking class the highest rating possible. Oddly, almost all students rated themselves as having "average" knowledge of homelessness. Of the four women, including the alternate, only one graduated, while of six men, four graduated. We don't know why.

Following a graduation at city hall with comments by the mayor, the five graduates began their six-month internships. Near the end, most were doing well. These are Patty's comments from her records:

John was completing his internship on the board of an emergency shelter and transitional housing agency. He was living in transitional housing at the time his internship began, but he had to leave due to medical problems that left him unable to work and pay his rent. He's staying in a men's shelter now. He has been clean and sober for a year and is doing additional volunteer work in the community. His board internship has been successful and he's been asked to stay on as a full board member. He has agreed to.

Thomas is completing his internship on the Mayor's Select Committee on Homelessness and has been accepted as a full member. His board mentor hopes he will begin to speak out more in meetings. He has remained in the apartment he had when he started classes and has taken a part-time human services position, thanks to the increased confidence he's gained through the Leadership Project, he says.

Danielle continues to live in a supported housing complex and is thinking about doing additional volunteer work. She has been clean from drugs for three years. Her board mentor reports that while she's quiet in meetings, she's an enthusiastic member and other board members are pleased with her involvement.

Robert is living in a nursing home recuperating from major surgery. He continues to do work there related to his internship with the board of an agency that dis-tributes food vouchers. Unfortunately, he'll have to find a new place to live when he leaves the nursing home, since Yale University has bought the rooming house where he was living. His board mentor gives him high marks for his internship and its positive effect on the board's work. [Robert would become one of the first peer mentors for the Citizens Project, the next major citizenship effort.]

James has been an intern on the state antihomelessness coalition for about three months and has also joined the Mayor's Select Committee on Homelessness. These activities conflict with his handyman and landscaping business, though, which has grown during the class and internship period. He has stopped attending both groups.

Board members, as Patty's comments suggest, were pleased overall with their experience with the interns and their contribution. This comment from a board member and longtime grass roots worker on homelessness is consistent with others we collected:

John [an intern] knows the life on the street and the people who live there. He offers the information in a dignified way and is clear and instructive. I think the board members feel comfortable with him. I think it has to do with his quiet and warm personality. He's teaching them things they wouldn't learn anywhere else.

The major shortcoming of the *Leadership Project* and our evaluation of it is that we lacked the time and resources to measure the impact of interns on board or agency practice or on the local Continuum of Care process that inspired it. The project seemed to have been personally empowering for students, but empowerment practitioners and scholars look for evidence of an intervention's consciousness-raising for participants and its impact on practice and advocacy. Lorraine Gutierrez writes that involvement with similar others on socioeconomic or political matters of concern to all can reduce people's stress, give them the opportunity to develop skills while learning about the social and institutional underpinnings of their individual and collective life trajectories, and engage collectively in social change.[63] Of these, the *Leadership Project* did not measure changes in levels of stress, gave what might be called an introductory course to some aspects of political and socioeconomic issues that affected students personally and collectively, and did engage them in the initial stages of collective change.

The 50% dropout rate is an obvious problem. Still, the five graduates were almost uniformly positive about their course and internship experiences, and board members gave favorable reports as well.

We learned some things. A longer class period, with more emphasis on public speaking, the legislative process, and advocacy would have prepared people better for their internships. Class instruction in how to become a board member should be balanced with instruction in how to be an effective advocate on or outside of boards and committees. Internships should begin before the end of the class period, with support and discussion on the experience built into the remaining classes. In addition to being hospitable to interns, a meaningful internship requires placement on a board that's grappling with important policy issues. Pre-existing relationships between the Project Director and agency directors or board members are also important, as these are likely to increase the organization's willingness to participate and see interns through rocky periods. If this lesson learned looks like a form of paternalism toward interns, it's worth pointing out that "non-peer" board members often are recruited by friends or business associates and have a high level of comfort with fellow board members upon joining, even setting aside the advantages that their working lives and social capital give them as the new kids on the block. They're not really new to the boards they join. Instead, board membership is kind of extension of the work they do.

We learned that it's important to bring together a group of students who are ready to learn, not only for the obvious reason—so they will learn!—but also to create the right conditions for developing mutual group support. Group cohesion and self-governance are not necessarily an unalloyed good, as groups can create lowest common denominator expectations that discourage their more capable and adventurous members. Instructors and class members, then, must balance encouragement of group identity with encouragement of individual efforts and "identity work."[64]

"Creaming" carries the negative connotation of producing successful interventions by recruiting those most likely to do well without it and excluding those who need the intervention most but are most likely to struggle in it. Of 10 students, as noted above, only five graduated. Graduates were not currently homeless, had higher levels of education, and had more support systems in place than non-graduates. Yet placing people with large gaps in education, social support, and greater need to focus on day-to-day survival may, in retrospect, have been a set-up for students. Projects like this one may be most appropriate for those for whom it represents a step in their lives that they're almost, but not quite, ready to take without the support the project could give them. That said, *Leadership Project* graduates had by no means "made it" in terms of personal stability or material well-being. Four of the five graduates had histories of serious psychiatric disability or substance use disorder or both, and none was far removed from being homeless.

Advocates and service providers who want to start leadership projects would do well to consider the funding they will need for ongoing support both during and, preferably, after board internships. They should also consider the need for ongoing commitment to the progress they help to foster. We were surprised, but shouldn't have been, by how much interns' experiences motivated them for paid work or more intensive volunteer work. Having a taste of what they could do, students wanted to go further. This fact points to the responsibility of planners to take next logical steps that come with projects such as this one—more courses and internships, paid work, or other valued roles following completed internships.

Summing up *Citizens*

Our evaluation of *Citizens* supported our first working hypothesis that there would be a tendency for members of social service organizations to dominate the development and governance of the project at the outset and that council members would need to make concerted efforts to shift the relative locus of power from them to the community and homelessness representative domains. During the first six months of the project, more than three-fourths of all program contacts that staff and council members made were with social service agency staff. At the start of the third year, though, *Citizens* embarked on an effort to strengthen the council by keeping members better informed of the day-to-day work and calling on them for networking or other direct help or consultation. During this year, contacts with social service providers steadily decreased compared with those with non–social service representatives until they represented fewer than 40% of the total, while contact with non–social service persons and groups grew from one-fifth to more than three-fifths of all.

Our second hypothesis was that there would be tension between the process of trying to gain general community acceptance of people who had been homeless, on one hand, and developing projects to help individuals who currently were homeless, on the other. The relative proportion of planning and actions during the first year reflected a process orientation. The majority of discussions were internal, and council consensus-building activities far outdistanced contacts with external parties regarding specific projects. As predicted, differences of interest and perspective among consumer, service provider, and community sectors influenced early development. A social service provider who, briefly, was a council member, complained that the council was being divisive, ignoring the community inclusion efforts that some service providers were making on behalf of their clients. "Homelessness" council representatives thought the project was moving too slowly toward helping currently homeless persons. And a "community" member of the council, a business executive, said that social service providers and evaluators were "academic gasbags"—all talk and no action.

These critiques prompted some changes. The agency administrator's criticism of the project's divisiveness influenced a relative shift from facilitating community members' involvement in helping people who were homeless to building bridges between community members, people who were homeless, and social service folk. "Homelessness" representatives were influential in the project's efforts to create a jobs project, even though the project didn't come off. And the business executive became a key player in the project's contacts with area businesses and neighborhood councils regarding that same jobs project.

Reflecting on our efforts, both successful and halting, it seemed to us that the citizenship framework resonated with commonly held values of individual rights, responsibilities, and contributions to society. These values have historical and cultural capital that, in theory, could help people who are excluded to enter into the fabric of community living. Homeless people's ability to survive in the most difficult of circumstances, for example, could be seen as exemplifying American values of independence and self-reliance. The citizenship framework could also be a guide for addressing gaps in policy and programmatic approaches to the community inclusion of people with mental illness, homeless and not. It might also encourage partnerships between peers, service providers, and community members and institutions to close those gaps. And it added a social level to "person-centered" approaches in mental health care.

The citizenship framework might encourage mental health organizations and those that fund them to collaborate with community organizations and civic associations to extend the range of opportunities available to their clients. Such collaborations might also serve as mediating structures between individuals and government to help people make contact with churches, civic groups, neighborhood associations, and others in their communities.[65] And the framework might help in shifting public discourse about people who were homeless, or had mental illnesses, or both, toward the contributions they could make to society rather than the burden on society they represented.

We had some ideas about future community-level citizenship projects. One had to do with leadership and representation. Allowing for the fact that different circumstances and objectives might qualify this strategy, citizenship projects should consider a representative balance among peers and advocates, mental health and other social service providers, municipal officials, and other community folk. Mental health and other service providers are used to running programs. They need to learn how to share power and honor other forms of expertise. Peers could become involved with citizenship projects at key points in their own recovery and personal citizenship building, and as part of both of those projects. Community participants may become disillusioned or impatient with the process of building links among diverse actors and delays in action. Each group needs to educate the others about which approaches can work and which need to be jettisoned.

Citizenship projects should be linked to such foundational human needs as living-wage jobs and affordable housing or they risked foundering in a directionless idealism. The challenge of managing the tension between grand themes and ideals and positive change on the ground might be described as that of integrating a "power-based" model of community development emphasizing a broad-based approach to "systemic change" and more modest programs aimed at providing access to specific resources.[66] Citizenship projects, we recognized, would need to vary with local constraints and opportunities. Successful projects were likely to be those with representatives of traditional sectors, such as the director of a local business district organization, who become advocates themselves while retaining the credentials to champion the case for change to their peers.

It was the business of resources, jobs and housing, the tools and supports, and the capabilities and capacities that help people "make it" as citizens that we were thinking about most as *Citizens* wound down. Here's Lezley once more:

> *Nothing grand happened. We were just getting started, trying to figure out how to be with each other. At the time we started, people were afraid of homeless people. Cross the street, hold on to your pocketbook, don't look at them. Each homeless person was isolated by him- or herself. We made a place where people could meet. But our process was so open. We were too intent on bringing people together to be the engine for specific projects and interventions. We thought we'd discover them as a group, but we couldn't focus our efforts and make things happen. So the best we could do was to get people together and not interfere too much with what went on. And the benefits from it, or not, would become evident. As for next steps, it was too soon for that.*

It's best to be careful with Monday morning quarterbacking 13 years after the fact. And in truth, we were no better equipped to develop a citizenship intervention for individuals at the outset than we were to develop a community-level project. The *Leadership Project* was a start, albeit a comparatively narrow one, on the way to a robust intervention to support the citizenship of *individuals* who were struggling on the streets or isolated in SROs and apartments.

Citizenship started on a grand scale by taking on the community-level pathway to citizenship. In this pathway, the community has a responsibility to welcome in from the margins excluded groups that are denied the full benefits and expectations of citizenship. Having such a responsibility, however, doesn't mean that society will act on it without a strong push from excluded groups and their supporters. This was true even in a socially liberal community, which also happens to be a community in which many people live in poverty. Thus we could have used a stronger dose of the social conflict model of change. That said, neither a social activism nor a social acceptance model had much of a chance to succeed this early on in the development of the citizenship model. And in fact, *Citizens* might more fairly be described as combining social activist, if not social conflict, elements with appeals to the democratic ideals of its local community. In addition, *Citizens* gave us a trial run at a community-level approach to full community membership with mental illnesses who were also socially and economically excluded.

Citizens touched on the 5 Rs as well. It supported the *rights* of people to be represented on the boards of agencies that governed a part of their own lives. It provided training and internships that required people to accept *responsibility* for their part in services provided to themselves and their colleagues. It involved taking on the valued *role* of being a board member. *Resources* were represented modestly in the work experience that came with the training and internships. And participants developed *relationships* with fellow students working toward a common goal and with fellow board members. Helping people become full, valued, and participating members of their communities and society lay outside the scope of the *Leadership Project*. But it whetted our appetites to do just that.

3

Citizenship and Individuals

THE *CITIZENS PROJECT*, EARLY

The opportunity came with a telephone call from Madelon Baranoski, Director of the Jail Diversion Program at the mental health center. This is from her description of jail diversion programs:

> *People with mental illnesses often get arrested for petty crimes related to symptoms of mental illness and complicated, destabilizing life circumstances including homelessness. Courts, however, often don't have access to mental health services without pursuing statutorily-mandated treatment related to "state of mind" defenses and "competency to stand trial." This forces judges to use incarceration to contain and ensure treatment for defendants with disruptive symptoms, a high risk of recidivism, or a lack of resources to be released without court oversight. Jail diversion offers courts an alternative to incarceration by providing mental health services, with the defendant's agreement. The court agrees to accept the mental health agency's clinical assessment and treatment plan, the mental health agency accepts responsibility for providing appropriate treatment, and the defendant agrees to engage in treatment and allow the clinical agency to report his or her compliance with treatment to the court. People who engage in treatment and complete required court monitoring can avoid incarceration. Some will have their cases disposed of early without a criminal record. If the court chooses incarceration over the mental health plan, jail diversion programs assure that the defendant will be assessed and offered services upon release to the community.*[1]

Jail diversion can get more complicated than this, with people in and out of community mental health treatment and jails or prisons in close sequences and with more serious charges involved. Still, the process follows this general outline. Jail diversion takes place in the context of a criminalization of mental illness so extensive that jails and prisons can be called contemporary replacements for state psychiatric hospitals of the past.[2,3] People with mental illnesses represent about one-fourth of inmates in state prisons and 14% of inmates in federal prisons,[4] and prisoners with major psychiatric disorders are more likely to have had previous incarcerations than those without.[5] Once released, their successful return to their communities is often thwarted by lack of access to mental and physical health care and disqualification, by various means, from housing and employment.[6–7,8,9,10] People with mental illnesses and criminal histories have high rates of co-occurring existing substance abuse disorders,[9] amounting to a "triple stigma" of mental illness, incarceration, and substance abuse.[10] Mental illness and incarceration are also associated with high rates of childhood trauma and traumas associated with arrest and incarceration. These conditions further complicate people's community re-entry following jail or prison stays.[11]

Christopher Uggen and his colleagues write that civic reintegration, along with work and family, are key elements of successful community re-entry for released criminal offenders. People released from prison after felony convictions, having technically paid their debt to society, continue to pay with loss of parental rights, voting rights for various lengths of time depending on the state, and difficulty finding work and building non-criminal social networks. These barriers lead in turn to social isolation and loss of economic opportunities and valued roles. Given the facts that almost one-fourth of African-American adults, including one-third of African-American male adults, will be incarcerated during their lifetime, and that eventually almost all criminals stop committing crimes, Uggen and colleagues argue that we should shift our attention from recidivism to the reintegration and restoration of full citizenship of released offenders. Doing so would be good for ex-offenders, communities, and society as a whole.[12]

Creating the *Citizens Project*

We met in Madelon's office, of modest size for most places of business but near-priceless real estate in New Haven's crowded mental health center. Documents and books were piled on her desk and bookshelves, a stand to the right of the chair for guests, the extra chair for guests, and here and there on the floor. It could have been a typical absent-minded professor's office, but with Madelon it seemed to be a function of her working on the run, doing competency assessments in one part of the state, rushing back to New Haven to teach a seminar at the law school, dropping by New Haven Superior Court to check in, confer, and troubleshoot with the jail diversion clinician there, checking in with colleagues in the Law and Psychiatry Division of the mental health center, and off to the medical school's institutional review board to review applications for human subjects research.

I moved some documents off the chair, balanced them on top of the others on the stand, sat down, and took notes, fast, as Madelon talked. She had long admired the work of the outreach team, she told me. She'd also heard about our citizenship work and had an idea she wanted to talk about with me. It turned out that she loved the jail diversion work as much I did outreach work but that, like me, she had grown frustrated with its limitations. She gave me examples of what she meant.

Jill was in her mid-thirties. She'd been homeless this time for about six months. She'd received care at the mental health center on and off over the past decade, off at the moment. Jill was walking down a residential street in New Haven on her way to a friend's new apartment where, he told her, she could stay the night. Any more than that would get him in trouble with his landlord. A foglight shining down from the second floor of a house she was passing by showed loose bottles and cans spilling onto the ground from a garbage can at the side of the driveway. They'd be going out with the trash, since there was no recycling in New Haven at the time, so Jill walked up the driveway and began to fill up a large plastic trash bag she carried with her at all times. Minutes later she was arrested for trespassing on private property.

Aaron, in his fifties, had also been in and out of mental health treatment and homelessness. He had medical problems, too. One morning he was arrested for disorderly conduct for urinating at the entrance to a local supermarket. He was insulted and outraged, more by the idea that the store manager would call the police on him than that he was being arrested. He expressed these feelings in a less than calm and coherent manner to the police officers who responded to the call. Later in the day at the local jail, he told the jail diversion clinician that he'd been walking *away* from the supermarket, not *standing* in front of it, when he'd lost control of his bladder. "I would never do that at my store," he said.

Ron is one of those people almost everybody at the mental health center knows, even if he might not be seen there for months at a time. Lots of people in town knew him, too, and so, knew he wouldn't harm a fly. Unfortunately, the dozen or so people waiting at the bus stop across from the New Haven Green as Ron walked by one afternoon were not among them. He went up to one, then another, and then another of the group, standing about three inches from each face and offering his analysis of the relative contributions of Sigmund Freud and Carl Jung to contemporary mental health practice. A police officer driving by noticed a commotion. He stopped, saw Ron intruding on the personal space of a third person, and arrested him for breach of the peace.

In each of these cases, Madelon said, jail diversion worked, as the "offender" was successfully diverted from the criminal justice to the mental health system. This was a good thing, she said, far more enlightened than locking people up for petty crimes that were directly related to their mental illness, life situations, or other difficulties such as reading social signals in Ron's case, knowing when to stop talking to police officers in Aaron's, or poverty and a loose understanding of private property in Jill's. But two things, Madelon said, qualified the success of each of the jail diversion program's interventions.[13]

First, Jill, Aaron, and Ron each could be seen as attempting to contribute to society, but neither the criminal justice nor the mental health system had any such expectation of them or any way to acknowledge their efforts. Jill, arrested for trespassing, was working for a living, a key factor we associate with being a citizen. And she was recycling. Aaron, arrested at the supermarket, saw himself as a member of that establishment and adhering to clear standards of behavior, in this case trying to move away from the store entrance, when he lost control of his bladder. Ron committed his "crime" not out of disregard for society, but in an attempt to make contact with his fellow citizens.

Second, jail diversion clinicians acted in each of these three situations, in part, on the correct understanding that Jill, Aaron, and Ron had run afoul of the law not out of criminal intent, but out of difficulty negotiating an acceptable niche for themselves in society. Yet in their own actions the clinicians, with their clients' consent and legal approval, had contributed to redefining criminals as mental patients, leaving no room for them to define themselves as people who could make a positive contribution to society.

Helping people manage their mental health symptoms and reduce their contact with the criminal justice system was something that mental health centers could do fairly well, Madelon said. What they didn't do well was help their patients build a life in their community and become valued for their contributions to it. The criminal justice system, she said, mediates the relationship between the state and the individual, public and private rights, and citizenship representing individual rights and status and citizenship representing one's relationship with, and responsibilities toward, one's fellow citizens and society. Yet the jail diversion response to this critical point of action was essentially a negative one—to get criminal charges dropped or stayed in exchange for taking the person as its charge. Substituting jail time for mental health care did not help people acquire valued roles in their communities and acceptance in society.

But opportunity had knocked. The Connecticut Department of Mental Health and Addiction Services, or DMHAS, had given the mental health center funds to expand the jail diversion program. Madelon suggested that we propose to use these funds to start a citizenship program. The mental health center and DMHAS signed off, and Columbus House agreed to administer the project. Madelon and I thought it best that a citizenship intervention we now had the task of creating take place outside the dominant institutional presence of the mental health center while still drawing on the center's considerable resources and expertise. Patty, Lezley's assistant for *Citizens*, was hired as project director. Eventually, she would entice Lezley, who had moved to North Carolina but was coming back to work full time for another agency, to be her part-time assistant. Three peer mentors, Madelon's administrative assistant, researchers and research assistants from my program, and I rounded out the planning group.

In 2000, we knew of no models for what we were trying to do. A few evidence-based mental health practices, including forensic assertive community treatment (FACT),[14] illness management and recovery (IMR),[15] and supported employment[16] were being adapted to work with people with both mental illness and criminal charges. These were good programs, but we were looking for something broader than supported employment, less illness-focused than IMR, and less "clinical maintenance focused" than FACT.

We met once a week. Madelon educated us on the criminal justice system. Peer staff educated us on their experiences with mental health and criminal charges. I talked about citizenship. Patty talked about her work with *Citizens* and as an advocate. The researchers talked about citizenship's relationship to concepts such as social capital. The research assistants drew upon their vast experience of living in New Haven and working with mental health center clients who participated in our studies.

We had a definition of citizenship with its 5 Rs. We had *Citizens* as a community-level intervention under our belts. We had developed community connections that we could call on. We knew there would be a group basis for the project, although likely with individual attention and support as well. There was plain practical sense in this. How, otherwise, could we work with enough students to justify even the modest funding the jail diversion enhancement funds allowed for?

There were other reasons for choosing a group-based intervention, too. *The Citizens Project*, as we decided to call it, would not be a clinical or even, from our perspective, a psychosocial intervention, but would draw from their examples, and groups are a primary method of treatment in many such interventions.[17–19] They can reduce members' sense of isolation as they learn that others struggle with similar problems. They can help them cope with mental illness and addictions by seeing how others do so. They can help them build self-esteem based on mutual support for each other's worth and abilities and support their efforts to reconnect and make reparations with family members. They can also help them build social skills by giving them a chance to try them out in a supportive environment.[20–25] We could look as well to non-clinical sources such as Alcoholics Anonymous and other self-help groups that help people achieve and maintain abstinence.[26–31]

We hoped the *Citizens Project* would be distinct from other group-based interventions, but to echo Lezley's comments about *Citizens*, we probably knew more about what it would not be than what it would. First, it would not be a clinical program. Staff and peers were not clinicians and we did not have a clinical charge or aims, although the project would benefit from the insights of clinicians such as Madelon. Second, it wouldn't be a skills-building project, although participants would learn some concrete skills such as those needed for job hunting and job interviewing. Third, the project would not be located at the mental health center but at a non–mental health site, which turned out to be the community room of Christ Church at the confluence of Whalley, Goffe, and Dixwell Avenues, named after the three judges who fled to America after playing their parts in the execution of King Charles I. The Community Soup Kitchen, the largest soup kitchen in town, had served breakfast and lunch in the community room for years. We would use it in the afternoon. The site would be familiar to most of our prospective participants, but more than that would be a place where students would, simultaneously, be citizens and citizens in training, not patients or clients.

Fourth, the *Citizens Project* would not position itself as an alternative to mental health treatment. It was about citizenship, not about being antitreatment. It's true that the citizenship framework came into being from an object lesson in the limitations of a particular mental health program, yet its purview largely fell outside of clinical practice. Citizenship set out to do things that mental health care did not do well, did not have the tools or orientation for, and in many ways, even at its most community-oriented, *should not be* a main provider of. This is a critical point that, a dozen years and a few citizenship projects later, we would revisit in contrarian fashion by staking a good part of the future of our citizenship work on the notion of "citizenship-oriented care" and the hypothesis that citizenship supports and community opportunities linked to clinical care would enhance people's citizenship and clinical well-being, both.

Fifth, the *Citizens Project* would not report on participants' status in the program to students' probation or parole officers and would speak to them only with the students' consent. The same ground rule would apply to speaking to clinicians, except in an emergency. This is not to say a citizenship project can't happen under conditions of constraint such as being on probation or having a trustee appointed to take control of your money. In fact, citizenship, recovery, and capabilities approaches arguably are even more essential under conditions of constraint.[32] Still, we didn't think it wise to, nor did we take kindly to the idea of, undertaking our first citizenship intervention for individuals, under the constraint of reporting to criminal justice officials.

We *would* be a *citizenship-building* project, one that should embody and reflect citizenship in its processes while supporting individuals' citizenship efforts. We just had to figure out how. After weeks of meeting, with revelations that were found to be wanting, arguments and faction-forming to advance one or another strategy, we came to a consensus. The *Citizens Project* would be a four-month group intervention with a 10-week course based on the 5 Rs of citizenship followed by a 6-week community valued role projects incorporating planning and doing. Participants, who would be called students, would also receive individual and group "wraparound" peer mentor support throughout. Criteria for participation would be be receiving public mental health care and having criminal charges within the previous two years. Participants' criminal charges would, as we learned from applicants for our first class, range from the petty such as Jill's, Aaron's, and Ron's, to the felonious including drug convictions and breaking and entering.[33-35]

THE GROUP COMPONENT

The objectives of the group component, comprising the course and valued role projects, would be to increase students' knowledge of community resources and their confidence in using them, help them build their social networks, and give them a chance to reach personal and collective goals based on mutual trust and shared interests. The group component would also give students a chance to demonstrate to themselves and others their ability to take on valued roles in society. They would be paid $10 for each two-hour session, with two sessions a week. Each class, or cohort, would average 10 to 15 students each.

THE COURSE

The course would focus on practical topics of community living and knowledge of community and institutional resources and tips on how to use them. Thus it would share some similarities with social rehabilitation and social skills programs. It would differ from them, though, in its combined emphasis on fostering a strong and supportive group, making contacts with community members outside students' usual circles of influence, and the 5 Rs of citizenship. Students would be treated as individuals with unique strengths and skills who are capable of exercising the citizenship rights and responsibilities and developing identities as valued members of society. Ultimately, these new identities would flower or wither under society's positive or negative regard for their value and worth as unique individuals, even if the project could provide a brief, though challenging, refuge for engaging people in citizenship identity work.[36]

Outside speakers—realtors, employers, public officials, and others, along with mental health and other social service staff—would teach many of the classes. The project director and peer mentors would teach others. As with the *Leadership Project*, students would develop group rules and norms and help shape the content of the classes by requesting additional topics and outside speakers. Following the first two classes on neighborhood, community, and citizenship and the impact of race, gender, class, cultural, racial–ethnic differences, and stigma on each, the classes would be categorized by single or paired Rs, albeit recognizing that there was overlap among the Rs in practice. A relationship, for example, can also be a resource for information, introductions, or advice. Likewise, some class topics, arguably, could have been taught under a different R, and elements of training under one R might be brought up in discussion under a class topic placed under another R.

Under *rights and responsibilities* would be classes on the *criminal justice system*, with presentations and discussion on the court system, stages of arrest, and personal rights and responsibilities in court. In a class on the *Americans with Disabilities Act*, students would learn about their rights under the Act and identify problems they'd encountered for which the Act might have provided protection, and might yet in the future. Another class, *sabotaging success*, would help them identify ways in which they had undermined themselves in the past and how they might take responsibility to change that going forward. A *patient advocacy* class would teach them about their rights and responsibilities, including grievance procedures and self-advocacy while receiving mental health or addictions care. A legal assistance attorney would explain family and child, housing, consumer, benefits and employment, and disability law in a *legal issues* class.

Classes in *personal responsibility and empowerment* would have a strong over-lap with relationships and the Rs of *recovery*. One would be *healthy alternatives* pertaining to feelings, thoughts, and behaviors that lead to drug or alcohol use, and alternatives from a recovery perspective. The strengths and drawbacks of *self-help groups* would be discussed in another class. In another, Mary Ellen Copeland's *Wellness Recovery Action Plan* for self-management of mental health symptoms would be introduced.[37]

Five classes would be grouped under *roles and resources*. The first would describe *entitlement programs* and how to apply for them. Two *jobs and education* classes would review vocational and educational programs available locally, with discussion on the benefits and restrictions of working while receiving entitlement benefits. The classes would include résumé writing, filling out job applications, and role-playing job interviews. *Housing and community inclusion* classes would review local housing options, including independent and supported housing pro-grams and sober housing, and tenant and landlord rights and responsibilities. They would also inform students about local social and recreation events and the comforts and challenges of trying out new activities. The group would then take a community outing.

Relationships classes would constitute the most exhaustive treatment of all the 5 Rs. An *assertiveness* class would outline differences among passive, aggres-sive, and assertive styles of communication, with role playing of interactions with community members and service staff. A *relationship-building class* would include a presentation on social skills followed by student identification of rela-tionships that are important to them and common problems they face in social situations. The class would also review listening, observation, and communica-tion skills. An HIV/AIDS educator would teach an *HIV/AIDS prevention* class to dispel common myths and give factual information on HIV/AIDS. Students could talk about their personal experiences if they wished. In an *intimate rela-tionships* class, they would reflect on individual rights and responsibilities in such relationships, develop a list of needs and wants, and identify ways that intimate relationships had affected their lives. *Stress and anger management* classes would review the emotional, physiological, and behavioral manifestations of anger and stress management tools such as breathing exercises, music, aromatherapy, and writing.

Two *public speaking* classes would stand on their own and, unexpectedly, come to serve as a transitional point from the course to valued role projects. Students would learn how to organize their thoughts and speak formally in front of others by developing and presenting four successive speeches on themselves, their com-munity, their goals and plans for achieving them, and what they'd learned from the project and other students. Their speeches would be videotaped and they would critique each other on them. The classes would help them learn more about each other and how to take and give constructive criticism, and would also help them prepare for employment, housing, and other interviews.

COMMUNITY VALUED ROLE PROJECTS

The classes would teach, and the community valued role projects would challenge students' low estimation of themselves while, at the same time, teaching other community members that people with mental illnesses and criminal histories can take on valued roles in society. Students would draw on their life experiences and class learning to design individual and group projects. The "community" in "community valued role projects" could vary for different students, but attention to community as the local form of society as a whole would be present during development and performance of the projects. Staff and peer mentors would advise and support students and help with project logistics.

PEER MENTOR SUPPORT

Peer-to-peer work in self-help groups has been around from the time of the founding of Alcoholics Anonymous, and even earlier. Peers as staff in mental health care is newer, beginning in the early 1990s.[38] Peer work on the Citizens Project would be a hybrid of sorts—not self-help, since the help would be unidirectional from peer mentors to students, but not standard clinical care, either. Brian Christens has described the relational process of mentorship as an expression of psychological empowerment, embodied in and practiced by the mentor, that facilitates the empowerment of the person being mentored.[39] My own and some of my colleagues' work with peers as staff began with ACCESS and SAMHSA's push for peer support work in the mental health field. Ron, a peer outreach worker, is the co-hero of the Jim story. The clinical director of the outreach team, Deborah Fisk, became an early innovator in peer mental health services, hiring part-time peers for the team, including people who were current patients of the mental health center.[40]

Almost simultaneously with the launch of the Citizens Project, we conducted a randomized controlled trial, or RCT, of peer specialists on four intensive case management teams across Connecticut. The Peer Engagement Specialist Project was a prospective alternative to court-ordered mental health treatment, including coerced medication compliance, of people with serious mental illnesses who were not engaged in treatment and had a history of violence or the threat of violence against themselves or others.[41] Findings from the study, thanks to David Sells' prescient lobbying for inclusion of a questionnaire to measure aspects of the client–worker relationship,[42,43] were that peer specialists have a special ability to motivate the people most unengaged in treatment. Participants receiving peer specialist care perceived higher positive regard, understanding, and acceptance from them than did participants from their case managers during the early stages of engagement. Positive regard and understanding positively predicted greater motivation for psychiatric, alcohol, and drug treatment and attendance at AA meetings at 12 months after enrollment in the study. Participants receiving peer services saw their peer staff as being more accepting, or "validating," of them than participants who received case management services saw their case managers to be.[44] Even *invalidating* experiences with peer staff were associated with higher quality of life and fewer obstacles to recovery for those receiving peer services. This association was missing with clients who had experienced invalidating communication from their case managers.[45] This might be called an example of "tough love" working when it comes from peers and falling flat, or worse, when it comes from other staff. Peer providers, then, could play valuable, and special, roles in mental health treatment, especially in motivating people for treatment.

Peer mentor work with people who had criminal charges is now called "forensic peer work,"[46] an inelegant term, but no better is available at the moment. Peer mentors' ability to instill hope and serve as role models may have a special meaning for people with criminal involvement, given the dual stigma and discrimination they experience as ex-offenders and people with mental illnesses. Peers can help people re-enter their communities after release from incarceration, get treatment and support services, and deal with the emotional and social challenges of re-entry. They can also encourage them to keep to to conditions of supervision such as probation. And they can share their own experiences as returning offenders and model the way they coped with theirs.[46]

For the *Citizens Project*, mentors would be people with knowledge and experience of living with a mental illness and, for most, have a criminal background. Working part time, they would support students in face-to-face meetings by helping them identify goals and set priorities for achieving them, sharing their own perspectives and coping strategies as people who have "been there," and advocating for them to gain entrée to social services, employment, education, and housing. They would encourage students to maintain their sobriety by offering the examples of their own struggles and recovery work. With students' permission, they could attend clinical sessions to support them in talking about their housing needs, criminal justice obligations, and other topics. Sometimes they would go with students to appointments with their probation officers.

Peer mentors with addiction disorders as well as mental illness would have at least a year of sobriety behind them. They would complete an eight-module course with information about people with mental health problems and criminal charges and training on topics such as setting boundaries and goals with students, respecting their choices, safety policies, and local resources available to students. They would be matched with individual students during the intervention. Patty and Madelon would meet weekly with them to review their work with students and support them in their own recoveries.

GRADUATION AND POST-GRADUATION

Graduation would be held at city hall for each class. Family members, friends, and mental health and other professionals would be invited to attend and mark the students' "rite of passage" from marginality toward full citizenship.[47] Students would choose a main speaker and would also address the audience. Graduates could continue to meet, more informally and as agreed upon, with their peer mentors for support, advice, and friendship. They could also attend weekly pizza parties at the mental health center and visit project sessions occasionally to reconnect with old friends and encourage new students. Some graduates would also go on to participate in the *Leadership Project.*

Starting Out: Ned's Story

Students share the experiences of living with a mental illness and having criminal charges. Most also have alcohol and drug problems. Beyond this, it's hard to talk about a typical client. One, Ned, who had been a client of the New Haven ACCESS project, was an early student of the *Citizens Project.* Ned is African American and was in his early forties at the time. He is divorced, with a young son for whom he wants to be a good father. And he is a talented musician and composer. Ned has served time in prison and has a history of drug addiction. He's one of the few outreach clients or students from the Citizens Project I've interviewed individually—focus groups are an exception—to connect his personal problems with race and politics, if obliquely and with a twist:

> *For a homeless person that . . . gave up on themselves, there's not much hope 'cause that's what they see every day. I'm free, like Martin Luther King said. I'm free at last when I'm dead and buried. That's my freedom, when I'm thirteen feet under, in the ground, with the plants on me. I'm free 'cause I don't have to wake up to face the negativity that's out here.* [48]

Patty talked with me about how Ned would sit, expressionless, "scoping things out" during the early part of the citizenship intervention:

> *He'd learned that from years on the street. That was one of the ways you survived. Also, I think the years of meds had flattened his affect. "How are we going to get through to this guy?" Lezley and I would say to each other. He was slow to build trust. Watching and listening, seeing how things worked with the class, that was his thing. But he warmed up after a while. He became talkative, likeable. He joined in on discussions and sometimes had to be reminded that we had limited time. Even when he was stressed out he was good natured and had a good sense of humor.* [49]

Music was something that kept him going during the bad times, Patty said:

> *He's a self-taught musician. He writes music, too. And he talked about playing the piano. He really warmed up then. And we heard him sing, too. One time I was driving a group of students back from Hartford after a visit with state legislators and seeing the new legislative building. He got everybody doing doo wop. He was*

directing and singing at the same time ... I'd never heard him laugh so much. The others, too ... He would talk about his love of music keeping him company when he was really sick and unable to relate to anything else but his illness. He became part of a group of students that was very connected and he sucked up wellness wisdom like a sponge.

Women and drugs were his biggest weaknesses, Patty said. On women:

Ned was always hooking up with women who were as unsettled as he was, and that made for stress and chaos. He would talk to people about it, including Robert, his peer mentor. Ned has a good heart. He cares about others. He has an inner sense about people. He knows when something's going on with them. One day before class he came up to me and asked, "What's wrong?" "Nothing. I'm fine," I said, but I wasn't. It was family business. And he knew something was wrong ... He just doesn't always make good choices about relationships.

With drugs it was selling, scoring, becoming addicted, and getting off and back on. It was also the street culture of drugs with its own set of norms, accoutrements, and consequences. Here's Patty again:

One day he didn't show up for class. He called me. He'd been arrested for holding up the Dunkin' Donuts downtown the day before. He got caught when he came back the next day for coffee. They called the police.

We agreed that Ned toting a gun was out of character for him. We also agreed that he was too smart to do something so stupid. There must have been a purpose behind it. Patty asked him about it later:

He needed to get off the street. He owed money to drug dealers. He never came right out and said it that way, but he as much as admitted it when I asked him if that's what it was.

Ned had talked to me about his sense of negativity and how that started early for him:

I grew up having a mad at the world attitude. My mother said, "The world doesn't owe you nothing. What you are being mad about, the world don't owe you nothing. You go out there and do something and make it happen, there's all kinds of opportunity out there. There's all kinds of things out there for you." I used to ask my Ma, I said, "Ma, why did you have me? The world is bad, there's all this negativity out here, there's all this war, people getting killed, there's diseases." I was sensitive to the ways of the world and what I heard on the news or what I might have read in the paper that was negative, killing and stuff. That wasn't the world I cared to be in and I realized that I had to be on my own out in that world.[50]

In a later interview, Ned talked about his experience with the *Citizens Project* and of still feeling like a part of that community. He didn't see himself as "a community type dude" before he joined, but Patty reached out to him, he said, and pulled him in. At the outset, he saw his fellow students as being "real straight and sober and [they] had jobs and stuff like that." He felt more comfortable with people on the street who were homeless. Through the "what's up?" discussion that started the citizenship meetings, though, and informally in smoke breaks, he learned how much in common he had with other people:

> *I didn't know there were people out there that could help you if you needed help. I didn't know who to go to and talk to. I wasn't guided anywhere. I didn't know opportunity was out there if you knew where to go and reach for it. They taught me how to hold my head up and stride and just keep going and try to make something happen positive.*[51]

The public speaking and valued role projects helped him get back to his love of music:

> *It makes me happy when people are happy when I perform. I like the adrenaline I get when I get into something I'm playing. I like the rush from the audience when they appreciate it, when they clap at the end or something. When I get a handshake or something like that.*[51]

Ned did a solo act for his valued role project. I went to Fellowship Place, a social club and provider of psychosocial services in New Haven, one frigid afternoon, probably in early 2002. There was a good-size crowd in the community room. Plastic folding chairs were set up in rows facing the far wall with a piano set on a narrow, slightly raised stagelike platform. I sat near the back. I don't know how it is for Ned, but when I'm nervous before giving a talk, that is, before I give a talk, I'm happy not to see people I know parked in the front rows.

Ned came in from a side room, barely acknowledging the audience. I know, man, I know, I thought. Then he sat down at the piano and played, brilliantly, for 20 minutes straight.

THE CITIZENSHIP COURSE

Many students hadn't done well in school growing up because of an early onset of mental illness, chaotic family lives, drug use, or other reasons. Thus the course might be an outsider's prediction for the most challenging part of the *Citizens Project*, given many students' lack of success in formal schooling. It would put a premium on topics that spoke to student's everyday lives while also emphasizing the foundational 5 Rs of citizenship. The give-and-take of class discussion, with students drawing on the examples of their own lives, would be as, if not more, important than the didactic presentation. We hoped these elements would not only make most sense for the citizenship work, but would engage students by playing to their strengths as adults with adult experiences of the world and topics of most interest and use to them.

Still, the course was the most structured part of the *Citizens Project*, and this seemed to help students focus and acclimate themselves to the project as a whole. There were occasional class disruptions or inappropriate behavior, but Patty and the peer mentors dealt with these as Patty had with *Leadership Project* disruptions, by asking students to agree on and enforce class norms of behavior.

A study led by Stacy Brown, a psychologist, yielded some interesting findings about students' learning and perceptions.[52] The interviews had a dual purpose. First, we wanted to understand how students perceived and ranked their needs for different categories of community-based resources. Second, we wanted to evaluate their learning. Unfortunately, end-of-course interviews weren't conducted due to Sharon's absence.

The interview consisted of 54 questions on housing and on vocational, educational, and social supports. Stacy asked students questions such as, "How would you go about looking for.... " an apartment, a job, an educational program, support and so forth, and code their answers as one of four other categories—community, mental health system, family or friends, or "non-normative." Responses coded as "community" meant the student demonstrated knowledge of how to gain access to resources by going outside the mental health service system, such as looking at newspaper ads or bulletin boards in stores or at local job training programs. Responses that referred only to the mental health system, such as, "I'd ask my clinician," were coded as "mental health system." Responses that identified family members or friends as sole resources were coded as "family–friend." Responses that reflected either a complete lack of understanding of normal means for gaining access to resources or socially inappropriate methods for doing so, or both—"I'd go around my neighborhood ringing doorbells to ask if they have an apartment I could rent"—were coded as "non-normative."

We wanted to understand students' knowledge of community-based resources within a citizenship framework. One of our goals was to help them learn more about New Haven and what its institutions, businesses, and associations could offer them, and so we wanted to learn about their connections to the community at large or the mental health system in their responses. This didn't reflect a judgment that, say, going to a community center for help finding an apartment was necessarily or always a better strategy than to ask one's clinician. Rather, it reflected our interest in the citizenship question of whether or not students knew about the resources that were available to them outside the mental health system and would consider using them to achieve their goals.

Interview questions also included perceived personal and community elements that students saw as getting in the way of their housing, vocational, educational, and social goals. They would rate their prospects of achieving these goals on a 5-point Likert Scale ranging from 1 for highly likely to 5 for highly unlikely. Stacy also asked them about past behaviors that led to their criminal activity, their awareness of rights and responsibilities in relation to the legal system, and behaviors they might change to reduce the likelihood of their involvement in criminal activity in the future. She then asked them to respond to such statements as, "I know what my rights and responsibilities are if I'm arrested" on the same 5-point Likert Scale, and talk about these as they understood them.

Stacy completed 43 baseline interviews. About 60% each were male and African American, with an average age of 40. One-third were homeless and one-fifth were employed. Almost everyone who didn't have a job wanted one and had good ideas about community resources they could tap for help. Three-fourths of those housed wanted better housing and most knew of community resources that might help them do that. Three-fourths said being involved in social activities was important to them, but less than half knew where they could go for information on them or for the activities themselves.

Three-fourths yet again were able to list personal behaviors that led to their criminal charges, including drug use and drug-related activities such as theft to get money to buy them. One said:

> It's been the drug and alcohol abuse and the street life. I've put the drugs and alcohol down, but I still think I can get involved in selling once in a while and hanging around people who use drugs.

Just less than one-fifth of the students identified personality traits or attitudes as factors in their having criminal charges. Some, like this student, linked personal and external factors:

> The police keep harassing me because I am on probation and happen to live in a drug area that I have to walk through to get to my apartment. They are always on my back and I don't take their crap and will tell them so.

A few connected money problems to their criminal histories:

> It was getting to the point where I became desperate. People need money to survive and I wanted to make more money the fast way without patience. Now I want to learn to make money the right way, with patience.

More than 90% of the students identified steps they could take or behaviors they could change to keep clear of the criminal justice system in the future. Abstinence from drugs and alcohol and avoiding people, places, and things associated with street life were mentioned most often. Other students, though, talked about changing negative personal attitudes that contributed to their criminal activities. Only five mentioned involvement in behavioral health treatment as a support and strategy for avoiding arrest.

About 40% of the students identified a worsening of mental health symptoms or increased drug use, homelessness or unemployment, and personality characteristics or attitudes as barriers to changing their behavior to avoid arrest and incarceration. One who was living in a homeless shelter, having been turned away from several housing programs due to past felony convictions, said it was "being homeless, jobless, depressed and lonely" that put him at risk of getting arrested again. Few identified any barriers to their avoiding criminal activities in the future. Unfortunately, it's not clear from the interviews if this means that people were confident about their ability to stay out of trouble, lacked insight into their criminal backgrounds, or were optimistic in general about the future.

Seventy percent of the students said they knew what their rights were if they were arrested. When Stacy asked them what they were, they mentioned being read their Miranda rights, making a telephone call, and having legal counsel. Half said they agreed strongly or somewhat with the statement, "I know what my rights are in court," and most gave correct answers as to what those were—to a fair trial, to be heard, have an attorney, plead either innocent or guilty, and be presumed innocent until proved guilty.

Students identified five types of personal barriers—psychiatric symptoms, physical disability, addictions, lack of money, and personality characteristics or "bad attitudes"—and two types of community barriers—past criminal records and mental health stigma—to reaching their goals. Many, like this student, said psychiatric symptoms interfered with their ability to work:

> The side effects of my medications and my depressive symptoms. I get deeply depressed and don't want to come out.

Surprisingly, given the high percentage of students who reported substance abuse problems, only two said these interfered with their ability to work. More than one-third identified no personal barriers standing in the way of achieving their employment goals. On finding better housing, more than 60% reported no personal barriers.

Fewer students identified community than personal barriers to attaining their employment or housing goals. A community barrier they *did* identify was having a criminal record. One, speaking of his chances of finding a job, said:

> I used to be a drug dealer and I have an extensive police record. People don't want to hire you after that no matter what you can do.

Only two students identified mental health stigma as preventing them from finding work:

> If people know I am a schizophrenic they won't want to hire or keep me.

> It is because I have a psychiatric disability and people don't want that type around, they would rather have people who are stable.

Almost all students who spoke of community barriers to achieving their housing goals identified their criminal records as the cause. One woman living at a local shelter said:

> My record. They hold your record against you for housing and I don't want to live in a crack area again. I can't go back to that.

Given the high percentage of people who were homeless at the beginning of the classes, it surprised us that two-thirds of all students described no community

barriers that interfered with their ability to find housing or move to better housing. In fact, most spoke optimistically about their community prospects. Even
though many of them identified personal and community barriers to employment, almost 80% said it was likely they'd find jobs. About 70% said they were
likely to find and keep housing, and 60% said they were likely to achieve their
educational goals. About the same percentage said they were likely to participate
in social events and activities, and more than four out of five said they were likely
to avoid future arrests.

Our research interview was a blunt instrument in some ways. In-depth,
open-ended questions on the same topics would have added depth and might have
resolved some questions, such as the apparent disconnect between barriers that
students saw to achieving their social goals and the optimistic assessments they
offered of their ability to achieve them. Still, the interviews do point out that disconnect and identify students' robust knowledge about community resources for
jobs, housing, and employment, as well as their lack of knowledge of social and
networking resources.

VALUED ROLE PROJECTS

It was the valued role projects that turned out to be the most challenging part of the
citizenship intervention, for students and staff alike. The relative lack of structure
of this component compared with that for the course, students' difficulty coming
up with meaningful individual projects or reaching consensus on collective ones,
and their anxiety about "life after the Citizens Project" that the valued role projects
signaled were part and parcel of the challenge they posed. Patty's notes on some
early projects and a few students' participation in them will serve as illustrations.

> *Staying in School I. This project involved a presentation and discussion about the
> importance of education for residents of a group home for youth in New Haven.
> The students [Citizens Project students] also presented "I'm staying in school"
> key rings to the residents. The theme was the importance of "staying in school"
> for success as an adult. [In preparing their project] The students had been learn-
> ing how to work as a team but I became ill, and they resented Lezley and Stacy
> taking over. There were some outspoken students and several others were experi-
> encing serious psychiatric symptoms.*
>
> *The project skidded to a halt as the students banded together to show their
> displeasure. They acted like a bunch of disorderly adolescents, which is ironic
> since the goal of the work was to encourage a group home of adolescents with
> severe behavioral problems to stay in school. Some students dropped out and oth-
> ers lost interest in the project. The group's work on honing their public speaking
> skills and learning computer graphics and research skills for the presentation hit
> the wall. When I came back I confronted them on their behavior. Several who had
> dropped out returned to the project and completed it.*

The presentation went well and the residents and staff were thrilled. The group came away feeling confident and valued. They had felt very strongly that they needed to reach out to children who were facing difficult times because of unstable family situations. They wanted to help them and felt protective toward them. They had "been there." In retrospect I think the intensity of their feelings had something to do with their difficulty focusing on the task as hand, and my being away had been almost too much for them to deal with.

All told, then, this was a highly successful first valued project. But beware the urge to repeat the experience. We all learn this, no doubt, many of us more than once. Here the urge, or fantasy, involved bringing the same passion to bear on the same project in the same way that the previous class had managed to do with theirs. Lezley and Stacy had again taken on leadership of the valued role projects, but these are Patty's notes.

Staying in School II. The project started small, with only three students, since some of the ones who had expressed an interest didn't show. The students talked about this, and took the others' absence to be a comment on the lack of importance of the project. It was turning into "a bitch and moan" time. Lezley and Stacy struggled to keep them upbeat and positive. But then some new students joined with a more positive attitude. They made group rules and worked hard to follow them. Then everyone began to focus and become supportive of each other. But one member, Peter, started coming in drunk or high. The staff confronted him and he left the program. He had been attending at the same time as his live-in girlfriend and this caused problems with their ability to stay connected and be honest in class. [Couples in current relationships were not allowed to join the subsequent cohorts, based on this lesson.] Then two female members, one rebellious, young, active, very intelligent and vocal, and another, older, less articulate but equally vocal, began circling each other to establish a pecking order. Jessica, the younger one, began to be seen as the leader. As Andrea, the older one, lost ground, she became less cooperative and often disruptive.

The presentation at the group home did take place. Thus this project can be called a qualified, though painful, success. But the thrill was gone.

The next valued role group took a new tack. Only a few students participated throughout, but it was one of the more successful of the collective projects and is my personal favorite. The students wanted to explain to police-in-training what it felt like to be homeless on the street with a mental illness and be approached by police officers, marked as an outcast and a suspicious character, and afraid of being arrested for simply being who and where they were.

The Police Academy Presentation. Only two students, Alfredo and Bernice, participated consistently in this project. Others attended more sporadically. They chose to write letters about the difficulties they had encountered with police officers and the general community after they had begun to clean up their lives. They worked on refining their public speaking and writing skills by practice-delivering famous speeches and trying out different body language, tones, and styles. They learned to identify the different parts of a speech, how to choose the presentation based on the audience, and how to craft a speech. They wrote about their feelings and then rewrote them until they thought they'd got it right.

One student, Manuel, really poured his heart and soul into his letter and became overwhelmed when he heard it read out loud by another student. He didn't attend the presentation at the police academy, but asked that his letter be read to them. It invoked strong feelings among both students and cadets. Because of this letter, there was a lively, frank, often difficult discussion between the students and cadets. In discussing these experiences with the cadets, the students became their teachers and educated them on the capabilities of people with mental illnesses.

The unwanted and feared "others," then, became the experts and instructors for officers-in-training who, soon would be approaching people who were homeless on the streets, having learned something about these others as persons with needs, desires, and fears not so different from their own.

Individual students' work on valued role projects give a feel for the opportunities they offered for growth, the difficulties some had in negotiating them, and a glimpse of their place in the context of students' lives and priorities. Some of Patty's notes, written in the present tense, refer back and forth to classes and valued role projects or to the gestalt of the students' participation in the project. Jessica and Andrea, the younger and older students competing for leadership in the Staying in School II valued role project appear again, this time in Andrea's story:

Jonathan is very quiet and withdrawn. He'll say he understands what you're saying but often he doesn't. If he joins in during class it is with a word or two. He's just starting to trust us and let us know what he's uncomfortable with and what he feels he can do. He's not comfortable with people and fears that being in contact with them will trigger a crisis. He can work on a valued project as long as he doesn't have to be a part of the presentation. When he relaxes he has a ready smile and if given a few moments to process a discussion, he gives good responses. He wants to learn to read but he already has a good understanding of the written word. He asks if he's correct after reading some material out loud and so far he always has been. Jonathan will work with the maintenance person at [a social service agency] by cutting the lawn as his valued role project.

Alice shifts personalities often. One minute she's outgoing and encouraging but on a moment's notice she becomes closed off or angry without giving a clue as to what's bothering her. At times like these she would find it necessary to leave class. But she praised the classes. She said she saw them as a foundation for building a new Alice. She loved the speeches part of the course and she presented her letter well to the cadets. She talked about a particular officer who had treated her with dignity even while he was arresting her, and the positive effect that had on her recovery. Alice won't allow herself to be photographed but she loves being the center of attention. She dresses in high fashion and changes hair style for every class. She's heavily involved with her church where she reports that she's a star. Alice plans to attend classes at Gateway Community College and enter human services.

Charles slept through a lot of the classes. He was in the Methadone program but he was on a high dose, or managed to get more than he should have been taking. He was on other medications, too. He moved to New York in the middle of the classes but returned to complete his treatment and withdrawal from Methadone and attend classes. Even when he was nodding off he tried to keep up with the topic and discussion. He didn't participate in the valued role project planning until the very end of deciding what it would be [a food drive], and he picked up a few boxes of food for it. Charles explored with his peer mentor what support he'd need to stay clean and get him over the rough spots after returning to New York. He talked in class about keeping his head on straight and dealing with barriers. He finally decided to complete the weaning process from Methadone on his own in New York, with little if any support. The class tried to talk him out of this but he was determined to do it. Charles says he knows it will be tough. He has talked it over with staff at the Methadone clinic. He has age and hope on his side, he says. He completed the classes but not his valued role project.

Andrea started out very interested and opinionated. She was judgmental and very blunt, but also extremely sensitive. She was the star of the class until Jessica, a younger, very intelligent student joined. There was a war of wills, which the younger student won. Andrea became bitter. She lost interest in the class but entered the valued roles portion [Staying in School II] with the agreement that she would complete classes she had missed later on. But only, she said, because "the 10 dollars is useful." She did not help in developing the presentation to the teens or in making key rings. She said that if she was not the center of attention she would not participate, and she did not. Andrea didn't complete the class and didn't graduate.

Carlos was very active in the classes. He was helpful and supportive. He was living in the Salvation Army Shelter and although he was struggling with his symptoms and legal troubles he was managing pretty well. He gave a presentation to the teens [Stay in School Project I] and they and he loved it. Toward the end of the course he was about to go to trial for drug sales. The tension was hard on him, but he spent time talking about his situation with his peer mentor. Carlos completed the classes and valued role project and then served six months of a one-year sentence. He said he would spend his time in prison building a firmer foundation for his recovery. He returned to us after his release for help in moving forward. He's in community college now and looking for a job. He's leaving the Salvation Army shelter to go into an emergency shelter so he can qualify for a housing voucher.[53] Carlos is working hard at not giving up on the system when he hits barriers, and doing a good job with that.

Since a person's community may include sub-communities and contributing to them can be part of a person's path toward full citizenship, some students, like Ned playing the piano for his community at Fellowship Place, chose individual valued role projects. Nancy was one. Her brush with the law had been just that—a brush, not a collision. She had a long history of mental illness, hospitalization, and treatment at the mental health center. What Madelon said of jail diversion clients—that they are not expected to take on valued roles in their communities and thus stood outside the door of the room where citizenship is being served—was true of Nancy among her family members. She wasn't expected to give gifts at Christmas time, only to receive them. She didn't have the money for such things, and family members didn't want her to go to a lot of trouble making something. She decided to cook Thanksgiving dinner for her family for her valued role project. She planned it with her peer mentor and Patty, found recipes, and practiced. Thanksgiving dinner was a success, as her family members confirmed in praising and thanking her.

Joe's community for his valued role project was his fellow students. He had a mental illness and previous criminal charges, but he'd never had a drug or alcohol problem and couldn't understand why people who did couldn't "just say no." All that was required was a little willpower, he said. And if you couldn't muster that, it was your own fault. Students and staff both suggested he had a lot to learn about empathy. He thought this would be a great idea for his valued role project. He went to the library and online, took copious notes, studied, and reported to the class on what he had learned. His colleagues suggested teaching a class on empathy as part of his valued role project. He thought that was a good idea, too. He taught the class, and it went well. Then his colleagues and staff suggested that he could polish off his valued role project by starting to practice empathy. He thought that was a pretty good idea. According to Patty, he made some progress.

Valued role projects gave students the opportunity to step outside of the relatively closed system of relationships they had developed in treatment settings or while incarcerated, and into the larger community. During the valued role process, they also identified up to three people who had helped them in their recovery and community living, then wrote letters and presented them to these people at the graduation ceremony. Many of them said the letter writing helped them to realize that there were people who cared about them, and they were glad to have the opportunity to thank them.

Most valued role projects went well, but participants sometimes felt their community audience didn't respond as favorably or quickly as they had hoped, not donating as generously to a food drive project as initially expected, for example. Yet experiences like these also became a source of group support and learning about the frustrations of translating personal growth into positive action and acceptance in society. Sometimes, in fact, "failing" became a catalyst for personal growth, or community building, or both. Doing the food drive was harder than students had thought it would be. They became discouraged, frustrated, angry, and wanted to give up. They didn't like the fact that there they were trying to give back and do some good and few people seemed to care. This experience led to some discussions about how you can live a positive life when others make it difficult or try to pull you down and learn new ways of coping in the face of their negative messages or behaviors.

Individual valued role projects offered their own opportunity for social growth. Daniel, an African-American single male in his late thirties, had spent much of his adult life in and out of jail or homeless. He was staying at a local shelter and struggling with his drug addiction and mental illness. He contributed at times in the class, but mostly was closed off. One day he commented that he was a poet. His valued role project, he decided, with his colleagues' encouragement, would be to give a poetry reading for people with traumatic brain injuries at a nearby rehabilitation facility. His reading and teaching were well received, and he was asked to come back to read for other patients.

The valued role projects, Stacy observed, transformed receivers of help into givers by placing them in roles that *required* that they give help. Doing so fostered hope, a future orientation, and responsibility. Public recognition bolstered these sentiments and perceptions.

WRAPAROUND PEER MENTOR SUPPORT

Patty and Madelon trained the peer mentors and gave them weekly supervision. Of six peer mentors hired at the beginning of the project, all were diagnosed with serious mental illness and were in treatment. The three who worked most intensively with students also had co-occurring drug or alcohol problems, and two of them had previous criminal charges. These three, who also were on the planning team that designed the *Citizens Project*, deserve brief profiles here.

Tim had a history of alcoholism but had been clean for years at the time he became a peer mentor for the outreach team. He had medication-related symptoms that led to his rocking back and forth in his chair in staff meetings, and his work for the project—mainly administrative—was erratic at best, partly, it seemed, due to his anxiety about getting things right. After a staff meeting in which Tim's rocking had been particularly noticeable, one of the project evaluators, Liz, a psychologist in training, asked to speak to Debbie Fisk and me. Why, she asked, were we putting someone in a position that he clearly could not fill? He was obviously deeply impaired. Wouldn't this be unfair to him in the end? And didn't it undermine our efforts to advance the cause of peers as staff in mental health care? Debbie patted her on the arm, smiling, and said, "It's ok, Liz. Tim will be all right. It will work out."

Tim was well educated, had a knack for making friends with renowned psychiatrists, and became learned on many subjects, such as the great cathedrals of Europe. He also had strong views on recovery from substance use and could be judgmental. He struggled at first with students he was assigned to help and resisted criticism in his supervision with Patty and Madelon. In some ways, Tim was better suited for the *Feeling Good with the Blues* seminar, a combination recovery and blues music appreciation group he developed a few years later and taught at several venues in Connecticut. With the right match, though, Tim was able to help students. He died a few years ago from symptoms related to his kidney disease.

Denise's main expertise was in helping students get connected with behavioral health and social services, or going with them to talk to their case managers about their needs and wishes in treatment. In that, Patty says, she was a good complement to Robert, next up, who excelled in getting people into housing. Denise was also a nurturing and supportive presence and counselor to the other peer mentors, all male. She had troubles of her own to take care of, with severe depression and self-mutilating behavior for which she'd been hospitalized many times, but not in the past few years. She was divorced, with two teenage daughters at home. Every once in a while she'd get a simultaneously tough-as-nails streetwise and at-the-point-of-tears look about her. This meant she was hurting and needed some time away from other people's troubles. But not too much and not without contact from Patty or Robert, because she had a tendency to become isolated. More often, though, Denise was a source of stability on the peer team, with a good sense of humor and a welcoming and wise manner with her clients to go with a robust knowledge of local agencies and programs. After her work with the *Citizens Project* she was routinely sought out to join advisory boards of projects involving peer services and was a member of the research team for development of an instrument to measure individual citizenship, coming up in two chapters.

Patty met Robert while recruiting for students for the *Leadership Project.* Later he would tell her, "When I first met you I thought, 'Look at this white woman [she's Native American] promising to do good things for this community. I think she's full of shit.'" He decided he'd enroll, but wouldn't stay if he didn't like it. He did stay, and Patty hired him, along with Tim, Denise, and other peers, to help design and then become a peer mentor for the *Citizens Project*. Robert had a long history of mental illness and drug use. He had a couple of brief relapses during his time as a peer mentor, but stopped using and came back each time. Robert also had serious heart and circulatory problems that, eventually, led to his having open heart surgery and, later, having both legs amputated above the knees. He came back from all to mentor new groups of students until his death a few years go from his physical health problems.

Robert was a fierce advocate for students and knew a lot about tenant rights and subsidized and supportive housing programs. His passion for getting people and keeping people housed was fueled by his own experience of having lost his housing after a heart attack and hospitalization when Yale University bought his building. Robert eventually got a HUD Section 8 apartment through the local housing authority. He didn't go through proper channels for that, nor did he, necessarily, in his work with Citizens Project students. He went to the source whenever he could.

The peer mentoring component had growing pains. There were personality mismatches of peer mentors and students that led to reassignments. Not all the peers were as strong as Denise and Robert, who between them spanned the mental health system and housing domains, or Tim, who specialized in the alcohol addiction and recovery domains. Then, too, we were all learning what peers could do and how to bring them into the group component of the project along with their individual counseling duties. We did some focus groups with them and found that their roles and relationships with students entailed benefits as well as obstacles and challenges for them. The benefits included being part of a team, helping students, and supporting their personal recovery through doing the work. The obstacles and challenges included problems fitting in on a team with seasoned advocates, clinicians, and researchers, and feeling "used" when students didn't accept their help. They also worried about their job status. "I've never been happier on a job than I am now," said one, "but it's not really a job, it's a study." By the time the randomized controlled trial we conducted got started, though, they had settled into their positions. Along with counseling and support for individual students, they had joined the group meetings and helped to stitch the intervention together.

GRADUATION

Class graduations, as planned at the outset, were held at city hall, the symbolic and practical local center of community life and citizenship for residents of New Haven. Graduation also was a marker point for the intervention as a rite of passage for helping people move from non- or second-class toward the goal of full citizenship.

INDIVIDUALS ACROSS THE CITIZENSHIP INTERVENTION

Most of the individual snapshots of students are linked with different parts of the project, especially the valued role projects. Here are three snapshots of students across the span of the project from classes through valued role projects and graduation.

Carl grew up in a large public housing project where drug use and sales were rampant. He used and sold drugs and learned how to express his sadness, fear, and anger through violence toward others. In the *Citizens Project* he began to learn and try out some other ways. One day outside the mental health center an old acquaintance walked by, taunting him and showing the knife he was carrying. Carl walked away and found a police officer, a response he would have scorned in the past. Other situations, including the death of a close childhood friend, tested him, but he brought them to the group, even dropping in on a class a year after graduating to ask for help. Carl had held down two part-time jobs during that time and told students that the *Citizens Project* had helped him stay clean, out of jail, and off the streets.

Sandy found new uses for strengths she brought to the project. She'd been in and out of drug treatment programs and jail for years. Although she was a strong participant with creative ideas about making good community connections, she didn't talk at first about herself, the recent death of her brother, or her father's sexual abuse of her. As she attended the classes and got support from her peers, she began to tell her fellow students about herself and her needs. She decided to research family support programs in Connecticut for her valued role project and talked to other women about their successes and setbacks in intimate relationships. Sandy spoke eloquently at her graduation on building community starting with family and others you're close to. She made plans to attend community college for an associate's degree in human services.

David struggled with a mental illness and alcoholism. He'd been jailed a few times, mostly for petty crimes. The first time he came to the Citizens Project he attended only a few classes. It was clear, from what he said in response to student and peer mentor advice, that he wasn't ready to deal with his substance use. David was back in jail a few weeks after dropping out. After being released to a residential program, though, he asked Patty about coming back. This time he attended classes regularly, "to catch up on all the time I missed because of my drinking," he said. He was intent on the personal and citizenship tasks he wanted to accomplish, at times even seemed to be driving himself too hard. His fellow students talked to him about slowing down, relaxing a little, and he took their advice. "This program taught me how to speak with people and have empathy," he said. "It also taught me how to deal with my depression and anger." David graduated. A year later he came to a pizza party and talked with people about his plan to go into inpatient drug treatment. He'd made all the arrangements and was waiting for a bed. He had started to slip again, he said, and wanted to stop before he ended up in jail, or worse.

There are plenty of less cheerful stories from the *Citizens Project*, and this chapter has offered a glimpse of some of them. Even the success stories aren't tied up with a bow and hand delivered. Often, people's struggles go on, or wane and return, and wane again. Some people who did well may have been ready to change, and the *Citizens Project* gave them a vehicle. And how do people do over time? We don't know, not yet, apart from what we hear or from graduate visits, sometimes from graduates who are doing well, sometimes from those who need a boost. We need to know more about the messy lives of citizenship students over time that are messy in their own special ways like most lives, but messy, too, by the particular patterns we may find among them. This kind of research takes time, is expensive, and usually does not yield easily quantifiable results. Short of that, we do have some initial findings from more focused and quantifiable research over a manageable period of time to point to for clues, after a word on "What comes next?" following projects like this one.

POST-GRADUATION SUPPORT

"What comes next?" is a question we've struggled with for years. Informal and limited peer support has been an option for graduates, along with occasional visits to the class and an open invitation to the weekly pizza party lunch at the mental health center. Now, years later and with additional resources, we've increased peer mentor support to graduates but continue to wrestle with the question of how the mini-community that the *Citizens Project* becomes for each class, and seems to become across time for all of them, might metamorphose into a community of citizens that moves beyond, and independently of, the project.

We had a first try with one-year funding from the Carolynn Foundation for a *Citizenship Council* that would support just such a group or association, but the sentence betrays itself. Its "we" was Patty, who guided the group to and through a "photo voice" project in which participants sketched their community through photos for the purpose of better understanding themselves and of representing it to others.[54] But another question suggests itself. How do we know that such next-step "non programs" are needed by how many graduates, some of whom may have moved on to new support systems, solidarities, and life projects? A reasonable question, even if it doesn't let the citizenship framework off the hook of the "What comes next?" question. And, as we say, a topic for further research, part of which we're doing now with in-depth "life story" interviews that are happening too late for reporting on in this book.

A Randomized Controlled Trial of the Citizens Project

Our first major test of the *Citizens Project* was a two-year randomized controlled trial, or RCT, that we conducted with research funding from the Yale Institution for Social and Policy Studies. Here and elsewhere I refer interested readers to our published articles for more detailed and technical accounts of recruitment, research methods, and data analysis on the study in question.[55,56]

Study participants with mental illness and with criminal charges in the two years previous to enrollment were randomly assigned to either the citizenship intervention plus standard clinical care at the mental health center or another public-funded clinic, or to public mental health care only. Standard care was individual or group treatment, medication monitoring, case management, and jail diversion services, as appropriate. We hypothesized that participants in the experimental condition—the citizenship intervention—would have more positive clinical and other outcomes than those assigned to standard care, as demonstrated by the results of baseline, six-, and twelve-month research interviews we would conduct, and controlling for, that is taking into account and thus neutralizing, any baseline differences in sociodemographic and clinical characteristics that there might be between the two groups.

One hundred fourteen people were enrolled in the study. Their average age was 40. Two-thirds were male, about three-fifths were African American, and 15% endorsed Hispanic ethnicity. Participants had either a primary or secondary diagnosis of mental illness. Seventy percent had "co-occurring" psychiatric and substance or alcohol addiction diagnoses. Almost 90% had one or more felony convictions such as robbery, burglary, assault, or drug possession or sales, during the two years prior to entering the study. Others had misdemeanors, or so-called "quality of life crimes" such as trespassing and loitering.[57]

Thirty-six percent of students were randomly assigned to the control, or standard care, condition, and the rest to the experimental, or citizenship, condition. We used this roughly 2:3 control–intervention ratio in order to be able have a sufficient number of students—around 12—in each citizenship intervention group. We conducted baseline interviews with all participants, including sociodemographic information and standardized instruments on drug use, quality of life, psychiatric symptoms, and social capital, and repeated these interviews at six and twelve months.

Our analysis showed that citizenship intervention students had statistically significant greater increases in quality of life from baseline to twelve months than those in the standard care group. Citizenship students also had significantly greater increases in amount of, and satisfaction with, the activities they engaged in from baseline to six months and baseline to twelve months than those in the standard care group. Of people who were working within the six months prior to enrolling, citizenship intervention students had greater satisfaction with work from baseline to both six and twelve months than the standard care group. Citizenship participants also had a higher increase in satisfaction with their finances from baseline to six months than those in standard care. Finally, citizenship participants had a higher decrease in drug use from baseline to six month and baseline to twelve months, and in alcohol use from baseline to twelve months, than the standard care group.

Not all was rosy, though. Students in the citizenship intervention had significantly higher increases in levels of anxiety and depression and higher increases in levels of tension, excitement, and distractibility from baseline to six months, than those in the comparison, or standard care, group. This finding disappeared at twelve months, and may not be surprising at six months, given clinicians' longstanding observations, and research findings, that socially positive life changes are often associated with anxiety and agitation.[58,59] It's also possible, based on "self-medication" theory,[60] that these symptoms were related to decreased substance use among citizenship participants, since decreased drug use can exacerbate such symptoms initially. Yet we didn't find increased anxiety and agitation among citizenship participants at the twelve-month follow-up point. This may suggest that the six-month finding reflects a short-term effect associated with a new approach to community life and participation.

At the twelve-month follow-up, though, citizenship intervention students reported higher levels of disorientation and emotional withdrawal than those in the standard condition. This could be associated with the removal of the intervention, but if so it's unclear why it would occur at the twelve-month and not six-month follow-up. Our working hypothesis is that providing more post-intervention peer mentor support than citizenship participants received will help to alleviate these symptoms among participants. Gaining, or regaining, one's citizenship can't be all about protecting people from its struggles as well as its satisfactions, but a little extra post–*Citizens Project* support might make sense, nonetheless.

Ours was a small study and both groups received standard care, so it's possible that the additional support and activity citizenship participants received, and not any particular strengths of the intervention itself, led to the positive results we found. This is a standard caveat for a research design such as this one, aimed at first-stage evaluation of a new intervention. Such a design suggests, as before, the need for further research, such as comparing a citizenship intervention not only to standard care but also to a similarly intensive additional intervention, to eliminate the "just did something extra" possibility of our positive results.

But there was more research, in any case. During and after this RCT we studied the *Citizens Project* through participant observation, in-depth interviews, and focus groups. We also modified and added to the intervention, which continued as a state-funded citizenship intervention. These are topics for the next chapter.

4

Citizenship and Individuals

THE *CITIZENS PROJECT*, ONGOING

The *Citizens Project* has continued for more than a decade since the end of the study I reported on in the last chapter. The student population has been fairly consistent across time, but the program has gone through some changes, and we've identified some additional themes that, over time, grew large enough to be seen.

Program Changes

FROM FOUR TO SIX MONTHS

The number of people we'd need to enroll during our two-year RCT supplied the most compelling reason for us to start with an intervention of no more than four months. Of course, a four-month intervention also had to make sense, and it seemed to us that it did, although we had no particular models to guide us for a citizenship-based program in mental health. Having settled on that length, though, two years with the study taught us that, while the intervention was effective, it was also too short. Students agreed. Their comments fell into "too short" or "next steps" categories, both pointing to a deficit in time, arc, and content:

> *It's not long enough. You're doing well and then it's taken away.*[1]

> *More is needed after the intervention. People are headed in the right direction and then it stops. There are more challenges to be met. People need the opportunity to work on a project [i.e., beyond the valued role project] and say, "This is what we did." It's a set-up to learn, to conform to the program, and then there's no more. People hoped for more. They need the project.*

To a naysayer in one focus group who scolded his fellow students for clinging to the project when what they needed to do was "get a life" another student responded:

> *[The Citizens Project] gives you a life because you now have knowledge and skills. We have a life for the two hours we focus on what to do and how to work in the community.*

Not long after the RCT ended, we expanded the intervention from four to six months. This would give us more breathing room for both classes and valued role projects and, we thought, be more conducive to students' gaining familiarity with the project and each other, building community and growing individually and then preparing to move on, albeit from a community that, over time, transcended its cohorts and considered its alumni to be part of it.

STUDENT SPEECHES

Part of the additional time was taken up by doubling the public speaking classes from two to four. As before, students were asked to prepare four short speeches, give them in front their fellow students, and listen to their comments on their speeches. Here is a brief version of Patty's instructions to the students[2]:

> *First Speech: Tell your audience a little about yourself. Who are you? What is your background? You can tell your audience about your family or some of your life experiences that have shaped who you are today. Also, tell us how you came to be a student in this program. Remember . . . only share what you're comfortable sharing.*
>
> *Second Speech: Tell your audience about your community. Who are the people in your community? Where is it located? Your community can be family, friends, church, people who provide you with services, neighbors, and so on. Describe your community, what you receive from it and how you contribute to it. If your community has recently changed, you could compare the new one to the old, stating the ways it has changed. If you feel that you don't have a community, tell us what your ideal community would look like.*
>
> *Third Speech: Tell your audience about your goals. Talk about goals you're working toward in the coming months or at most a year from now. Remember to include goals that are fun as well. For each area, talk about how you plan to achieve it, what steps you'll be taking, and who will support you in achieving it.*
>
> *Fourth Speech: Your final speech should tell your audience how you feel about this program. What, if anything, did you learn from the staff, presenters, and your classmates? And most importantly, tell us what you learned about yourself.*

For each of the four, the instructions reminded the student that the speech should be no longer than five minutes.

It seemed like a lot of time to spend on speeches, I thought, and one day said as much to Patty. Why so much emphasis on the speeches? They now took up four times as much space in the syllabus as most other topics. If the *Citizens Project* were a training course for advocates, I said, then fine, but it wasn't that, or only in a modest way. Given the ground to be covered even with an expanded intervention, wouldn't two sessions, as before, be enough? Patty told me it wasn't just about public speaking, that other things were involved. Keep watching, she said in effect.

I did, and she was right. Think about it—to give a successful public speech you need to choose a topic of interest to you or others or both, do some research on the topic or draw from personal experience or both, consider points to be made with supporting examples, shape these points into a coherent form while keeping in mind the time limit for your speech, practice giving it, make modifications to time and content as practice instructs, then stand up in front of a group of your peers and deliver it, take in their critiques without becoming defensive, and apply the lessons you've learned from the experience and critiques to future speeches, board or action group membership, job interviews, formal and informal social interactions, and other situations that draw on similar skills and finesse you will be expected to demonstrate in those situations. Patty said the public speaking classes also contributed to the development of trust relationships in the group and helped the more withdrawn students open up to their peers. We've come to think that the learning and skill development inherent in successful completion of the public speaking classes may also help students take on broader roles such as those of teacher and leader.

The speeches had a powerful impact on students, even if many resisted and feared them, forgot to do their homework for them, and had stage fright at first:

> *I could find myself. The public speaking and other classes gave me confidence to speak in a setting and helped me be more comfortable.*

> *The speeches are a big difference. Doors open that were closed. [They're about] how to speak out, advocate for yourself. Like telling my clinician I think I'm on the wrong meds.*

These classes also took on another role, migrating over time from the latter third to the tail end of the course schedule, just before the valued role project period. This new placement highlighted their hybrid status as kin to the classes in being vehicles for learning and kin to the valued role projects in being a first public demonstration of their learning. As such and in their new slot, they prompted an earlier outbreak of anxiety among students over the project's impending end and, at four classes, offered them a longer opportunity to prepare for it as they made their transition to the valued role projects.

WHAT'S UP?

"What's Up?" began spontaneously, instrumentally, and contingently not long after the end of the study, and evolved to become a core component of the *Citizens Project*, of equal standing with the course, the valued role projects, and peer mentoring. Transitioning from the course to the valued role projects was vexing for the first few cohorts. True, the course held its own challenges. Some found the material difficult or had trouble focusing on the topic at hand. Some taking certain medications, or most during the dogs days of summer in a community room with no air conditioning, had trouble staying awake. But the course had structure, and that seemed to work for most students most of the time. The valued role projects were different. There was no "it" to it to start with beyond its name and stated purpose. This was new territory, as unfamiliar to the staff and peer mentors as it was to the students.

There was a rash of goofing off, playing hooky, and side-talking in the early days, reflecting the uncertainty that students felt. Generally this phase passed as ideas for group or individual projects began to take shape. Not long after the end of the RCT, though, a new group was particularly disruptive at the outset. In what started as a concession, Lezley said, "All right, we'll take a few minutes at the beginning of each meeting for everyone to talk what's going on with them. And after that we'll get down to business. Deal?" It was a deal. It took the form of each student talking about what's up with him or her and getting comments—advice, encouragement, empathy, offers of support—from others. It worked.

A new class meeting in the adjacent main community room of the Christ Church annex got wind of the fact that the valued role group ahead of it was doing something new and interesting. They told Patty they wanted to do it, too. Soon, the groups merged at the beginning of each class to engage in what came to be called "What's Up?" One of the secondary impacts of this move was that through this exercise, veteran students in one class were able to mentor and socialize incoming students one cohort behind them. In addition, the exercise seemed to foster the growth of trust among the students in both groups and across the two.

"What's Up?" has evolved through mutual student–staff experimentation. Topics of discussion include current issues, dilemmas, and goals or other topics in individual students' lives. "What's Up?" is seen not as a therapy session but a way for students to connect with each other and get feedback on a wide range of personal interests, successes, and failures. The support and advice that group members give to each student who speaks is the second, and equal, half of the exercise.

Not limiting "What's Up?" to a narrow set of treatment- or recovery-related topics gave students a place and time to talk about all areas of their lives, not just mental illness, addiction, and criminal charges. This approach came about in part as acknowledgment of some student complaints that their clinicians seemed to be interested only in their symptoms, and from the recognition that how well people managed their recovery was about more than how they coped with psychiatric symptoms, how much clean time they had, and how long they could stay out of jail. Students took turns leading each "What's Up?" session, learning group facilitation and leadership skills in the process.

Five rules structure "What's Up?" The first, confidentiality, came from students who had experienced a lack of it in some 12-step and other programs:

Other groups, you have to hold back, be careful. Your confidentiality is not respected. Here it's important. There, I'd always wonder if I'm going to hear about my business on the street… We know we're respected here so we give more, we can open up, talk about serious issues. You can give of yourself, so others can, too.

It's good, Patty has said, for people to open up, but also to have some rules to fall back on. The confidentiality rule and its enforcement through group norms and values helps students learn how to trust while being trusted by others. This is an experience, she notes, that many students rarely experience and have the opportunity to practice outside the project.

The second rule is that everyone speaks. Staff instituted this rule during the early stages of "What's Up?" but had strong support for it among students who talked of a feeling of dislocation or loss when they took the risk to speak and others did not. Students who are unable, emotionally, to speak in the moment can take a bye, but are given another chance to speak before the session ends. When students are new and having difficulty with the exercise, staff and students will support the person's gradual inclusion, celebrating their participation as it increases. When a student is familiar with "What's Up?" but is balking at it or being disruptive, students or staff will comment on this. The same response applies when a student tells what's up with him but offers no personal content beyond trivialities. Student interventions in such situations give people practice in taking risks and expecting accountability of each other.

The third rule—keep the focus on yourself—was put in place when it became clear that, often, students were more comfortable talking about a situation or event than how it affected them personally. Thus they avoided "feeling their feelings" or skated over their role in how what was up with them had played out in what happened. "War stories" that glamorize addiction and allow students to downplay their personal responsibility in drug use were also banned. Also regarding this rule, students sometimes have trouble staying in the moment, and this can lead to things spiraling off into crisis for them. The "focus on yourself" rule can serve as a mnemonic to help students steer clear of this opportunity for a setback. Staying in the moment as they map out a life situation that they fear coming, or see as inevitable, also may help them and their listeners to witness its likely development and do some prospective problem solving.

Rule 4 is "No cross-talking;" that is, no responding to feedback after telling the group what's up with you. At first blush this rule may seem counterintuitive. Why not respond to others when they've given you advice or commented on your behavior? Or maybe better put, isn't it odd *not* to? This rule, like the others, came out of early experience with the exercise. The speaker talks about what's up with him, and his listeners comment. "No cross-talk" forces the speaker to mull over what others have said about his "what's up," and prevents him from responding too hastily. Consider a quick read of an e-mail or text for how affect-laden it can appear in the moment and how mild in tone later on, assuming you've passed up on the temptation, built into the medium and to human relationships, to return fire when, in fact, no fire may have been given. "What's Up?" is not a conversation.

Feedback can be supportive, celebrative, critical, and more. Receiving it without comment teaches students how to accept all forms of it, or at least to consider them. Even praise can be hard to take for people who are not used to receiving it or have learned to automatically question the motives of the person giving it. A peer staff member in the Program for Recovery and Community Health (PRCH), where I work, made exactly this point in a recent staff meeting in regard to her suspicion of a new colleague's helpfulness toward her when she started working at PRCH. On the street, she said, that kind of friendliness sets off alarm bells. What other shoe is about to be dropped? Sitting with one's discomfort over others' support and caring can be a way to begin to accept and be cheered by it, Patty says. Finally, rapid-fire exchanges on the street can lead to devastating outcomes. Being asked to listen silently constitutes a picking up, a weighing, and a turning over in your hand of a tool that may serve you well elsewhere.

Rule 5 is to keep the focus of feedback on the person who just spoke in the present place and situation, not on your interpretations of what her words would have meant to you if spoken on the street, in front of others, with your boyfriend at your side, and so on. In addition, the world of mental illness, as Patty notes, can isolate people, and the world of addiction can be selfish and self-centered. Listening first, then giving feedback pushes students to reach out beyond themselves and learn that others struggle as they do, sometimes over the same things. It may also help them to recognize, in the spaces that prospective rejoinders would have taken up, that the advice they give others may apply to them as well.

Students have talked in focus groups about the difference between "What's Up?" and other self-help groups they've attended. It's possible there's over-emphasis in some of their responses, given that they were discussing the question with staff who had an interest in the success of the *Citizens Project*. Or there may be a "fallacy of comparison," in which comparing distorts the "itness" of the experience being compared with another and encourages you to dig for the commonalities or dissimilarities between it and another program when the likeness, or the distinction, may be illusory or trivial. A partial response to such a caveat is to accept the discount it suggests, but focus more on the *type* and *nature* of the difference described. In the focus group comments below from students regarding "What's Up?" and the *Citizens Project* as a whole compared with AA and NA groups, the emphases are on dialogue and the individual's place in relation to the group. DTR below stands for Double Trouble in Recovery for persons with mental illnesses and addictions:

> *It is a "we" program, not an "I." The sharing and feedback is more personal than in NA or AA. You have lots of strangers there that come and go.*

> *In DTR it's your recovery against yourself. Here you get to know others and everybody can help each other... This ["What's Up?"] is about life, not about drugs. There, it's about recovery, one's recovery. Here's it's about life and supporting each other, not about support within recovery.*

> *Getting feedback without a response is distinctive, it's different to have no back and forth. You get to analyze what people say to you, to take it with you. You take it in, see how others see you.*

"What's Up?" encompasses teaching, practicing and modeling of a variety of social situations and skills and helps students nurture a sense of community, some even say of "family." Skills learned in it can be adapted for other areas of people's lives while also giving them a place to come back, week after week to get more practice after what may be halting early attempts "out there." "What's Up?" as Patty notes, is also a vehicle for putting the 5 Rs into practice. Students are encouraged to exercise their *rights* as members of a voluntary community. They also learn they have a right to their feelings and views and to be treated with dignity by others. Through their discussions they learn how to practice *responsibility* as members of the group. They examine current and possible *roles* in telling what's up with them and make decisions based in part on their colleagues' advice. They share information on community *resources*. And they learn and practice skills that help them develop and maintain a variety of *relationships*.

STUDENT CHARACTERISTICS

Gender, race and ethnicity, mental illness and substance use, crime, age, and poverty are facts for citizenship students. Their profiles have become a bit clearer over time.

Gender

Men have outnumbered women by more than 2 to 1 since the *Citizens Project* started in 2000. That difference has widened with recent classes, leading to new efforts to recruit females. Our current work to bring "citizenship-oriented care" to our local mental health center, including those without criminal charges, will draw from a much larger group of female clients and more equal in size to males than has the *Citizens Project* in the past couple of yearsat this writing.

Race and Ethnicity

African Americans are overrepresented among citizenship students compared with the general population, although the African-American percentage of the New Haven population is closer to that of the *Citizens Project* population. The experience of having grown up African American, often male, and often in New Haven, has helped to shape the project over time. This makeup may suggest questions about the relevance of the intervention to ones that might be started in other areas, even as it may provisionally, and partly, support its relevance in settings with similar ethnic–racial characteristics in other urban settings. Students identifying as Latino have represented a sizeable part of the student population over time as well.

Mental Illness and Substance Use

A serious and disabling psychiatric disability or substance use disorder or both, along with lack of insurance to cover the costs of private mental health care, constitute eligibility for public-funded behavioral health care in Connecticut. *Citizens Project* students meet the mental illness criteria, and most meet the addiction criteria as well.

Crimes, Trivial and Felonious

The original *Citizens Project* target group was to be jail diversion clients with profiles along the lines of Jill, Aaron, and Ron. Students, that is, would be people who committed low level, "nuisance" crimes directly related to their mental illnesses or to associated difficulties such as reading and responding appropriately to normative social signals, or to their living conditions, such as homelessness. Any thought that members of this group would fill our citizenship classes was soon dispelled. We could not recruit enough of these folk at any given time to "make our numbers" for our RCT. We changed the criteria to criminal charges within the previous two years of enrollment. No charges were automatically ruled out, although there have been very few students with serious sexual offenses. There have been many with convictions for breaking and entering, physical assault, drug use and sales, and other felony charges including manslaughter. A few have been on parole, though many more on probation. Many have spent a decade or a good deal more in prison.

Age

Citizenship has not been a young person's game up to now. Nor an old one's, if we use, say, 60 as the cutoff point. The vast majority of students have ranged from thirties to early-ish fifties. The younger students have not been shunned and more often are adopted and doted upon, but they have had a different kind of citizenship experience, for that. The most obvious significance of the age factor is that it means we're trying to support the citizenship efforts of people who've had enough time to lose it or, if they never had it, face a long road to reach it after many years of marginalization, as opposed to trying to *prevent* the loss of budding citizenship in a class of younger students, or give extra support in the face of early warning factors of its impending loss for other young people. We see this group as one of our next-stage obligations for our citizenship work.

Poverty

Poverty and lack of upward mobility based on lack of advanced education, training, work experience, social networks, and other factors are so commonly known among people receiving public mental health services that often they are scarcely talked about. They are also among the most difficult conditions and situations to address. Of the 5 R's, *resources* may be the toughest one to help people change appreciably.

Core Themes

Many themes have surfaced and re-submerged over the years in the *Citizenship Project*. A few have proved durable. Among these are the dual themes of skill and citizenship building and the intervention as a mini-community, being a student as a valued role, the citizenship intervention as "something to do" and shared values in interaction, religion and spirituality, money, peer support, the citizenship intervention as a speech community, citizenship work as a rite of passage, and "next steps" linked with the tension between citizenship as a program and citizenship as a community. Some of these themes surfaced early on, some later. All have legs. Another, more recent and more speculative theme I've identified may well have been present long before I detected it. I'll call it "the possibilities of place."

SKILL AND CITIZENSHIP BUILDING AND THE INTERVENTION AS A MINI-COMMUNITY

The *Citizens Project* focuses on knowledge and skill building regarding institutional and community resources, requirements, rights and responsibilities in relation to an institution or one's community, and the opportunity to take on valued social roles. The sociologist Ann Swidler's idea of culture as a "toolkit" of ideas, ways, and mores that people draw on to understand and make their ways in the world[3] comes close to capturing the melding of practical skills and knowledge with a broader sense of belonging and becoming a valued community member that the *Citizens Project* tries to offer.

Soon, though, observation taught that, in addition to bundling tools for facilitating individual citizenship, the project was facilitating, or students were forging, a strong sense of community among themselves. This seemed to be a positive development, but I did wonder if the intervention we had designed to prepare people for more successful community living was at risk of devolving into a soup kitchen form of group therapy. Further observation and discussion with students, however, showed that they rarely talked about symptoms of mental illness during "What's Up?" and other discussions, but talked instead of finding housing, rebuilding bridges burned with parents, friends, and lovers, and other relational- and resource-based themes and projects. This in itself was not unique compared with topics that might be raised in clinical groups, but the relative emphasis and air time these topics got in the *Citizens Project*, as well as the evolving group ownership of the process that we observed, seemed unusual. The *Citizens Project*, then, was becoming a small supportive community for students, oriented toward the community at large and, at the same time, giving students an experience of belonging that they sought in that larger sphere.

We then returned to the tool-kit idea as exemplified in classes such as "negotiating the criminal justice system," "relationship building," and public speaking. These topics seemed too specific, and to bring with them another risk, that of turning the course and the project into a skills-building group. There were a variety of those already, valuable in their own rights, in the mental health system. But more observation and discussion changed our minds here as well. Toolkit and community building seemed to meet, and find themselves to be compatible, in the *Citizens Project*. Public speaking, for example, was a way of connecting with others while offering the valued role of one's experience *and* teaching students how to speak in front of others who might, at another time, be landlords, judges, or neighbors. Supporting students' ability to gain access to the community resources and social networks involved, as it turned out, supporting the growth of a small community that helped students develop personal identities, valued roles, and membership in the larger community.

There was tension between the project as a way station for individuals on the way from non-citizenship to citizenship and the intervention as a citizenship community that also pointed to what would come after it. My favoring the "way station" metaphor at the outset came from my zeal to put the citizenship framework to use in helping *individuals* after three years of coalition and community building through *Citizens*. But the two halves were inseparable, or should be. Perhaps I had made, at the local and contemporary level, what the sociologist Robert Nisbet saw as a flaw in the extreme Enlightenment view of the individual as the center of creation, unshackled from old prejudices and social and religious dogma. In advancing this view, Nisbet argued, its proponents forgot that the "new person" had emerged from thousands of years of society, religion, and culture, and failed to see that walking away from the foundation for the new person would have disastrous consequences for modern societies, separating people from the associational life that is required to sustain and nurture them.[4] People still need to "make it," but they don't make it by themselves. Or, if they manage, initially, to overcome their status as a "surplus person" for whom society lacks a valued role,[5] they will soon enough find themselves facing the need to be recognized by others as persons of worth in order to develop and maintain a sense of self-esteem.[6] This lesson seems to be embedded in the citizenship work.

BEING A STUDENT AS A VALUED ROLE

By design, the classes involved students' participation in learning with others followed by putting their learning into action through a valued role project. In fact, we learned that being a student was, itself, a valued role for students. Many students had not done well in formal education and saw themselves as being at a disadvantage in life because of this. A related theme was that of finishing something of value to the person:

> *I finished something that means something.*

> *It makes you feel that you're about something. That you're not just a loser. You get the stigma off. You're about something.*

> *I felt like somebody. It's a stepping stone.*

Graduation, then, was not only about having made one's way through a six-month intervention. It was also about being a student and graduating from school, for some the first, or at least the most important, project they had completed as adults.

SOMETHING TO DO AND SHARED VALUES IN INTERACTION

Tom, who had been homeless, was a guide to me for all things homeless when we were building the New Haven outreach team. On my first time out on the streets with him he told me, "Homeless people don't know how to have fun." This was because they spent so much time surviving, he said, that they didn't have time to learn or practice the art of having fun. I think Tom's point can stretch to reach the one here. There are good things to come from getting together with others for shared and constructive, rather than destructive activities, even if the connection to citizenship is not immediately apparent to the observer. This aspect of the *Citizens Project* emerged as a theme in recent interviews:

> *We as a community did something so that we didn't have to go to jail, instead of running downtown with nothing to do. It helped us to stay off drugs. You know what they say, "Idle hands are the devil's workshop."*
>
> *A lot of people coming out of incarceration…this gives them something to do. If I did not know about this I would still be out there* [on the street].
>
> *There aren't that many opportunities for people with mental illness and criminal justice problems that you can do something positive.*
>
> *Some people were on the verge of going to jail, of getting in trouble, but they ended up in this program… This helped me stay out of trouble, helped me better myself. I look forward to this group.*
>
> *It's fun. It gives you the opportunity to express emotions. Having people to talk to one on one is important, too. But they are the right people.*

Something to do that is benign may be enough by itself sometimes to keep you going, but over time you need something better than that. You need something of value that, in the best scenario, is also seen as valuable by others. Sharing value, and values, hinted at in these students' comments means that the overarching purpose and goal of citizenship is likely present in varying degrees in all student, peer mentor, and staff interactions because it is built into the structure of the situation that is the *Citizens Project*. The setting is one in which people are not only seen as students and citizens but as equals deserving of equal respect. If—and this is speculative, an inference from observation, not a clear cut theme emerging from it—if, as Immanuel Kant wrote, people must never treat each other only as means to an end but also and always as ends in themselves,[7] and if Axel Honneth's idea of recognition[8] involves immediate mutual acknowledgment of the basic dignity and worth of the other as the proper default setting of all human interactions, then something of these ideas should be present in all *Citizens Project* interactions. The 5 Rs are doomed to extinction without them.

RELIGION AND SPIRITUALITY

Many African-American students, as well as others, have grown up with a strong religious and church presence in their lives, and almost all citizenship students are familiar with the language of a "higher power" from attendance at NA and AA meetings. It's not surprising then, that biblical and AA-like references—surrendering your ego to the Lord, looking to your "higher power" for help and guidance—are fairly common, especially during "What's up?" There have been a few times, probably no more than two or three across the span of the project, that Patty has had to remind the group that people have different religious views, a fact that should be understood and respected in group discussion.

The presence of religious themes and language is stronger or weaker with the attendance or absence of different students in a given class and across classes. That said, it's interesting that religion and spirituality are alluded to far less often during individual interviews than one might expect based on listening to the same students during group meetings. It's true that religion and spirituality have not been core questions to guide our interviews. Yet even the demographic forms that students fill out before their interviews report little regular church attendance or other involvement with organized religion or spiritual discipline.

Most people working in the field of mental health would probably agree that we haven't done a great job of connecting with people's religious beliefs and spirituality. This is partly due to the separation of church and state, partly to faith being seen as a private matter in such settings, partly because staff with religious beliefs do not want to "push their religion" on clients, or be seen as doing so, and partly because many staff do not have strong religious beliefs. For many *Citizens Project* students, though, the language of religion may provide a kind of cultural glue in addition to, or outside of, the religious beliefs and practices it refers to.

MONEY

A recurring verbal motif running across the project from the beginning to the present is a variant of one of the following:

> *The money was one thing but the people in the group made you want to come to the group.*
>
> *The stipend helps. It's not the main issue, but you can use it. People down and out want money, but it's easy to hustle $10 on the streets … It helps, but you have to be interested in the program.*
>
> [Asked why he decided to participate:] *At first for the money. But then that changes and the program ends up being important. Now the support and the information is worth more than the $10.*

The easiest, and probably most accurate interpretation of these statements, is that they are true. There may also be a bit of showing one's union card in them—you "get" what the *Citizens Project* is about when you recognize that it goes far beyond the $10 that drew you to it. I hear something else, though, in these statements and their delivery, a sort of amazement and pride that, poor and broke as they are, the *Citizens Project* could come to mean as much to them as it has. Comparing that impact to the money they so desperately need, I think, is part of making that point, and reminding themselves of it.

PEER MENTORS AND PEER SUPPORT

The surprising thing about the peer mentor component is how little students talk about it in interviews or focus groups. This is likely due, in part, to the fact that some of both were conducted at times when peer mentor presence in the project was reduced because of budget problems or mentor departures and lack of timely replacements. It may also be that the distinctive nature of the course and valued role projects during a time when peer staffing was becoming more common in mental health and psychosocial settings naturally turned students' attention to them when asked about their experience of the *Citizens Project*. When students *do* talk about the peer mentors, they generally give them high marks. The following comment is typical when peer support comes up.

> *The peer mentors are helpful. They can relate. You can open up to them. You can be honest with them. I can let them know if I screwed up. We can talk, give a hug …*

New funding has enabled us to hire more mentors, including for more one-on-one time with student and graduate support and for assuming greater leadership of the project as a whole. We'll see if they start getting more press.

THE CITIZENSHIP INTERVENTION AS A SPEECH COMMUNITY

A "speech community" is a group of peers that share a set of rules and principles regarding dialogue and the use of language as part of that dialogue.[9] In Jurgen Habermas' theory of communicative action, autonomous and equal members of what might be called a "speech community" or "speech group" make truth claims that are subject to questioning by others, with the goal of reaching consensus leading to action guided by that consensus and mutual understanding. For Habermas, communicative action acts as the intersubjective "lifeworld's" check and balance on, and defense against, the overweening power of systems of governance, finance, and administrative systems in the modern world. Communicative action supports a reassertion of democratic control over systems, including mental health systems of care, that threaten democracy and individual autonomy.[10,11]

Now, I doubt that the *Citizens Project* as a whole and "What's Up?" in particular would be what Habermas has in mind for his ideal speech community. Speech in "What's Up?" is as a thing as much of emotions as of reason, and the use of rote phrases and colloquialisms such as "fake it 'til you make it" and others, along with appeals to faith, might disqualify a good deal of the speech in it for Habermas. Yet I'm struck by how the "What's Up?" exercise, involving the speaker's comments on his or her current challenges, accomplishments, self-assessments, and appeals to the group, and the assessments and support given by fellow students, embody agreed-upon speech rules, assume participant investment and sincere speech given in the moment and based on "speech as given," not on outside considerations or personal motives. This process, as Patty has pointed out, goes against the grain of "street speech" with its different considerations of saving face, one-upmanship, and not merely for performance's sake but for the sake of coping's and, sometimes, even of survival. This is not to say that face saving and getting over never occurs in students' performance of "What's Up?"—all social interaction has an element of theater, and buy-in may differ in degree among students—but that participation in "What's Up?" involves acceptance of basic premises of speech and shared citizenship.

RITES OF PASSAGE

Shadd Maruna and Thomas LeBel describe re-entry after release from incarceration as a negative rite of passage with no positive ceremony to mark the person's having paid his debt to society and being welcomed back as a member of his community. They propose a strengths-based paradigm focused on the contributions that ex-offenders can make and the valued roles they can take on in society.[12,13] Jonathan Simon writes of a dominant criminal justice paradigm of control based on risk that overwhelms any carrot that may be offered with its stick. Effective community and social re-entry, he argues, requires moving to a "restorative" paradigm involving reintegration of relationships with one's fellow community members, rituals that replace disapproval with forgiveness, and the contributions the person can make to society.[14] These theories resonate with the citizen's intervention as a whole, its classes in which participants take on the mantle of student, its valued role projects that mirror and prepare students for new roles outside the project, and its graduation ceremony, a classic rite of passage in our society.

THE POSSIBILITIES OF PLACE

This is the most speculative of this set of themes. Studying transcripts recently of interviews with students and graduates, I was struck by the fairly frequent appearance of "refuge" and "haven" in people's description of the *Citizens Project*, and by the apparent contradiction between fostering citizenship and refuge from the world outside the community room where the group met. Could the *Citizens Project* offer both refuge from and entrée to the community at large, and society? If so, did refuge come first and citizenship follow? Returning from a conference and thinking about the people I'd met there and a longtime colleague I'd reconnected with, I remembered the old saying that it's not the formal presentations that make a conference memorable, but the meetings that take place in the interludes between them. In these, you meet new people, catch up with old, exchange ideas, and talk about future collaborations. When people recite this saying, however, they often seem to be forgetting that no spontaneous encounters would have occurred at all in the absence of the structure and fact of the conference, the travel it took to get there, and the people who gathered there around topics of common interest.

The analogy to the *Citizens Project* can only go so far. The classes, valued role projects, and peer mentor counseling sessions would be the formal presentations and colloquia, and the informal conversations would take place before and after the meetings, during smoke and snack breaks, and the like. But unlike a conference, the *Citizens Project* lasts six months and its components cover enough time to be called ongoing. And I hope the classes and valued role projects mean as much to students as their conversations during smoke breaks. Still, I wonder if something in the structure of the intervention might support the apparent dichotomy of refuge and citizenship work, a rough pattern of effort and surcease, pressing and letting go, and the gaps between the two in which surprises happen. It may also be that the real tension associated with the *Citizens Project* is less its structure and its gaps than the project as a whole and its place in comparison to the world "out there," in relation to which the *Citizens Project* is a haven from negativity and dim prospects and, at the same time, suggests to its students that they can have a different relationship to the world outside than they've had for much of their lives—that of participants not mental patients, ex-cons, or other such ascriptions that are conferred upon them and that, often, they internalize and render core parts of their identity.

NEXT STEPS LINKED WITH THE TENSION BETWEEN CITIZENSHIP AS A PROGRAM AND CITIZENSHIP AS A COMMUNITY

The "Now what?" question came up earlier in this chapter. It continues to be an important theme for the citizenship endeavor that reflects a larger gap in mental health care in general, in which promising interventions come and go, often in association with research funding that comes and goes, disappear from systems of care, and sometimes return years later in a different form. Another problem with such interventions is that, typically, they don't have time to weave themselves into the fabric of local systems of care or beyond them, but may, instead, leave their participants feeling all dressed up and empowered with no place to go. Said one student from an early cohort:

> *[The Citizens Project] opens up doors—to Fellowship* [a local service agency], *other resources...[But] we need to continue, to know that we're not just castaways.*

And yet there's a question as to whether or not the citizenship defeats its purpose if it solves the problem in the last paragraph. A contradiction at the heart of the *Citizens Project* is that the citizenship framework, which began as a critique and response to the limitation of programs as to the community integration and social inclusion of people with mental illnesses, has put much of its mind and muscle in the past decade into developing and perfecting...a program. This particular program may stretch the meaning of the term, yet it retains many of the trappings of one. Perhaps the most telling fact in favor of the *Citizens Project*'s distinction from clinical treatment and traditional psychosocial programs is that you won't find a chart on its students. The next best argument in favor of its difference is that within and across individual classes and over time, the project has come to have the feel and character of a small community that is simultaneously a training ground for participation in the community outside the annex doors. A hybrid community, perhaps, but one that may belong as much to the community of New Haven as it does to the mental health system.

People do need structured support beyond the *Citizens Project*, but services researchers tend to know programs better than they do communities. We should pause before settling on the obvious means of follow-up support—a continuation or scaled-down version of the program that people are leaving—especially when we know so little of how people live outside of the programs we create for them, how-ever much some of those programs push the margins of what we understand social service or mental health interventions to be.

Individual Students

"Diversity" is a term that conjures a response to race-ethnicity or gender inequities in hiring and promotion in the workplace. The diversity I'm thinking of with the *Citizens Project* is prompted by a series of interviews we've conducted recently with students past and present. It has to do with the range of their talents, challenges, traumas and, not least, their resilience. The challenges are cognitive and addictive, bridges burned in any direction, it seems, that a person could possibly turn to set a new fire, and can seem so overwhelming for some as to make you wonder if it's fair to put this citizenship student in the same class as that other, who seems so much better equipped to take advantage of what the project can offer. Looking below the surface, though, the troubles that other student has come through become more apparent. Even with the *Citizens Project* it's possible to fall prey to a variety of the "clinician's illusion," in which your dim prognosis for your clients is a function of seeing them when they're sick, not when they're well.[15] From another stance, I might say that, whatever the core commonalities and differences among students in a given class, almost all come to constitute a class and small community that strives to support its members.

BOBBY

Bobby is a mid-forties Puerto Rican man who has lived almost all his life in Massachusetts and Connecticut. He is the former president of the Latin Chiefs in southern Massachusetts that started as a community and self-help association and devolved into a notorious gang known for drug dealing. Bobby came up through the ranks and was involved with both the good and the bad seasons of the Chiefs. When the federal and state crackdown came in his late teens, he did his first stint in prison. Since then he has spent more than 20 years inside across three sentences. Bobby has a history of depression and addiction, and contracted Hepatitis C in his early twenties from dirty needles. He has a girlfriend now and lives in a supervised cooperative apartment with supportive housing funds. He gets food stamps, but does not have SSI.

Bobby was the father figure of a male-dominated citizenship class that was the most nurturing group of males I've ever seen. He has a quiet sort of charisma, and is the student who initiated the closer line, "And with that I pass," with which most speakers end their "What's Up?" His valued role project was a speech to an assembly of high school students about his experiences, his ongoing recovery, and his sense of having turned his life around. Bobby and I met in a quiet area of a local coffeehouse.

> So I found a new way of life, you know. I'm just glad that I'm a productive member of society now, so. That's about it, you know?

Bobby attributes much of his new way of life to the *Citizens Project*, although he was also involved in a day program for people with behavioral health problems on probation that meets at a social club near Christ Church. Patty supervises the peer mentors for this group. Bobby met Patty there, and decided to join the *Citizens Project*:

> Oh yeah, it was a life opening experience. It taught me how to be myself and not to be afraid when them doors open to walk right through. I was the type that always used to run all the time and jeopardize my success and I tried doing that in Citizens, but it didn't work... My drug of choice was heroin, [but] I ended up picking up cocaine...so I went to Citizens and told everybody what was going on and everybody just supported me and you know I just jumped right back on the saddle and just rode into the sunset.

Bobby still struggles with depression and to stay off drugs, but it's hard to doubt the sincerity of his sense of having been given a second chance, and taking it:

> Citizens, it just saved my life... I was able to take Citizens with me to the community, you know to the schools and I was able to talk to the kids about the dangers and the pitfalls of falling into gangs and...how important it is to protect yourself from [diseases] and stuff like that.

A question that comes up for me, given the prime citizenship age group that Bobby and many of his colleagues have occupied over the last few classes, is whether or not age and time on the street, time with drugs, time in prison, time to get "tired" as students say with both metaphorical and literal meanings, contribute to a readiness for change as much as the motivation and tools that citizenship or other projects may provide for them. Or whether or not people are ready at particular times in their lives to take advantage of such opportunities. John, who comes up next, made a reference to this:

> *I...look at myself in the mirror and say, aren't you getting too tired of that stuff? All the stuff you've done played you, played itself out. I mean you can't do the same thing you used to as you get older.*

Allowing for personal readiness doesn't negate the project's contribution. If anything, it might help it hone its tools and increase its impact. It also suggests the question of the project's fit, or the modifications that might need to be made for its use, say, with a younger group of students.

Citizens wasn't a picnic for Bobby. It was hard work, although he refers in the following not only to his work in the *Citizens Project* but his work outside it as well:

> *You have to take criticism and you have to really take inventory of yourself, daily inventory of yourself, you know, 'cause you have somebody looking and seeing something that you're not seeing... It's a lot of responsibilities that goes with life, you know. It ain't just laying down in a cell watching TV and just letting years go away, 'cause that's what I did with my life. Society is not a...it's not anything that you can play with. You're either going to do the positive thing or you're going to do the negative thing. You can't straddle the fence because you're going to get yourself in big trouble....*

The positive side of Bobby's message is that you can change your life and, in his case, help people rather than harm them. The negative side is that you'd better change your life, because if you don't, society will take you down in the end. The citizenship way seems to steer a course between these two messages, albeit with an overall bent toward the positive. As before, the *Citizens Project* does not report on students to probation officers or share information with clinicians without the student's permission. Patty and the peer mentors' focus with students is on learning, honesty, and constant reminders to yourself about what you need to do to continue on the new path you've chosen, with society looming over all, and the "or else" message there even when it's not being spoken.

Citizenship, for Bobby, seems to be about his sense of a changed personal identity that is linked to taking on the role of a helper in society, especially for people with struggles similar to his:

> *I represent* Citizens *everywhere I go, so when somebody sees me and they look at me, they say, okay, "There goes Johnny, he's a productive member of society. I can go talk to him about this or I can go talk to him about that."... You know, a lot of people calling me up [too] and telling me what they're going through, whether it's problems with the wife or problems in jobs or stuff like that. And I'm there two, three o'clock in the morning when they call, I'm there. It doesn't just stop, you know.*
>
> *You represent something, I represent something. I represent* Citizens. Citizens *saved my life.* Citizens *showed me how to live.*

When I say that I'm a productive member of society, it's because I earned that and I'm living it now. I'm not just Bobby the Latin Chief, I'm Bobby the citizen, the Citizens *graduate.*

A recurring theme in Bobby's story is that of turning away from an overwhelmingly negative self and personal narrative to a positive self and narrative:

Citizens *brought out the good Bobby, the Bobby that's supposed to be, the Bobby that was always there. That I was always afraid to take them chances and do positive things.*

I heard this in some other interviews and am of two minds about it. One is that when you are undergoing a life changing experience it is natural to divide your life into a before and after because it feels that way, and naming it makes it that way for a while, and is a way of making sense to yourself of a new life you see unfolding before you. The very extremity of the language used to separate the old and the new suits the nature of the drama you are enacting. Moderation would not do justice to the thing, and pushing at the gates of language helps propel you on the new road you're traveling.

A second thought is that the language of the old and new lives, as Bobby and others speak it, is so powerful that the acolyte may neglect to notice, or may not have time for his old self to demonstrate to him, that in being admitted to his new life he has not completely left himself—either his foibles or his strengths—behind. And this suggests two other thoughts, the first being that citizenship interventions may need to help people attend to the fact that change has its long jumps and its hobblings, the second that there was a little bit of a good Bobby during his bad life and that some of the strengths he made use of in that life—organizational, for one, as president of the Latin Chiefs!—have followed him into his new life. At some point these things may need to be acknowledged and called upon. This can take some of the air out of the initial lift of things, but it may also offer some help for the road.

Bobby did look back with affection and nostalgia on an earlier life than the one he had with the Latin Chiefs:

Well, I just got started talking, you know, having a relationship back with my mom. My mom lives in Florida and she loves me to death and everything and because I was incarcerated all this time I couldn't really get in contact with her. But I now I pick up the phone and call her and we have a good time on the phone and we talk about things that happened when I was little and she was telling me stuff, how I used to be when I was little. You know, it just brings things into perspective, it puts it into perspective for me.

Bobby saw *Citizens* as challenging and orienting him to a different way of living his life, but also as being a place of refuge:

Citizens *is a safe haven. It's a place where you can come and spill the beans, so to speak, and get feedback that will save your life.*

A refuge or safe haven may be more easily associated with a place of retreat, of safety, and of a momentary pause, but Bobby seems to link with it change and transition, as well. And he also sees *Citizens* as helping him make a social as well as a subjective and spiritual transition. After saying that *Citizens* showed him how to live, he added:

> *It eased me into society, didn't just throw me out there and say, "Here's your bags, see you later. The* [Citizens] *family was there and the family taught me the morals and respect and the responsibilities that I had.*

The spirit-filled flavor of Bobby's account of his new life involves more than seeing himself in a new light. His is a life of doing, like talking to students who are facing some of the same challenges he faced. He met the incoming mayor of New Haven, Toni Harp, at his graduation at city hall and told her he wanted to become an alderman. Interestingly, when I asked him about "rights" in relation to his citizenship, he didn't describe them as inherent or guaranteed to him:

> *I don't know if I have any rights… I have to earn everything that I get. You know, I have to work hard for everything. Nothing comes easy… Everything I do is a project… It's work.*

Bobby wants to own a house, adopt a child with his girlfriend, and help others through teaching. Like a few others, he used the image of walking through a door that the *Citizens Project* opened for him:

> *You walk through that door when it opens up and stop sabotaging things [and I] can bring other people with me. It ain't just me makin' it and then just leave the guys.*

And if he had enough money to live on, and more? What would he do with it?

> *I'd open up a house for people that are HIV positive. If I was a millionaire I'd do that. You know, open up a few houses and let them live there and give them a chance, don't kick 'em out, when it's cold outside, you don't kick 'em out.*

If all this sounds too rosy, it is, a bit. Bobby still struggles with temptations, and he has some health problems. For people like Bobby, too, the buffers that keep an accident from becoming fate are thinner and less absorbent than for many others. Yet he's resilient, too. He strikes me as someone who might benefit from a next step after the *Citizens Project*.

Bobby had told me when we started that he had to keep an eye on the time. He had a meeting with his probation officer on the other side of town. He leaned back, looked at me, and said:

> *You know, today people ask me what am I? And I tell them I'm* Citizens, *a productive member of society, that's what I am. And with that I pass.*

JOHN

John and Bobby arrived at the coffee house together. Annie Harper, an anthropologist, interviewed him. John is African American and in his mid-forties. He has a 12th grade education. He has been homeless half a dozen times, but not for some years now. He's also been incarcerated many times for drug use and sales and was headed to the same office as Bobby to see the same probation officer. John lives in subsidized housing. His diagnosis of a psychotic disorder would likely classify him as having a more serious psychiatric disorder than, say, Bobby, or Rita later in this section, although suicidal depression in both Bobby's and Rita's cases are serious enough.

John gets SSI. He recently got married, although from his comments and the form he filled out on his housing, it seems he is not living with his wife. He is subdued, shy, polite to the point of self effacement. He has a tendency to repeat certain catch phrases—"taking it slowly," "keeping my focus on me first before I try to help others"—that may serve as guideposts for him for navigating the day. They could be dodges, too, but with John I think they're the former:

I'm living at [a New Haven Street] in supported housing and right now I'm going through some problems with that, but I'm all right, I'm just taking it slowly but surely.

Citizens had a big impact on him. Talking to Annie, whom he hadn't met but who is good at drawing people out, may have helped him overcome his shyness and reserve to talk about his experience:

Citizens, *it helped me a lot. It changed my perspective to society. Helped me grow and [so, if] people be talking to you and you listen and then they get aggressive and stuff like that, then you just know [from* Citizens*] how to walk away and tell them, "You know, I ain't got time for you" [if they say] you're ignorant and crazy.*

Knowing when to walk away from a brewing conflict of any sort, whether physical, emotional, or intellectual, is something many of us can use help with. If you have a criminal record, though, the need to learn the lesson is more acute.

John, like Bobby and others, used the metaphor of a door opening into a new life and out of an old one. Like Bobby, too, he spoke of his old, bad life, and the new, good way he had found, of, in effect, being a wrong person in the past and having become a right person now. Unlike Bobby or most others, though, John gives God the credit for showing him the way:

Citizens *opened a door, gives a view. The life that I was living was crazy, selling drugs, running the streets. Oh God I mean, I'm glad God took me outta that. He changed me.*

John has paid attention to the 5 Rs and, like others, puts personal touches on them. Annie asked him if he thought he had any particular responsibilities:

> *My responsibilities as a man are to keep a roof over my head...keep a house and*
> *have a nice car...I have to take responsibility as in...be responsible for yourself*
> *and taking care of yourself, getting a job and doing things that you want to do*
> *instead of listening to other people taking you down. ...*
>
> *I learned things through* Citizens *and* Citizens *taught me how to, you know,*
> *be responsible, be productive, be on time, respect others and they'll respect you,*
> *and respect yourself when you're speaking to people. And don't get out of charac-*
> *ter just because somebody says something bad to you.*

I'll admit that I was thinking more, at the outset, about the responsibilities of paying taxes, obeying the law, and contributing to the common weal when it came to
responsibility in connection with citizenship, but John is right, too. Taking care of
yourself instead of leaving it to others or giving the whole thing up for a lost cause
resonates with citizenship. And with John as with most, though not all, of his fellow
students, responsibility to himself did not stand in opposition to his responsibility
to others, but was a prerequisite for it—you can't do good for others if you can't do
anything good for yourself:

> *[And] taking care of my mother and taking care of my little brother and my*
> *sisters and her man, just being responsible, growing up and being an adult, and*
> *everything is good and keeping on that order and telling them things they can do*
> *and what they can't do besides getting in trouble and going to jail. And there's*
> *better things out there in life and they know it, if I teach them before it happens,*
> *then they will understand me.*

Responsibility for John also means reaching out to those in similar circumstances
to his before he began to turn his life around:

> "What do you feel would be most helpful that you haven't done?"
>
> *Running a group, running like a* Citizens *group. And getting them to understand*
> *what they really want in life and how would they go about doing it and stop, you*
> *know, acting like a kid, stuff like that and just respecting, think about your future.*
> *What's going on in life, not just let your life pass you by.*

As to *roles*, John has a different work role in mind for himself than dealing drugs.
As with Bobby, turning your life around and becoming a citizen means not only
having a change of heart, but changing what you do:

> *I'm going to go back to school for truck driving and I want to do a lot of things*
> *that I didn't do when I stopped and...fell down the wrong path and got hooked up*
> *with the wrong people. And my life just went... [it] went. I'm 46 years old now.*
>
> Citizens *taught me how to get up, go to school, do things, you know, you normally*
> *wouldn't do, but you're supposed to do.*
>
> *To act right is to be right...*

John could use the Rs loosely or improvisationally, mixing the subjective, the inter-subjective, and the external, but his seeming-loose way with citizenship also captures something of the way the Rs can fade into each other at their borders—the rights in responsibility and responsibility in rights, for example:

> *My rights are to vote...be a productive citizen, just carry myself in a respectful way and don't let nobody, you know, bring me down...*

Graduation and the diploma to prove it are also metaphors for the larger project of building a new life, and of the rite of passage the student has completed to get there:

> *I got certificates home...Citizens certificates and everything and so that I know that I'm doing something, and everybody can see that I'm doing something with my life instead of tearing my life apart.*

Family is important to John. His comments on the topic seemed to be heading for a description of close ties with those who lived nearby, of family reunions and parents who were or weren't alive and still together. Instead, his was a story of separation and disjuncture:

> *My family, they're all separated, sisters, brothers, some's in the Army and some just live somewhere. My mother died, my grandmother died, you know, everybody just went their way. The only time when people come together is on funeral nights, funeral days and I told them that we got to make some kind of arrangement so that we can be...a family reunion so that we all can see each other as we grow up, you know.*

Citizens is a replacement family for John, a community of reference and identity:

> *My real family is* Citizens, *they keep me going every day. You know I miss them, 'cause they were supportive...They give me feedback and explain it to my knowledge that they're trying to help me, you know, instead of doing criticism...They're giving, you know, the nice feedback and tell you that you can do things if you really put your mind to it.*

RITA

There's a tendency in social service programs for staff to designate certain clients as models for what people can achieve through them. Often, this is not a good thing for those clients. The pressures of stardom are fierce at any level of fame. Rita, who graduated from the *Citizens Project* more than 10 years ago, is in no danger of suffering such a fate, partly because Patty is careful not to single out people for this crushing honor and partly because Rita's accomplishments are quiet and have come over a long period of time, not the stuff of stardom.

Rita is Latino, in her mid-forties, and is single with three children. She receives SSI. She has her own apartment with her children and has contact with her family and a few close friends. "I talk to people as friends," she told me, "but not too much. I'm by myself. I stay by myself." Rita heard about the *Citizens Project* after her last release from prison after five years of being in and out on drug charges. She started going to a social club for people with mental illnesses. She met Patty there, heard about *Citizens*, and thought she'd try it. Rita had highly practical and pressing needs. She had ended up at an emergency shelter the day she was released from prison, and her children were living with family members.

I asked her if she knew of the 5 Rs of citizenship. She did. I asked her what she thought about the R of responsibility:

> *I was not good with financial and then I was on drugs myself and then I was doing this, a little bit of that. But then when I joined the program [*Citizens*] over here I started changing...and I wanted my own place and I had got this thing called Shelter Plus [a HUD housing certificate program for people who are homeless with disabilities]. And then I spoke to Patty and Lezley... They helped me and I had no other choice but to get my act together because I have kids.*

"How many kids do you have?"

> *Three. Two girls and a boy. So I have taken responsibility.*

I wrote earlier about the sometime-synchronicity of the right intervention or approach and the person who's ready to change. Something snapped into place for Rita with *Citizens*:

> *To be honest with you I just started taking responsibility like 10 years ago, you know, it's been 10 years...I haven't been homeless. I'm more outspoken with people. I do what I have to do, and the program taught me that. They taught me responsibility. They taught me to talk to people correctly because I had like a bad attitude, you know, towards the whole world. They taught me things. I really liked it. If I could [go] back I would go back... It's what you get out of it. And I forgot what you call those people when you go to jail and you're trying to expunge your [criminal] record... They helped me out with that.*

Rita's comment about going back to the *Citizens Project* if she could suggests again the question of what might or should come after the program to help people build on what they've got started. It may be that the weekly pizza party lunch, open to all students but focused more on new ones and graduates, has been something of that for Rita. She has attended for a decade since her graduation, a record I think, and Jeff, the peer mentor who coordinates it, continues to counsel her.

In asking people about the 5 Rs, we've also asked people if there are Rs—responsibilities and roles especially—that they wouldn't mind doing without, in hopes of trying to understand what the caveats to "becoming a citizen" might be and how people cope with them. Rita talked about a responsibility she wouldn't mind taking a break from:

> *My house. It's too much, you know. I'm not going to lie right now. It's too much. I mean, the rent is not so high. It's cheap. I'm on Section 8. But it's just the bills like the light and the gas, right.*

Rita's 18-year-old daughter and 15-year-old son live with her. Her 12-year-old son has lived with her sister since Rita gave birth to him in jail. They are a responsibility she takes pride in having. Still, having prospectively forgiven them for the demands they place on her life by noting that "they didn't asked to be born in this world," she went on:

Don't get me wrong, I take care of my kids. I've been taking care of them since they were small and then their father raised them when I was locked up. But then they just bum rushed my life when I came out, you know. And this is my first apartment. I had an apartment when I was married, but it didn't work out with the mental health issue and the selling drugs. So I ended up, you know, bouncing from house to house with my kids. But, I mean, now they're just like taking over the house...

Rita cleaned this up fast:

Which I don't mind. I love it. I love every bit of it and I love having my daughter and my granddaughter there and she's a newborn. She's two months. I like having them there now. I don't know what I'd do without them. Yeah.

But she needn't have. Want them as you do, plan for them as you must, love them when they arrive, if you've never felt that your kids have "bum rushed your life," you probably employ a nanny or two.

Drugs weren't Rita's only behavioral health problem. She has suffered from severe depression and suicidality for years, had episodes of psychosis, and been in and out of the hospital because of these. "The thing is," she said, "I haven't been in the hospital in 10 years and I haven't felt suicidal in 10 years." She sees her children as a big part of her recovery. They sustain her. Many citizenship students have had children they struggled to reconnect with. That struggle can be an impetus, too, a sustaining force, but it carries with it the constant reminder of mistakes made that are associated with the original separation. For Rita, having and taking care of children is a gift:

It feels good, you know? I don't know what I would do if I wouldn't have had kids. And I'm grateful that God gave me kids because at one time they said I couldn't have kids, you know... I was literally off the wall because they told me I couldn't have kids and then when I found out I was delusional and going crazy and saying there's nothing in my stomach and my stomach was growing, you know, because of it. Because of what they said.

I asked her about other roles in her life. She was going back to school, community college, she said. She regretted having dropped out of college when she was younger, but she was going back in a month to learn auto mechanics:

It's not about the money for me. It's about what I like doing, you know, what I can do, show my kids you're never too old to go back to school... My kid looks up to me, my son... He's proud of me and... not to say nothing bad but he's real bad. He's like me when I was a kid, but he really looks up to me so I don't want him saying, "Well, my mom's on drugs," or "She carries guns." I want him to say, "My mom is in school. She's doing something."... I missed out, you know, but I'm here now and that's what counts.

I wanted to get back to what she had said at the beginning of the interview about the *Citizens Project* making a difference in her life. "Is there anything else you have to say about being in the Citizens Project that made a difference in your life?"

It changed my life as, how I look at life right now is practically, and taking more charge of myself. That nobody else is going to do it unless I do it. And that's what they taught me, you know... It helped me a lot... Even though it's been 10 years, I still come here and do the meetings Monday that we have, the pizza party... .

"But you also have to be ready to receive it, too."

I was tired... Yeah, you know how they say you get tired and so I got tired. I said these people all the time work with me and I'm not working with them... I didn't say it worked right away... I guess it worked after me going to city hall and getting my certificate... We had to speak in a camera and I'm not really outspoken and... I got an attitude. I was like, "I ain't doin' this." But I did it... My family went. And it made me feel good about myself... That's the first time I received anything, you know, so I was proud. I was proud.

I interviewed Rita at the end of a long day in the only room I could get, one-half full of outdated audiovisual equipment in the basement of the mental health center, a rather dismal place at any time of the day. I was tired and wouldn't have minded being stood up. But I felt good now. Walking up to the first floor and out, I thought about something Patty had said to me about self-defeating attitudes that some students bring with them to the project and how they scare themselves out of being successful, or scare themselves when they start to succeed. She talked about how people limit their expectations and desires because they feel unworthy of receiving them, or fear that happiness or a moment of ease will pull their triggers and cause them to relapse. Some, she said, deal with all this by putting their success into someone else's hands and removing their roles in their own recovery. "I owe it all to God, my Higher Power, my case manager, my program, my wife, my children, my husband.... "

Then she talked about the messages she tried to give people, about staying in the present, talking about what you're doing, not what's happening to you, making what you're doing good enough for the day, taking one step at a time... "As tiring as it gets," she said, "those clichés mean a lot, and they work." She talked about repeating the same message over and over again with variations and lots of different examples and stories, and about asking people to think and talk about personal experiences that reflect whatever principle it is that's being stressed so they can see how it works in their own lives. She also talked about trying to help students have high, stated expectations and a plan to meet them, and about helping people building structure into their lives that reinforce that. She talks with them about how body language, tone of voice, facial expressions, and words all reflect whatever message you're giving yourself, and about being honest with yourself. And finally, about having a sense of humor about all of this because, after all, we're people, not machines.

All that had seemed true enough to me at the time, but more so now—how practice, of auto mechanics or writing symphonies, the doing of the thing lays down tracks in your mind and body and can put you in a place somewhere between routine and revelation.

Rita's getting the job done.

NICHOLAS

Had he been born 150 years earlier and in Moscow or St. Petersburg rather than a working class town well outside the latter, Nicholas might have served as a model for one of Dostoevsky's brilliant young men riven by the entanglement of their emotions and reason in an unjust world. Instead, Nicholas was born Nikolai in Russia in the mid-1970s and moved to the United States in the early 1990s. His mother had preceded him here by more than a decade, sending home money to his father. His parents did not reunite.

Nicholas may or may not be on probation—he's not sure—for a brief stint he did in prison for assault in another state. He's homeless, sleeping in a local park or, the odd night or two, in a men's shelter. It's not clear how he manages to keep his head shaved nub close to bald, unless it doesn't grow. But people who are homeless can be quite resourceful without the standard tools used for such mundane tasks.

Nicholas drinks and dabbles in street drugs. He didn't graduate from high school—he disdains formal education as it's taught. He has been diagnosed with a mental illness, but with an exception or two also disdains clinicians with their professionally and institutionally compromised knowledge and judgments. He has been suicidal many times. On his 16th birthday, two days after moving to the United States, "I played Russian roulette…It was a Smith and Wesson 38. I load that one with one bullet, spin that thing and pulled the trigger."

Nicholas is the youngest of four siblings, with two sisters living in the United States and one in Russia. His father died 10 years ago and his mother, an alcoholic, was murdered by her second husband in his alcoholic rage. Patty broke her own rule by letting Nicholas enroll in the *Citizens Project* even though he was not in treatment and refused to consider it. She worried about that decision, but something told her she needed to give him a chance even though his refusal might extend to his deigning to participate in any meaningful way in *Citizens*. Maybe he'd open up, she thought, and benefit from it.

By the time I met him, he had opened up a bit in class, if mostly about others' situations and problems, not his own. He would sit leaning forward, intent on his own thoughts to judge by the far off look in his eyes, until he commented on a fellow student's "What's Up?" and was invariably on the mark, straight, and empathic. We met at the same coffeehouse where I'd interviewed Bobby. He loved the *Citizens Project*, he told me:

> *So I went there and I did what I had to do to get into the group. I went there with wounded spirit and I was suicidal. I hated myself. I never hated the world. I never hated people. I hated myself for I don't know why actually... The Citizens group, they gave me sanctuary... As much as I went there for money which I needed to deal with my habits, I changed my mind very quickly. I just loved that group.*

I sometimes come back to an idea that I call "latent citizenship," a sense of citizenship that comes from being and feeling like a member of one's neighborhood, community, society that is basic, almost instinctual, tracks laid down to use the preceding metaphor, long ago and deep enough that they are just there, available to draw on consciously to reassure or encourage yourself but more often a substrata of belonging and membership that you don't need to think about at all. I came across something like this not long ago in Anthony Giddens' work. He calls it "ontological security," a "basic trust," a way of "screening off" the constant influx of data in modern life, and a precondition for establishing a positive personal identity and experience of "coherence, continuity, and dependability" of the world.[16] Both Bobby and Nicholas refer to the *Citizens Project* as a refuge or sanctuary, especially in their early days in the project. As previously, a sense of refuge and of challenge seem to co-exist for more than a few students with *the Citizens Project*.

Nicholas has a strong moral code if, perhaps, a quirky one. He wants to visit his mother's boyfriend in prison and forgive him face to face. He's "not a bad man," Nicholas says, and his mother was "a nasty drunk" and "a piece of work." Yet while he professes to have forgiven his parents for their separate moral lapses, his gut still churns with them, he told me, and "ambivalence" toward his mother is too pat an explanation for his ability to forgive her murderer. He still feels guilty about not having saved her life, and still feels the wound of her moral failure, which came after Nicholas defended her against her boyfriend's brutality at the boozy end of his 18th birthday party:

> *So my mother said, "Listen, I want to throw you a party." I said, "No, no, no, I will pass on that," because, you know, her second husband and her, when they get to drinking it's going to be shameful... So I said no, no, no. But she was insisting and you know it was my mother so I said I would let her do it. So I invited some friends who knew my situation... It was after 10:00 p.m. and there was a lot of alcohol and food left on the table. And my mother drug her husband to the bedroom to sleep. So my neighbor said, "Let's go to my apartment so we can party." So we did. And all of a sudden I hear screaming and shit like that from my apartment. My mother...knocks on my neighbor's door all beaten up and she said, "Oh this motherfucker beat me up." So I left my neighbor's apartment, went to my mother's*

apartment, beat the shit out of the guy. Then I saw him bleeding on the floor and I got him up, got him to the bed and I left because I felt sorry. That's how I always feel when I do something right and wrong at the same time… And you know what she said? She said, "Apologize to him." Oh my God, Mike. Oh my God, that was a stiletto straight to my heart. Oh my God, Mike, my mother did not hurt me more ever in my life than she did that day. "I'm defending you and you're telling me to apologize to the guy who beat you?" She lost my respect completely.

His father's moral failure occurred when Nicholas was seven:

My father… had [an] extremely kind heart. He will take stuff from his house and give it to other people, to his friends. And we in our house, we had enough [but] we were a poor family… Anyway, there was [the Russian equivalent of $5] in our house somewhere and I will remember the day for the rest of my life… They were building a new church and accidentally I went there. I was so proud of myself. I said, "Oh, I'm a good boy." [Then] I get home and my sister jumped on me, "Oh you stole $5!"… Five dollars was really a lot of money [then] and my sister said that I stole it. I didn't. My father was sitting next to me like investigating me… You what I found out later? My father took that money.

"What did he use it for? Do you know?"

No, I don't. You know what? It does not matter to me. Even if he gave it to some poor hungry lady with kids, I don't care… I'd love to say that I understand that differently. I honestly can't because it still hurts me even though I have the wisdom that God guided my father to give me hard experiences at that young age so I can carry in life later when I have stuff like that. If the man you love the most in your life, your father, your example which is supposed to be, treats you like that, you are prepared in later life… [But] even though I have that wisdom and understanding, it still hurts me. I still cannot let that go… How can a man sit and accuse his own son and seeing his self lying? [It's] like I have no father. I was an orphan.

Perhaps there's no real mystery in the world of Nicholas' moral values. Parents have a special responsibility to their children and so their sins impart a special hurt for a seven-year-old boy or an 18-year-old stranger in a strange land. Nicholas' values have a strong spiritual–religious bent and, no doubt, the influence of his native culture, but his code of honor seems also to have been nourished by his dream of joining the US Army Special Forces from the time he was four years old. He knew before long that he'd need Lasik surgery to correct his near-sightedness, but also knew he would come to the United States eventually and have the procedure done. He did, but the fact that he'd had it, he said, was enough to deny him entrance. His dream shattered, he went to California and started a pool cleaning and mainte-nance business. He has no respect for money:

Money was never important to me. Unfortunately we do need those stupid basics… [but] I have the talents to make money in any business.

He did make money with his pool business, but then started having problems with his girlfriend:

> *For some reason I was kind of in love with her, or whatever kind of energy she created, I was stuck with her. I tried to move out so many times my friends were making bets, how long it's going to take this time, one week, three weeks. And I was always coming back to her. I cheated on her because I thought it was going to help me to leave her forever. It didn't . . . [One day] I was cleaning a pool and there was two dogs behind the plants and there was a strong bigger dog and little dog and the bigger dog was biting the little one and I'm cleaning the pool and I'm looking and I'm with my girlfriend . . . She saw the bigger dog biting the little dog. You know what she did? It was so cute. It was like a little girl picking up the garden hose and tossing the water on the big dog. That day I said to myself, "This girl has my kind of heart, protective heart of the weaker." So I really fall in love with her that moment [but] my feelings didn't change her personality . . . .*

After she left him, Nicholas experienced another blow against his sense of honor in life with the disappearance of his friends after he became homeless for the first time. He drank heavily. At age 31 he was arrested for unlawful restraint and interfering with a police officer, and spent two years in prison. "I was devastated," he told me. "I was angry, pissed off at everything, God, humans, you name it." As hurt as he could be by others, though, his experience and understanding of human suffering connect him to others, too:

> *I had lot of people do things to me in my life . . . Some guys were molested by their father? Then that was the most biggest trauma in their life. I am built different. I believe that we are all suffering on scale one to 10. Every human suffers this scale 10. Every human suffers the 10. But everyone has different meaning of the 10. To some men their father molested them. That's the biggest suffering. To me the biggest suffering was my father lying.*

Nicholas came to New Haven sometime after his release. He was homeless again. Someone mentioned the *Citizens Project* to him. Like Bobby, he spoke of his early experience *Citizens* as being a "refuge" for him. I asked Nicholas about helping others, which he'd referred to earlier in the interview:

> *Listen, it makes me feel amazing. It's like food to me helping other people. It's like basic . . . it's necessary food to me, spiritual. I need physical food and spiritual food. Helping others is my spiritual food . . . Every day in the shelter . . . on the streets I talk to people every day and I build them. I show them who they are. I show them they are better than they think they are because we pulled ourselves down. So yes, I do help them every day and I do my psychology every day . . . It's possible to achieve heaven on earth like Buddha wanted, but he didn't . . . because he had nirvana as far to my knowledge and others didn't. And his goal was others*

have everything he has and unless I would have my nirvana, knowing that others have nirvana, I wouldn't be happy.

People who are homeless, and his citizenship colleagues, are Nicholas' community. He connected with the latter group about three months after joining the *Citizens Project*. The turning point, Patty says, came the day he told the story of another community he had found, at the park where he slept and spent time during the day:

> *I was sitting almost with my feet in the water and I was feeding the geeses in the water and there was a family, Mama, Papa and three geeses and a lot of others around them... I want to feed the little ones because they are weaker and they need more food to grow and blah, blah, blah. And other geeses were on the ground behind me or next to me and they start fighting. [On a later day at the pond] I had some meat... and I was hungry so I started eating the meat. The leader of the group, the greedy one which [the earlier time] was trying to grab the food from the family I was feeding was behind me and almost had my arm. I turned and... it was fear between us... I got up and I tried to chase him... He looked at me and started that geese's warrior dance with those wings, and I'm sitting and I start laughing. I said, "OK what are you going to do now?" I was looking in his eye and I was thinking in my heart, I said, "Listen, you attack me and I will break your neck in less than a second. I came here to feed you." I was honest, kind, and assertive in my heart. [Then] he peacefully ate every crumb from between my legs and I'm saying, almost touching my feet. [The next time] I'm holding the bread bag. All the gooses are away to the farthest corner. And all of a sudden my favorite family's swimming next to me—father, mother, and three puppies. They are swimming next to me and my first reaction, grab the bread and feed what I favored. I swear to God I felt that [other] goose... And they [the family] swim away. Then how did it happen that they came back to me? I started throwing bread and they came, all of them, but they dance in a circle before me. And then I started feeding them all together.*[17]

Nicholas acknowledged smoking K2, a street drug made of legal herbs and sprayed with a chemical with cannabis-like properties,[18] during two of his trips to the pond. For Patty, though, the story represents a marker point for Nicholas' full entry into the *Citizens Project*, not only for the sense of connection with a community that the story reflects but, more importantly, for the fact that he told it to a human community he was finally ready to join.

5

Going to the Source

CITIZENSHIP MEASURE DEVELOPMENT AND VALIDATION

We used a theoretical framework of citizenship rooted in outreach work and developed a community-level intervention aimed at helping people who were homeless gain a sympathetic hearing from the "housed community" they were trying to enter. Then we developed an intervention for individuals—this time people with mental illnesses who had criminal charges—that had promising outcomes. Thinking about next steps, we had come to worry about a few things in the work we'd done so far and in some critiques we'd received of citizenship as a way of thinking about full community membership for people with mental illnesses. On the first count, we worried about the gap between citizenship theory and practice. We had taken a "reasonable and sensible" approach to linking the five Rs of citizenship to distinct program components in the *Citizens Project*, but we needed more empirical data on the elements of citizenship to make adjustments and improvements to the current project and for starting new ones. On the second count, we worried about the occasional critique that citizenship's legal aspect overwhelmed all others and so, rendered it too narrow to support the ideal of "a life in the community" for people with mental illnesses. Another critique was that, since citizenship is an exclusionary as well as inclusionary title and status, it is not a happy term for use in supporting the social inclusion of people who stand at the margins of society.

My response to the "narrowness" critique was that citizenship's history and theory encompasses both political-legal[1] and civic-participational[2] realms and that public debate over citizenship's inclusions and exclusions did not disqualify it as a means of supporting the social aspirations and goals of the people we were working with. Still, there was that devil's advocate's voice, my own, which said that while the historical and theoretical traditions of citizenship might give a rounded portrait of it, we didn't know whether or not people, thinking about citizenship in everyday life, would see if that way. We had to wonder if, indeed, an overwhelmingly political-legal face would emerge from a study of people's views on citizenship. As for citizenship's dual inclusionary and exclusionary quality, that seemed to me to enhance its relevance. Debate over citizenship's inclusions and exclusions, I thought, over who gets to be a citizen under what conditions and why, would be a good thing to have. That is, assuming a good outcome from that debate for people with mental illnesses, people who were homeless, and people with criminal histories.

A different kind of worry was that, given an average of 12 to 15 students in each six-month class, freestanding interventions such as the *Citizens Project* could help two dozen or so people a year at most and might be difficult to get funding for on a large scale. This made us wonder whether or not citizenship interventions or citizenship supports could be integrated into treatment programs that, in a large mental health center like ours, see thousands of clients a year. But this worry brought us back to our first—the gap between theory and practice and the need to have more empirical data on the elements of citizenship that could help us develop a variety of interventions and supports based on them. What we needed, my colleagues and I agreed, was to develop an individual instrument to measure citizenship. The National Institute of Mental Health funded us to do that.

Measure Development

We wanted to "go to the source"—to hear from people with mental illnesses on their citizenship ideas and aspirations.[3] We were also interested in the viewpoints of people who had been excluded or marginalized in society for reasons other than, or in addition to, mental illness. To do this, we chose a concept-mapping research design proposed by my colleague Maria O'Connell. Concept mapping captures and integrates the views of many stakeholders to create "maps" or visual representations of the data collected from them.[4] Maria and another colleague, Chyrell Bellamy, a psychologist and social worker, proposed that we also enlist the theories of "off-timedness" and life "disruptions" for comparing the citizenship views of people with mental illnesses, people with other life disruptions, and "non-interrupted" people. Life disruptions are dramatic personal events, such as the intrusion of "first break" psychosis in the lives of teenagers or young adults,[5,6] that contribute to a sense of "off-timedness" in which people may not meet expected developmental milestones. An Iraq or Afghanistan war veteran's return to the United States after two years of putting his life on the line every day, only to find that the country has changed while he was away, his friends have launched their careers and are not particularly interested in hearing about his experience, and his veteran status gives him no special boost for catching up with them, may give him a felt experience of off-timedness that contributes to his difficulty in starting on his own career trajectory, attending college, getting married, or reaching other milestones of adult life.[7,8]

We also decided to adopt community-based participatory research, or CBPR, methods. In CBPR, with its roots in social justice and social change movements and its premise that knowledge is created in collaboration,[9,10] people who typically are subjects of study participate in all aspects of the research process, from conceptualization through dissemination of findings.[9–10,11] CBPR is well suited for exploring community- and individual-level socioeconomic conditions, community health, and disparities in care across racial and ethnic lines. The core of our CBPR approach was to recruit an eight-member co-researcher team, or CRT, of men and women with mental illnesses. Three were African American, three white, and two identified as white and Latino. We trained the group in protection of human subjects and HIPAA requirements and conducting focus groups and concept-mapping procedures. CRT member were involved in all stages of the research.

Study participants included people with life disruptions—those who were enrolled in public mental health services, were receiving medical treatment for a general medical illness that interfered with their daily lives, were on probation or parole, or who had returned from foreign combat within the previous five years and people with combinations of these characteristics—as well as people with none of these disruptions. In the event, we enrolled too few veterans to include their citizenship "items" in the measure.

We recruited 141 people for the overall study through flyers and phone-ins: 75 for 7 focus groups and 66 for individual concept-mapping sessions that followed. Fifty-eight percent 60% were women 65% were African American, 30% white, and 9% identified as Hispanic or Latino. The mean age of participants was early 40s. These and other demographic characteristics were similar across both interrupted and non-interrupted groups.

Since we didn't collect personal health information, we decided to treat focus groups and concept-mapping sessions as separate sub studies of the larger study. Thus focus group participants could also participate in concept-mapping sessions and concept-mapping participants could, but need not have, participated in a focus group. We conducted one focus group each with people receiving public mental health services, people on probation or parole, and people with a general medical illness, and two each with people with more than one these life disruptions and people who had not experienced any of these disruptions. Of participants in the individual concept-mapping exercises including overlap for those with more than one disruption, slightly more than half were receiving mental health services, about 30% were on probation or parole, and slightly more than a quarter each had a current general medical illness or did not have any of these disruptions.

FOCUS GROUPS

The research team talked about multiple terms for use as questions or statements to prompt focus group participant responses. "Citizenship" was the obvious one, of course, but we considered adding "sense of belonging," "social inclusion," and "community integration" for help in generating discussion. CRT members, though, voiced a strong preference for a "citizenship" prompt alone. Citizenship seemed broader to them than social inclusion and community integration, which they associated with the marginalized status of people with mental illnesses. We agreed on the prompt, "To me, being a citizen means..." for the focus groups.

CRT members and two other researchers conducted the focus groups. Participants were asked to speak freely and generate as many ideas and items as they wished. "Being included," "Feeling safe in my neighborhood," "Giving back," "Doing what I want to with my time," and "Having equal opportunities" were among more than 750 items generated. The only follow-up probes that focus group facilitators used were for clarification on some items as in, "Can you say more about that?"

SYNTHESIS AND REDUCTION OF CITIZENSHIP STATEMENTS

We met several times to reduce our 750-plus items to 100 for use with concept-mapping software. We eliminated duplicate or near-duplicate items, for example, and separated multithemed into single-themed statements.

SORTING AND RATING OF STATEMENTS

Individuals who identified with one of our participant groups were given lists of the 100 citizenship statements and asked to sort them based on similarity and name them—"doing things for others," "social services," and "civil rights," are examples names used. There were two ground rules for this exercise. First, individual participants had to create more than one group, that is, one group of 100 items was not acceptable. Second, each group they created had to have at least two items.

After the sorting exercise, participants were asked to look at the entire list of 100 statements again and complete two ratings of each item on a Likert scale of 1 for "none or very little" to 5 for "a lot or all the time." The first rating was the importance of the item to participants regarding their views on citizenship. The second was how they saw their degree of achievement of that item. So, for the item, "Feeling safe in my neighborhood," Joe, who lives in a safe neighborhood and rarely thinks about his safety might rate the item as a one for "citizenship importance" to him but a five for his "achievement" of it.

STATISTICAL ANALYSIS

We entered statement groupings and importance ratings into a database and analyzed them using concept-mapping software.[12] The software scores any two items as 1 if a participant sorted them into the same pile and 0 if she sorted them into different piles. A high sum for a pair of items across all participants means that many people sorted them into the same grouping, reflecting a strong perception of their being related to each other. We then analyzed the sorting of all items across all participants using multidimensional scaling analysis,[13] which creates a two-dimensional representation of the clustering of items, with statements piled together more often located closer together in the clusters than those piled together less often. We then performed hierarchical cluster analysis,[14] which places multidimensional scaling results into non-overlapping clusters. We also identified items that were rated both "most and least important" and "most and least achieved" by people in each of the five stakeholder groups of mental illness, on probation or parole, general medical illness, mixed disruptions, and no disruptions.

Hierarchical cluster analysis sorted citizenship items into a diagram, called a dendrogram, which arranged statistically significant clusters based on participants categorization of the 100 statements. This process yielded different cluster arrangements ranging from one to nine clusters, or domains. The research team then reviewed each of the nine domains to determine which provided the most coherent and distinct groups of items. We decided that the seven-cluster domain "solution" was the best for our conceptual model of citizenship, and named the domains "Personal Responsibilities," "Government and Infrastructure," "Caring for Self and Others," "Civil Rights," "Legal Rights," "Choices," and "World Stewardship."

We then looked at the results of individual item analyses and decided on the most appropriate items to include in our citizenship measure. We kept items that, overall, were most important to each of our stakeholder groups and had discrepancies between one or more stakeholder groups regarding importance or sense of achievement. We eliminated items that lacked discrepancies between stakeholder groups *and* were not rated highly by those groups. We chose 46 items for our citizenship instrument from the seven domains. For each item, participants would be asked, "Thinking about your life in general now, rate how much the item applies to you on a scale from 1 to 5, with 1 being least important and 5 being most." We piloted the instrument with CRT members of the research group and made minor adjustments to wording and items. Here are 11 items from the instrument, using every fifth item starting with the first:

> *How much do you feel that your personal decisions and choices are respected?*
> *How much do you feel that people would give you a second chance if you needed it?*
> *How much do you feel that you have choices in your mental health care?*
> *How much do you feel that you participate in social and recreational activities in your community?*
> *How much do you feel that you take care of the environment?*
> *How much do you feel that you have or could have access to emergency services (police, fire, ambulance, etc.)?*
> *How much do you feel that you are included in your community?*
> *How much do you feel that you are connected to others?*
> *How much do you feel that you have the right to protect yourself and others?*
> *How much do you feel that you or your family has choices in education?*
> *How much do you feel that you have or would have access to jobs?*

We now had a measure that we thought would help people working solo or with their clinicians or others to calculate their social and community progress and come up with strategies for working on weaker areas or building on stronger ones. The measure, we thought, would also help us assess *Citizens Project* students' progress toward full community membership, and perhaps help us enhance the impact of the classes and valued role projects or for use in discussions of individual goals in student-peer mentor counseling sessions. The measure might also be used for verifying the citizenship progress or lack of progress of people receiving services that were not specifically citizenship oriented but were oriented toward stable "community living," such as supported housing, supported employment, and others. It could also be used in advocacy and self-help groups as a measure or personal planning tool or both.

There were limitations to the study. Our categories of life disruptions were broadly defined. We didn't screen for types or severity of mental illness. This was deliberate, since we didn't want our measure development process to be diagnosis-based. Still, it's possible that looking at specific conditions could yield information on the relative citizenship strengths, challenges, views and aspirations of, say, persons with psychotic *or* affective disorders. Another limitation was that, having excluded veterans from the measure development process, we had only four life disruptions, including combined disruptions. In addition, our non-disrupted participants were so named only in relation to the life disruptions we singled out and, so, some may have been experiencing other serious life disruptions. Still, the study gave us an empirical foundation for our citizenship framework and showed that people with and without serious life disruptions, including those with and without mental illnesses and with and without current criminal charges, saw citizenship as a broad concept that went far beyond its legal status. Taking its possible uses together, having the measure, we thought, could help open up a new domain of study on how people with serious mental illness build a life in the community, and inform the development of citizenship-based interventions to help people reach that goal. But first, we needed to validate the measure.

Validation Studies

The classic form of validation is to compare the completed instrument to other, already validated instruments to see whether or not it measures something new, yet also has elements in common with other instruments in the same field. A new measure of "community integration" for persons with mental illnesses, for example, is useless to the field if it measures the same elements as a validated measure of social inclusion. Yet on the other hand, if the community integration measure is so different that is has nothing in common with the social inclusion measure, it probably isn't measuring what it set out to measure.

Measure validation is a process as much as a product, since further validation testing on a "population of interest" can be done, albeit eventually with diminishing returns. Validation studies can also be done for subsets of a given population, such as persons with mental illness who also are homeless or have criminal histories. We conducted three forms of validation for the citizenship instrument—a statistical validation study, a qualitative check of our instrument using focus group transcripts that captured participant conversations as well as citizenship items, and a study using the domain map with a related but distinct group of persons who were, or had been, homeless.

MEASURE VALIDATION: STATISTICAL

We conducted statistical tests to measure the internal consistency, convergent validity, and discriminant validity of our citizenship measure.[15] Internal consistency is the degree to which items on a measure that should be related to each other are, in fact, related.[16] If our participant above who lived in a safe neighborhood were asked, "Is your neighborhood safe?" he would reply yes. If later in the same interview he was asked, "Do you feel safe in your neighborhood?" and replied yes, there would be internal consistency between the two questions, or items. Convergent validity involves whether or not, and the degree to which, different measures that we would expect to be related are related. We would expect a measure of citizenship to have commonalities with a measure of social recovery or social inclusion, for example. Discriminant validity involves the opposite expectation. We would expect little commonality, for example, beyond an other-side-of-the-coin connection between a measure of citizenship and a measure of social isolation.[17]

We administered our measure along with several others to 110 clients of our mental health center whom we recruited at the center's cafeteria during the lunch hours over the course of a week. The additional instruments measure quality of life, social capital, sense of community, and social recovery. *Lehman's Quality of Life Scale* assesses what people with serious mental illness do and how they feel about what they do. Questions include living situation, leisure activities, familial relations, social relations, work and school, legal and safety, and health.[18] The *Social Capital Scale* is used to assess trust in the government, community involvement, and giving back to one's community.[19] *The Sense of Community Index II* measures this concept through the domains of membership, influence, meeting needs, and shared emotional connection.[20] Finally, the *Recovery Markers Questionnaire–Revised*[21] assesses important aspects of social recovery.

ANALYSIS

We analyzed data from the 110 interviews using SPSS statistical software.[22] We created scores for each of the seven domains of citizenship by computing the mean of all items in a given cluster and arrived at an overall citizenship score based on computing the mean of all 46 items. We collected descriptive statistics based on demographic characteristics and conducted correlation tests to determine the associations between the citizenship measure and other measures. We also conducted stepwise regression procedures to examine demographic, sense of community, and social capital predictors of scores on citizenship, individual recovery, and overall well-being.[23,24]

Results

Fifty-eight of our 110 participants were male and a majority were African American. Twenty identified Latino origin. The average age of respondents was 48 and the average level of formal education was more than 11 years. Fifty-five percent of participants reported a history of alcohol or substance use. Almost half had been on probation or parole at some point in their lives and more than half had been homeless.

Overall scores on the citizenship measure were positively associated with scores on quality of life in general and with individual recovery and overall sense of community. Citizenship was also positively correlated with trust in government and volunteering from the social capital measure. As we had hypothesized, citizenship was not correlated with the amount of activity from the quality of life measure but was correlated positively with subjective measures of quality of life, meaning that participants' satisfaction with their social contacts, family contact, and general activities was more important to them than the amount of those activities they engaged in.

We conducted three linear regression models to determine the total amount of variance, that is, the difference in scores between different groups, in well-being, recovery, and citizenship. The first model examined predictors of overall citizenship scores. Results were that having a criminal history accounted for 13% of the overall variance in citizenship scores. Satisfaction with social relationships, satisfaction with health, and sense of community social connectedness together accounted for an additional 40% of the variance in citizenship scores. The second model examined predictors of well-being. Almost half of the variance in overall well-being was accounted for by satisfaction with activity and with health. The third model examined predictors of recovery scores. A little more than half of the variance in recovery was accounted for by satisfaction with social relationships, sense of community influence, satisfaction with activity level, frequency of social contacts, and satisfaction with family relationships.

On average, participants had the highest scores on the domains of "Choices" and lowest on "Government and Infrastructure." People with criminal histories had lower citizenship scores than people without, and thus are likely to need additional citizenship supports. People had higher citizenship scores if they were satisfied with their living situation; family and social relationships; finances, safety, and health; if they had a sense of well-being and of making progress in their recoveries; and if they had a sense of community in their lives.

We found that the citizenship measure captures elements of citizenship that people experience but that, until now, have been difficult to specify. The CBPR and concept-mapping procedures we used to develop the instrument support the relevance of the 46 items in the measure to people with various life experiences and differing degrees of marginalization. The research process and findings also gave us a more nuanced understanding of citizenship as a multidimensional concept that is related to, but distinct from, recovery, well-being, and quality of life.

MEASURE VALIDATION: QUALITATIVE CHECK

Because we reduced more than 750 citizenship items from the focus groups to 46 items for our measure, we wanted to be confident that we hadn't missed themes that may have arisen in general discussion in the focus groups but not been named as citizenship items and so, not made it into the measure. Two members of the research team conducted a qualitative check by independently listening to and taking notes on the audio recordings of all seven focus groups.[25] They then compared their notes, looking for confirmation or contradictions and for themes that were poorly represented in the measure.

We concluded that the focus group transcripts supported the domains and items and that no major themes had been missed. We did identify comments, though, that added contextual richness to the measure. For examples, two of the seven citizenship domains are *Personal Responsibilities*: Domain 1, and *Choices*, Domain 6. Focus group discussions of the right to protest, the importance of second chances, and the right to protect yourself and others mapped onto the items captured under personal responsibilities. Participants also commented on personal choices and freedoms including family planning, abortion, choice of partner, traveling freely, and control of one's money and finances. Domain 2, *Government and Infrastructure*, deals primarily with access to services and government responsibility to provide them. Participants talked about the importance of access to resources such as employment opportunities and the use of parks and libraries as well as government aid and services such as garbage pickup, fire departments, and welfare, and about the importance of being able to influence the government through voting.

As we found through the concept-mapping process, citizenship included both *Civil Rights*, Domain 4, and *Legal Rights*, Domain 5. Regarding civil rights, people spoke of constitutional freedoms such as speech and religion. One participant said that citizenship means "having the right to say whatever you have to say. Nobody can stop you." People also talked about racism and racial profiling. One said:

> *Police really harass more black people and Spanish people... They see me driving a Mercedes Benz, a nice fly car. "Hey, what is he doing driving that car?" They are gonna stop me... If you're a white guy they ain't gonna stop you.*

Another talked about discrimination against people with mental illnesses:

> *They look at us like we're something really bad... We should get equal treatment.*

Legal rights included the right to fair treatment in the legal system, such as the guarantee of a fair and speedy trial. Participants also spoke of the need for accurate information to effectively exercise legal rights, since "knowledge is power," as one noted.

Two domains—*Caring for Self and Others*, Domain 3, and *World Stewardship*, Domain 7, involve the responsibilities of citizens to others in their communities and the world. People talked at length about the obligation to provide for the future by raising "our kids to be better than us for the next generation," and giving back to the community by "reaching out to the homeless and less fortunate," and other community service. There were also comments and exchanges about the responsibility to care for animals and the environment, to donate to foreign countries in need, and to contribute to world peace and national security.

Some interesting differences and commonalities among the groups emerged from reviewing the transcripts. The mental illness and mixed groups, for example, incorporated a global perspective into their sense of responsibility, both as to the need to take care of the environment and animals and as to the obligation to help people in foreign countries. One participant spoke about the need to "protect animals from cruelty and abuse." Another said, "The country wastes our money on things we don't really need...other countries need help."

Members of the criminal justice focus group commented, as might be expected, on being law abiding and being a positive force in the community. They often focused, too, on their personal shortcomings and their need for self improvement and accountability, but also talked about the difficulties of making it in a society that wasn't looking to give them second chances:

> *Society should be providing more programs for people coming out of jail.*

> *When you take an ex-con and throw him out on the street he's got nothing. He's going to go right back in.*

> *Being on probation, parole, whatever, most of the time you're restricted from a lot of things, when it comes to a job, loans... [But] everybody has a checkered past.*

The medical group did not talk about access to medical care, while the non-interrupted and criminal justice groups spoke about the right to refuse medical care. Members of the mixed group talked about access to mental health services and general medical care. One spoke of "having affordable and complete health care. Being on Medicare, they don't care if you have a dentist, because you won't get one if you're on [it]." The mental illness, medical, and mixed groups spoke of violence and the need for protection from it:

> *You expect the government to protect you, not to get in trouble and have the World Trade Center bombed.*

> *Everyday people [are] getting shot. It's harmful to the whole community. A war. There is a war in America.*

In the mixed and criminal justice groups there was discussion about the importance of being a role model for the next generation:

To be a faithful father, a faithful mother, being a good role model because a lot of us get tied up in drugs. These things are put there to distract us and we don't realize it.

Staying involved with your children's academics . . . going to school meetings, parent's nights.

Participants in both of these groups talked about not wanting to be the cause of problems in their communities.

In general, all the interrupted groups emphasized the responsibility of giving back and helping others more than the non-interrupted groups. Also, the interrupted groups appeared to put a greater premium on community membership and belonging, with comments such as the importance of "being included in the mainstream decision making, when things are thought of and decisions are made," than the non-interrupted group. Scholars such as Edward Portis, who writes that people define themselves in social terms and that social commitment is a universal quality in human affairs with normative value beyond the instrumental behaviors of individual citizens, would agree. People are social beings, and individuals fulfill themselves in large part as members of society.[26]

Non-interrupted group members gave greater emphasis to accountability for those who break the law than those in the interrupted groups:

People who do bad things still have the same rights and freedoms that others have even though they don't deserve it. They shouldn't have the same rights as normal citizens have.

The non-interrupted groups also sounded a more cynical note at times than other groups:

We're supposed to have laws that protect you . . . supposed to.

[Citizenship is] the right to live in the greatest country in the world. So they say.

Non-interrupted focus group participants seemed to place relatively more emphasis on their entitlement to citizenship benefits and less on responsibilities to others and society as a whole than did participants in the interrupted groups. Unlike those in the latter groups with their emphasis on civil and legal rights, non-interrupted group participants seemed to apply the notion of rights to a broader range of issues, such as "the right to file for child support and alimony" and "the right to be an organ donor." Their dialogue also included more references to the right to act in unsanctioned ways, such as "the right to be prejudiced."

The non-interrupted groups discussed preparations for death, such as wills and life insurance, more often than the other groups. They spoke more of the importance of ownership along the lines of pursuing the American dream and of financial success than the other groups. "If you want it, you can get it," said one. "All you have to do is work at it." Non-interrupted group members also appeared to be more focused on outward expressions of individuality—wearing clothes of one's choice, for example—than their counterparts.

It's possible that our qualitative check encouraged a search among the researchers who conducted it for similarities and differences from the citizenship items and domains that might not have appeared, or that might have looked less dramatic, had they, with knowledge of the completed instrument under their belts, simply been asked to review the transcripts and give their impressions. Thus it may be best to say that it *tends* to support the findings from our concept-mapping research method, and that it brought out additional subthemes and nuances that concept mapping is less well equipped to identify.

MEASURE VALIDATION: "WHAT IS THIS?"

At a symposium on social integration at Columbia University in 2011, Maria and I presented on citizenship measure development, including a PowerPoint slide of our seven-domain map of citizenship. In the discussion afterward, Kim Hopper mused about the idea of convening a group of people with mental illnesses, showing the map on the wall without explanation, and asking, simply, "What is this?" We were intrigued by the idea. Allison Ponce, the associate director of New Haven's local mental health authority, or LMHA, and a member of the citizenship research team, offered to take up Hopper's suggestion. She proposed that we conduct focus groups with people who were or had been homeless, had dual disorders of mental illness and substance use, were on probation or parole, and were receiving services from LMHA housing agencies. This was a group with multiple needs and high risk of criminal recidivism, homelessness, or both, that had been identified by LMHA agency staff as difficult to serve effectively.[27]

We were eager to bring a citizenship lens to bear on housing agencies that were attempting not only to provide a place to be *in* the community, to draw on Norma Ware's phrase again, but help prepare them to take their places as members *of* that community.[28] As before, we'd come to think that our measure would be useful not only as such—to measure people's citizenship—but also as a tool for developing interventions and supports aimed at helping people work toward full citizenship. For example, people with both mental illness and criminal histories scored lower in our validation research than all other groups on six of the seven concept-mapping domains of citizenship. In theory, modifications to current services and supports might help to address this fact. Before bringing citizenship to our local service system, however, we wanted to know whether or not the framework resonated with the people it serves. By showing people the citizenship map and asking them what they thought of it, we hoped to learn which, if any, items and groups of items were most meaningful to them.

We recruited 11 people. Although we'd hoped for more, the small size of each focus group seemed to foster individual participation while still allowing for lively discussion among all. Most participants had experienced more than one episode of homelessness. Seven were currently homeless, three were housed, and one did not respond to the question. Five were white, five were African American, three endorsed Hispanic origin, and one endorsed Hispanic origin but not a race. None had participated in the citizenship measure development focus groups or concept-mapping sessions. They were invited to participate in order to share their "ideas about ways to describe your experiences of living in your local community and society" and "ideas about how you might change things if you had the opportunity."

Each participant was given two documents—a copy of the citizenship map (Figure 5.1) and a separate list of the exact items that appeared on the map. The map was also projected on the wall.

The focus group leader's first question was, "What is this?" Participants were also asked what the image meant to them, what was missing from the map, and whether they had these things in their lives. We audio recorded and took notes on the focus groups. At the end of each one, we gave participants details on the measure development study and its citizenship focus.

Following the focus groups, we read the transcripts and listened to the audio recordings individually, coding themes in and across the groups, then met to discuss themes. We reached consensus on seven—responsibility, giving back and helping others, assaults on dignity, "being in the hole" and second chances, "help isn't always helpful," time, and employment and housing.

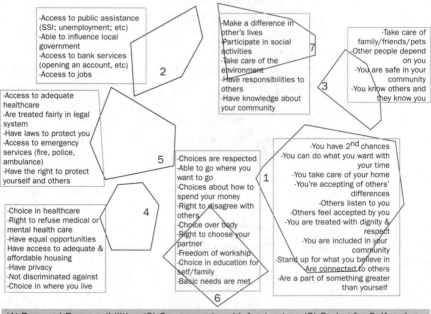

(1) Personal Responsibilities (2) Government and Infrastructure (3) Caring for Self and Others (4) Civil Rights (5) Legal Rights (6) Choice (7) World Stewardship.

FIGURE 5.1 Seven Cluster Concept-Mapping Construct of Citizenship.

RESPONSIBILITY

Responsibility meant different things in different contexts to participants. Some said they felt responsible for their homelessness and criminal behavior, and for taking charge of their lives now:

I am not perfect and I will be the first guy to tell you that I have made a lot of mistakes in my life, but I am trying to do things now to straighten up. I have made a lot of bad choices—drinking, drugging, fighting. I don't know what happened. I started going out and one thing led to another and I got off the path and made a lot of mistakes and lost everything.

Being homeless was difficult, several participants said, but it required less responsibility than maintaining a home, family, and work. Living in your own place, they agreed, was a "huge responsibility":

The more things you have going on, the more responsibilities you have. When you're homeless, you have no purpose.

When asked about the meaning of the citizenship map, one participant said it had to do with "regaining your self-worth and responsibility." Another said the items represented "the responsibilities associated with growing up right."

GIVING BACK AND HELPING OTHERS

People wanted to help others and contribute to their well-being. One said the map "is about making a difference in other's lives." He continued:

Sunday I usually go to my church. And afterwards we feed the homeless. It's a good feeling, you know? When people are helping me out, I want to give back to the community because I feel grateful and blessed that people are taking time to help me . . . It makes me feel good . . . that's kind of what it's all about.

Another said:

I think you get a sense of yourself back when you help others come up a little bit. You get that rewarding feeling.

When asked which group of items on the map was the most possible to achieve, one participant identified cluster 7—World Stewardship—and particularly the "helping others" item. Cluster 7 also includes items such as "make a difference in others' lives" and "have responsibility to others."

ASSAULTS ON DIGNITY

Loss of self-worth and personhood as a result of "assaults on dignity" was a strong theme across the focus groups. Participants talked about how the struggles they faced, from stigma and discrimination related to mental illness and criminal involvement to finding employment or housing, took a toll on them. Finding work, one participant said, was a way to "feel human" again:

> First of all, you got money coming in . . . [and] not just for yourself [because] you get a sense of yourself back when you help others come up a little bit. You gain a sense of self worth, responsibility. You feel like you are human. You feel like you are a man.

People spoke of ill treatment at the hands of staff members of various social service programs:

> They hurt your feelings. You are already hurting inside. While you are down they want to kick you and make you feel like shit. It's frustrating, you know?

They also talked about having to tell their personal stories over and over again in applying for jobs or mental health, case management, or other services:

> I get really crazy, man, when I am doing all of these intakes and I got to go through all this history again . . . Two, three times in a day . . . and that is something that they should really know about me . . . I don't have any employment. But when I see that and I got to fill that out, what do I do? Chronically unemployed . . . Then they want your criminal record. "How many times you been arrested?" God! I am 58, I was 14 the first time I was arrested . . . You got to go through this four, five times a week! It is depressing, man.

BEING IN THE HOLE AND SECOND CHANCES

People talked about being discriminated against in the workplace and of feeling as though the barriers to making it were next-to-impossible to overcome. They also talked about the anguish of having to check the "felony conviction" box on an application, forcing them to put their "worst foot forward."[29] One said:

> Once you tell them you have a felony, I have never heard back from any of them [potential employers]. Your chance is 100% no . . . Nobody wants you once you've made a mistake.

Having a felony carries with it stigma and discrimination that participants described as keeping them down both emotionally and socioeconomically. "Once you are in [the criminal justice] system," said one, "they don't want to let you go." The stigma that accompanies having a felony conviction "keeps you in the hole," said another. Still another talked about trying to turn his life around and having people gossip about his incarceration. "Once you get into a certain level [criminally]," he said, "it takes a long time to get out of that." And if you are lucky enough to get a job, you are still marked. He continued:

> There is somebody who works there who already knows your whole life and . . . the guy is telling everyone . . . "he goes to jail a lot." Gossipin'. It gets to the manager and your application is, like, torn in half.

People talked spoke about mistakes they made in the past and their responsibility for turning their lives around. At the same time, they expressed a sense of powerlessness to achieve their future goals because of their pasts:

> *I have made a lot of mistakes in my life, but I am trying to do things now and straighten up . . . Case managers tell us to do this and do that—you know—but the record is killing me.*

HELP ISN'T ALWAYS HELPFUL

Similarly to assaults on one's dignity, being offered "help that isn't helpful" left participants feeling used. One spoke of seeking help from a number of different organizations, sharing personal information with them, and then not receiving help he thought had been promised to him:

> *I have been a couple of places where they took all my information and they used me . . . They promised me, "Oh, I am going to do this and do this" and they didn't do nothing . . . They didn't even help me . . . I felt used. I really needed the help, you know, and they weren't there.*

People spoke of social service organizations taking advantage of them. Not only were they not offered the services they applied for, but they had to divulge personal information that benefitted the organization by allowing them to report on people they had interviewed. "They are getting all of this funding," said one man, "and they use all of your information . . . and they screwed me over." Feelings of disappointment and betrayal emerged as participants talked about their efforts to help themselves through signing up with social service organizations. One spoke of feeling betrayed by "free" job training programs:

> *It's frustrating. You feel used and you get tired of people doing this . . . Free training? No, I don't want no more. I ain't got no job . . . I knew [learned] all of that stuff for what? They ain't going to hire you.*

TIME

Time, like "second chances" and "getting started," was a pervasive theme. Time was not on their side, people said, and they were right in at least two ways. First, their histories of mental illness, homelessness, and incarceration involved life interruptions[5–7] that removed them from the mainstream for long periods of time. Second, these interruptions had rippling and long-term impacts on them. The stigma associated with incarceration, homelessness, and mental illness continued to interrupt their lives and present barriers to their getting started again.

One line of discussion related to time had to do with the difficulty of living by schedules and keeping appointments upon returning to the community from incarceration:

That is one thing, coming out of prison and being homeless, you don't keep appointments... That is one of the things that you got to get through. Keep your appointments and [get] help with scheduling because you overbook yourself. "Can you meet me Friday at 9 o'clock?" I say, "Oh, sure." And then I am like, "Oh no! I made the same... Oh God. ..." And then I got to call... You got to be on top of that because if you're not, it's overwhelming and you get really frustrated.

In prison, one's time—for eating, bathing, exercising, seeing family and friends—is controlled by others. The contrast between that way of life and the messiness of everyday life outside of such "total institutions"[30] is, no doubt, unsettling for many.

Time overlapped with the issue of looking for work. Hours spent in "free" job training is a waste of time when it doesn't lead to a job for people who've already fallen behind in a competitive job market. The participant quoted at the end of the "help isn't always helpful" theme continued:

Free training—no, I don't want no more. It takes up a lot of my time. Eight months, two and a half months...6 hours, 8 hours a day... [And then] they are like, "OK, where are we going to put you at?" And I am like, "You ain't got no job?!"

People talked about having lost time due to living for years with undiagnosed mental illnesses and trauma and then of being rushed into talking about these problems by untrained or half-trained clinicians. The first speaker below refers to a group treatment experience. The second responds with his thoughts:

I have PTSD. So now I come in...and from the first moment...I am just shaking and my jaw got super tight and I felt like I couldn't walk. I said I got to go. The walls are coming in...I was like, "Where did that come from?" It was pressed down so far and I had self-medicated so that I forgot what happened to me...He [the clinician] said more is gonna come out. Another topic comes up. Similar thing. I was like, man, I can't keep going through this. I am not ready for this... [They] don't know that feeling... I am not ready for it yet, you know what I mean?

I agree with you whole-heartedly... They can listen to you for an hour, hour and a half, but then after the break down, after you've been down that hole, how do you put it back together? They look and see it's 4:30... They got to go home to their family.

Such comments, which may stray from the text of the domain map, nonetheless speak to the context of people's struggles and the challenges of supporting their social integration and valued community participation as well as their mental health recovery.

Time spent homeless was time wasted, and worse, when it came to making it in mainstream life. "Time is precious, it runs out," said one participant. "You have to make the most of it, but that's hard to do when you're homeless, wondering where you'll get your next meal." Time in the moment, time in the long haul, and time taken to lead to next steps, especially employment, were tangled together for people, and they were hard to untangle.

EMPLOYMENT AND HOUSING

Participants spoke of the practical work of finding housing and employment and barriers they faced because of their histories and the current economic environment. On housing, one echoed a theme noted by several:

> *When you get out of prison... it doesn't matter how much you've done, even if it was something that was positive, trying to show them who I am now, and they say those things will not be held against you, and you tell me in an interview that, uh, "You the perfect fit," but ok, why didn't I get the job then?*

Trying to get an edge based on education or other qualifications, which might have helped participants during better economic times, proved fruitless when so many overqualified people were competing for the same low-wage jobs:

> *You spend all your time getting your GED and now you got people like, at Yale, who spend all this money and graduate and can't get a job. I couldn't get hired at McDonald's. They told me I was so-called "over experienced" or "over qualified." What do you mean about "overqualified"? But yet, someone who graduates from college, you got that person to work [there].*

This speaker, while noting the competition for work, also said that "overqualification" often was a code term for not being wanted because of your criminal record.

Barriers to housing appeared to be as daunting as those for finding work:

> *Housing is pitiful. They look at your credit or being a felon and you can't get housing. I know a lot of people who are in the shelters now who are still working, but because they have this on their record or their credit is not up to par, they can't get a house. And they need a second signature and nobody wants to do that because they might not want to risk it because they don't know if you have made that change yet, and they don't want to risk it because it might jeopardize them. So there is a lot of strikes against us.*

Even the most practical aspects of moving from the extreme social and economic margins to the mainstream, or close to it, involve affective elements as well. The link between instrumental and affective elements of exiting homelessness and becoming a full member of the "housed community" is, in fact, where citizenship began almost 20 years ago. Mental health outreach workers, we learned, could help people get housing, but having an apartment did not confer upon them the status of citizen, let alone that of neighbor or community member.

In the focus groups, we found that participants who were housed generally appeared able to stand back emotionally and consider the abstractions of participation, rights, and responsibilities represented by the seven domains and 46 items projected on the wall of the meeting room. Currently homeless participants, however, seemed more on edge and attuned mainly to in-the-moment meanings of domains and items, that is, to the reminders the map gave of their continuing marginalization. The difference between calculating one's activities on a given day in relation to food, clothing, and shelter or of having your own place that provides shelter, heat, and a means to cook your own food were dramatic. Those who had their own apartments had not necessarily achieved a high level of citizenship by virtue of that fact, but being housed seemed to provide a foundation from which, with additional support for their valued participation in society, they might set out to achieve it.

"Giving back" to others was a major theme for participants. The power of this theme appears to extends beyond the borders of the *Citizens Project* and the focus group participants in our measure development research. This suggests that housing and employment programs should consider ways to help their clients giveback to their community along with the support they provide for the goals of stable housing and competitive employment. It also suggests that their clients may be ready to take advantage of such help.

Educating providers of services about their clients' experience that "help doesn't always help" could help make them more sensitive to this reality for their clients, and take action to help them in ways that do help. It may also encourage them to go beyond this to develop better follow-through on service plans or, at the least, exit interviews and information about other resources when help, in fact, has not helped. This is not to say that providers of services are generally insensitive, but that new knowledge can changes one's understanding of others' situations, and that this understanding can have an impact on how one gives help.

The researchers who worked on this validation study have logged much time in providing and evaluating services for people who are homeless, but the compression of discussion and shared sentiments among our participants were bracing for us. This was especially the case for the theme of being in a hole and needing, but often not getting, second chances in their lives. Their responses and themes add a sense of gravitas, for us, to the further application of the citizenship framework in practice.

Participants' empathy for the struggles of others and their desire to give back may derive in part from their own struggles and a wish that others had given back to them, or their gratitude when people did. Recent studies by Jennifer Stellar and colleagues report that lower income people showed greater concern and compassion for the suffering of others than their upper income counterparts.[31] The authors suggest a possible explanation for this finding—that lower income people may "hear" and "see" other people's stress more readily than upper income people and are more attuned to other people's stress because of their own experiences with it. Our own findings from this more modest study appear to support this research.

With completion of our measure development study and validation we had reached the end of what, looking back, can be called a long developmental phase that paved the way for taking citizenship to scale through developing "citizenship-oriented mental health care" and making it available to larger groups of people than had been able to receive it through stand-alone interventions such as the *Citizens Project*. This work, along with a more in-depth look at what citizenship theory can offer to the mental health field and a prospective model of citizenship and mental health are topics for the remainder of this book.

6

Taking Citizenship to Scale

THE *CITIZENS COLLABORATIVE* I

Taking citizenship to scale was the next logical step for us, but logic didn't pave our way. We proposed a randomized controlled trial (RCT) to the National Institute of Mental Health that would put a modified *Citizens Project* head to head with Illness Management and Recovery, or IMR, a "psychoeducation" and relapse prevention intervention that educates people about their mental illnesses and has been effective in supporting decreased psychiatric hospitalization and severity of symptoms for people with mental illnesses.[1] The hook for our proposal was that evidence-based practices like IMR had a positive clinical impact for people with serious mental illnesses, but had shown no such impact on community and interpersonal outcomes. Individual skill development interventions, we argued, can't help people with serious mental illnesses navigate their way from marginalization to community membership. For that you need to help people take on valued social roles and make more contacts with their fellow community members. We went further, hypothesizing that community inclusion would lead to improved clinical outcomes. We had some initial hints from the RCT of the *Citizens Project*, such as improvement in quality of life, satisfaction with work, and successful community valued role projects, that this might be so.

It didn't fly. In retrospect we concluded that we'd missed an opportunity to build on our measure development study by proposing to use the citizenship instrument as both a measure and a tool for developing what we'd begun to call citizenship-oriented mental health care. In the meantime, the press of other work delayed completion of the validation study longer than we'd hoped. The measure was attracting some attention even so, but validation of it stood poised in hand as a period waiting to be put at the end of a sentence.

We did finish the validation study, but problems surfaced elsewhere. Lezley TwoBears had retired for good this time and gone back to North Carolina. Far more important than the loss of Lezley's dependable four or five hours a week with valued role projects, though, was that Lezley was both a close friend and advisor to

Patty. The peer mentors weren't able to pick up the slack left by Lezley's departure, as we were short on funding for them, with a lean budget that hadn't increased in years.

Rolling enrollment, a strategy we instituted when it became difficult to pull together a dozen students to start at the same time, had a downside to it, we learned. Using it, you could keep the group at a fairly steady census, and veteran students could help initiate the novices and encourage them to hang on through the rough patches. But rolling enrollment undermined the logical flow of classes, and fielding a cohesive group of students for developing valued role projects was difficult to maintain with people entering at different times. Also, problems maintaining group momentum with rolling enrollment seemed to have a negative impact on individuals' progress from marginalized person to student to valued role actor in society.

"What's Up?" came to the rescue to occupy the center of the project, often taking up entire classes and giving preeminence to the R of relationships but at a cost to the other Rs, particularly that of *roles*. Finally, the *Citizens Project*, always tilted toward males, had recently become a nearly all-male domain due to reduced time for recruitment and the availability of eligible clients from a mostly male day reporting program for people with behavioral health problems and criminal charges.

All this said, a culture of citizenship that spanned separate classes or cohorts after more than a decade of classes was in place. Returning graduates helped to maintain this culture by dropping in and, in effect, speaking to the commonality of experience between old and new students *and* to change over time that demonstrated the community's ability to adapt while maintaining its core ideals. They offered proof of the project's success, too, either as successful graduates who had built new lives based in part on what they'd learned from the *Citizens Project*, or as people in need of support and encouragement who knew where they could find it. And if "What's Up?" had come to dominate the project, time and experiment had given it a unique role that, if added to a revitalization of peer, class, and valued role elements, could help it become, not the center of the progam, but a supple underpinning to it. Finally, people as different as Nicholas and Bobby, and others, too, swore that the project had saved their lives, or changed them for the better. Something was still going right.

Yet it was undeniable that the tension and challenge of forward movement needed to make a full citizenship claim for the intervention had diminished. We needed more peer mentoring and leadership, more classes and presenters, and substantial and challenging valued role projects that stood up to earlier ones. And we needed to develop a full-fledged manual after a number of attempts that Patty and Lezley and I had made over the years. But citizenship might lie elsewhere, too, now that we had an instrument to measure its achievement in individuals. We were thinking of this as we began to talk about citizenship-oriented care that would reach more people, such as the thousands that received care every year at our mental health center.

We wrote a proposal to the Connecticut Department of Mental Health and Addiction Services, DMHAS, proposing to take citizenship to scale with its mental health center in New Haven as a pilot site for the state. We had two main objectives. One was to write a detailed manual for the *Citizens Project*. The other was to develop citizenship-oriented care on one or two treatment teams at the mental health center, with citizenship principles incorporated into clinical care and tangible connections to community resources. The citizenship manual would make it possible for others to develop citizens projects in Connecticut for people with and without criminal charges. Citizenship-oriented care would be for all people with mental illnesses, including those with criminal charges. Two key legislators liked the proposal, as did DMHAS. The project was funded.

The *Citizens Collaborative*: Foundational Ideas

Each of our two main objectives hosted a dilemma. The dilemma with the citizenship manual was how to capture in such a nuts and bolts document the gestalt of an intervention that was a hybrid of social service program and ongoing community. How could we help others create their own citizenship projects without bleeding the poetry out of the model?

The dilemma suggested by the notion of citizenship-oriented care could be traced back to the limitations of outreach when it came to supporting "a life in the community" for people who were homeless with mental illnesses. That is, even the most innovative mental health programs, in which work that was more than work, that went beyond the clock and even smashed the damned clock, could not make people neighbors, community members, and citizens.

The *Citizens Project*, a program that started to address the fact that programs were not the answer, partly negotiated its contradictions by coming to have the feel, and showing evidence of being, an enduring community. But "citizenship-oriented care," even with its promise of offering new avenues to community connections to clients and caregivers, had the nervous feel of, maybe, sending citizenship into the belly of the beast. Why not locate the whole effort outside the center instead, with liaison to it but with a main focus on activities in the community at large? Hadn't I coined the term "program citizenship" to convey what happened to people who managed to survive on the street but who, having signed up for mental health care, became isolated in their apartments and dependent on clinicians and case managers for much of their social contact?[2]

Program citizenship, as I described it then, involved the idea that the deals people who were homeless made with outreach workers might buy them only a ticket to "a new poverty niche, with substandard housing and social isolation in place of emergency shelters and homeless companions in misery, and second-class or 'program' citizenship in place of the non-citizenship of homelessness."[3] Program citizenship thus might take outreach team clients to a place in which, as Jacqueline

Wiseman wrote in the early 1970s about treatment and rehabilitation services for skid row alcoholics, "public institutions can become the only source of mainstream social contact in the lives of many marginal persons."[4,5]

Supporting clients' place and participation in their local communities is challenging for clinicians and case managers, due in varying degrees to the individually and clinically-focused care they provide for their clients, their administrative and rule-bound positions in place of more spontaneous community associations, their lack of access to community resources, and their protectiveness toward their clients who face discrimination and social stigma, extreme poverty, and often, gaps in mainstream social skills, work histories, and social networks. The tendency of public mental health institutions to provide a bare bones social world that may, in fact, help people maintain clinical and housing stability can, unintentionally, limit their access to community life outside the purview of mental health centers and associated programs. Kathryn Mackay writes of "conditional citizenship" in which poverty, difficult living environment, illness, and disability are exacerbated by people's contact with welfare agencies. These agencies encourage dependency and, through administrative processes and their relationships with recipients, distinguish "welfare dependents" from other citizens. Mackay's social citizenship model includes procedural rights such as information about gaining access to social and other supports, and participation rights involving the right to be present and be heard when policy decisions are being made about social and mental health interventions.[6]

"Program citizenship" was a provocation on my part and was useful for dramatizing the gap between entry into housing and the goal of full and valued membership in society for people with mental illnesses. It was also useful for trying to push systems of care to the edge of, and outside, their boundaries by holding up the ideal of "a life in the community" that had, after all, helped to spur the community mental health movement in the 1960s. I rarely use the term now, though, for several reasons. One is that the term could be offensive to clients of public mental centers who see these institutions as part of their community and who may both contribute to and benefit from the subterranean "underworld" of nonsanctioned help that exists in all structures and systems of care.[7] A second is that we don't know enough about how many people who receive public mental health care cope from day to day and over time, how they establish beachheads of community outside of their connections to mental health agencies, or combine institutional and programmatic resources with other supports and social connections, to confidently assert who suffers and who does not from the condition of program citizenship.

A third reason for moving away from the term is that, if mental health programs can't give people a ticket to citizenship and community membership, they may still be able to provide care that is supportive of them, in something like the way recovery-oriented care argues that, while you can't do people's individual recovery for them, you can provide care that is consistent with, and supportive of, their recovery.[8] Or so went the thinking we arrived at with the idea of "citizenship-oriented care," and so would a strict insistence on the idea of program citizenship be a contradiction in terms. For now, then, I'll use the term "bounded" in place of "program" citizenship. This term is far from perfect, too, since citizenship itself is bounded by nation-state borders and since the caveat of limited knowledge of people's lives in their communities still applies, but it will have to do for now.

There were promising reasons for bringing citizenship into the mental health center. Ours was a mental health center in a state of creative ferment, with a new CEO, a psychiatrist, Michael Sernyak, who liked the citizenship framework and its fit with his interest in promoting "customer satisfaction" to replace a "last resort for the poor" reputation that clung to public mental health centers. Some of his other interests—the integration of mental health and primary care long denied to people with mental illnesses, and community building both within the center and the New Haven community at large—also made citizenship-oriented care look like a promising venture. Robert Cole, longtime Chief Financial Officer of the center, played a leading role in building community, legislative, and DMHAS connections and communications, and figuring out how to keep a much larger ship than the *Citizens Project* afloat financially. A separate nonprofit associated with the center had a leader, Kyle Pedersen, who was funding food, health, and "financial health" projects, talking with community folk about citizenship, and introducing me to them.

Increased citizenship, we hypothesized, would lead to better clinical outcomes for clients, while citizenship-informed clinical care would support people's increased citizenship. In other words, clinical care, even though it struggled when it came to clients' social lives, might be a missing link in supporting their citizenship aspirartions, and supporting people's citizenship would also support and enhance their mental health. Citizenship-oriented care, as above, had a forerunner in Connecticut in "recovery-oriented care," and clinical care is at the core of mental health care, with psychosocial support, housing, vocational, educational and other supports arranged around and working with it. It made sense to link citizenship to the heart of the action, then, even at some risk to our founding narrative about the limits of formal care and services that people with mental illnesses must slip the bonds of in order to achieve full citizenship.

But there were reasons for skepticism, too. Rob Whitley and his colleagues write of the difficulty of integrating recovery-related interventions into mental health centers, what with burgeoning caseloads, staff burnout, skepticism, and high staff turnover. An alternative approach, they suggest, is freestanding peer-staffed recovery centers that focus on people's functional and social challenges.[9] We looked forward to drawing on our relationships with recovery centers, but were not opting for such an approach. In addition, the street-level operation of citizenship-oriented care—how it would be integrated into clinical care and where most citizenship-related activities would take place, in or outside the mental health center—remained to be seen. Only one operating principle, we decided, would apply across any set of citizenship components. This was that all clinical team members—team leaders, psychiatrists, clinicians, case managers, peers and others—would need to buy into the basic principles of citizenship and its relevance to mental health care, regardless of how much time some staff, such as peer mentors, or how little other staff, such as clinicians, might spend on specifically community-oriented planning and action. Otherwise, citizenship-oriented care would sink and disappear under the weight of the clinical mission and the regulatory and practice standards and requirements that defined, reflected, and maintained it in public mental health care.

We chose our name—the *Citizens Collaborative*—through generating ideas as a group, debating, and voting. The collaborative includes researchers, clinicians, peer staff, and administrators. A selection of key themes from our planning efforts to date will give a taste of how the *Collaborative* deepened and added variety to our citizenship palette.

THE CENTRALITY OF THE 5 RS

Our continuing discussions of the 5 Rs of rights, responsibilities, roles, resources, and relationships affirmed their centrality for us. Our communications guru, Lucile Bruce, thought the project's success hinged on staff and client familiarity with and endorsement of them:

> *The Collaborative needs a variety of visual means to represent what we mean by citizenship and the 5 Rs. Words are essential, but images are also key, especially as we think about how to explain them to clinical teams and outside the center. Why don't we choose images and objects that represent the 5 Rs? And examples of the 5 Rs in real life—what do they look like? How do we turn these abstract concepts into actions that people can take?*[10]

Lucile and Yolanda Herring, a peer mentor, began to design a project with the Yale Center for British Art and Yale Art Gallery to find paintings and photographs that would illustrate each of the Rs. These could then be used as part of a public relations and communications effort to bring the 5 Rs to the center and its satellite clinics.

My presentation to the planning team on another R—Axel Honneth's concept of recognition and of social conflict as the process through which excluded groups demand full political and socioeconomic inclusion in society, seemed to inject another level of meaning into our own Rs.[11] From Honneth our discussion moved to the R of legal, civil, and social rights. Kimberly Guy, a peer supervisor, asked, "Who gives you your rights? Who protects them when you're living in public housing and it's hard to get to the places you need to get to get all the 5 Rs?" Chyrell Bellamy, director of peer services and research for our parent program, added another, that of respect:

> *Seems to me that the "respect" R is needed for the other Rs to work. It can be applied by acknowledging people, saying hello, making people feel welcomed and affirmed throughout the center, not just clients but all staff from security*

> *to custodial to case managers to clinicians to leadership, etc. Inclusion begins*
> *with all feeling a sense of respect and belonging in the organization. I think in*
> *organizations we all have the "need to belong" and so that feeling that you are*
> *recognized and belong goes a long way.*[12]

To be clear, we did not change the 5 Rs to 7, but the concepts of recognition and respect enriched our understanding of citizenship and its considerations.

CITIZENSHIP FOR ALL

Chyrell argued that citizenship had to be for, and directed toward, everyone. It would fail, in fact would not be itself, if it were something we did for clients that was not reflected both in how we did our work and in the center as a whole. Allison Ponce suggested that we consider the 5 Rs of the mental health center. What would taking such a notion seriously mean for the center's operation? What were its rights and responsibilities? What would a complete list of its roles and resources include in relation to its clients, its staff, and the residents of New Haven? With whom were its relationships?[13] Chyrell, in turn, wondered what a self-inventory of one's personal citizenship might suggest for our project and the mental health center:

> *What about the different aspects of experience that affect your notion of citi-*
> *zenship, such as race/ethnicity, social class, illness status, gender, age, education,*
> *immigration status, language, incarceration experiences, sexual orientation? Or*
> *at least how society has defined and situated us based on these things. Citizenship*
> *is influenced by the intersectionality of these experiences and identities.*[14]

CITIZENSHIP IS HERE

I came into this new project, the *Citizens Collaborative*, with two cautionary tales in mind. The first was a lesson from what, eventually, would be a largely successful introduction of recovery-oriented care into mental health centers in Connecticut. During the initial training process for recovery-oriented care in the early 2000s, some clinicians, psychiatrists, and other staff felt that they were being blamed for not having provided humanistic care to their clients in the past. The need for a delicate balance comes into play with such new approaches as this one was. Change is often unpleasant, especially at first, and often meets with resistance. And innovators, who earn the title by identifying and offering new ideas and ways, may miss the fact that some staff are already thinking about and doing some of what they propose, and if they see it here and there, may miss the opportunity to endorse it as part of their efforts. What was the best mix of identifying citizenship-related work being done at present while forging ahead with what we had to offer? We didn't know, but we knew that a sister project had hit some snags. An interview with a psychiatrist on one of the clinical teams, more than a decade after the recovery-oriented care project began, gave us a lesson in how deep the feelings of being blamed or of being seen as "not getting it" could go, and how long they could endure:

> *Even this whole sort of...citizenship, which, I totally buy it. I mean I under-*
> *stand it. It makes perfect sense, [but] you know in the recovery movement, there's*
> *almost a sort of top-down, "You're doing it wrong. You better do it right." And I*
> *think some staff here for years have sort of known [recovery] and understood it.*
> *And I think there's really...this sense that nobody's doing this right. We have not*
> *just to be taught but we have to, I was about to say, "be shamed." I don't think it's*
> *quite that extreme, but there's almost this sense that, "Here comes another initia-*
> *tive that you tell all the staff, 'You're doing this one wrong, too. You don't know*
> *how to do this either.'" And certainly people could do better, but people who work*
> *with patients every day really often do know what they need even if they may not*
> *say it in the right words.*

A key factor in our success would be the support of the Director of Clinical Operations. Happily, she, Peggy Bailey, welcomed the project and joined the *Collaborative.*

A related cautionary tale is less specific and more chronic. It involves the intro-duction of any new project or new mandate to clinicians and clinical teams who already feel overwhelmed with high caseloads and are trying to "keep people alive," as one clinician said of her clients. As we went from team to clinical team talk-ing about citizenship-oriented care, I tried to reassure clinicians and others that we didn't intend to add new elements of care to what they were already deliver-ing without, at the same time, bringing in more staff resources to address them. Allison understood the reasoning behind this message, but did not find it to be an inspiring one:

> *We can talk all we want about this not being an "unfunded mandate," but unless*
> *we create a framework that allows providers to understand this as something*
> *they're already doing—which just needs a boost—or as something that will actu-*
> *ally make their jobs easier, they may see it as burdensome. It may be useful to*
> *paint the picture of how a person in recovery who is engaged as a citizen may*
> *be less in need of "clinical treatment" and "case management." It does seem*
> *that many clinicians view clients as people who need constant monitoring and*
> *who can't be accepted in the community because of their eccentricities or lack*
> *of social desirability. I think the reality is that if the mindset shifts and we think*
> *about how community engagement is different for each person and meaningful*
> *for different reasons, we may get some traction. It's unrealistic to assume that*
> *all people with serious mental illnesses will be readily accepted into the com-*
> *munity and be able to gain access to all civic resources given that stigma is a*
> *real barrier, but eliciting each individual's goals and hopes will be a step in the*
> *right direction. Given that the mental health center is basically on board now*
> *with person-centered recovery planning, this might be a platform for integrating*

citizenship. Encouraging clinicians to consider citizenship-oriented goals with clients when doing recovery plans, for example. This doesn't require any additional work, just a small shift in thinking.[15]

In talking about what clinicians were "already doing," Allison was clear that she didn't think all clinicians or case managers were equally invested in, or adept at, supporting their clients' social lives, but that some were and we should identify and encourage their work. She continued:

Citizenship-oriented work is already happening, but it may be "undercover," below the radar, not recognized. In fact, it may be somewhat discouraged in some circumstances because it is not focusing on medication adherence, symptom reduction, and attendance at clinical appointments. By naming the practices we associate with citizenship, we can frame and celebrate what providers are already doing ... We can support and encourage clinical staff and client thinking and stories about how this is so. This may include a citizenship story contest or awards that we could sponsor, [i.e.]: "You'll be getting a notice on a CMHC community building contest that will be starting soon." In doing [something like this], the process would shift from "coming up with" a citizenship-oriented care intervention that teams or programs would be asked to implement, to identifying and celebrating citizenship from the ground floor—direct clinical care—up. Citizenship supports, tools, components, and interventions will likely come out of this process, but more organically and building on/highlighting/supporting work being done now.[15]

After more discussions along this line, we revised our research protocol for interviews with clients and clinicians to a nomination process in which clients and clinicians would nominate clients whom they saw as making progress on their community membership, and clinicians who had a particular knack for supporting people in doing the same.

HEALTH AND SOCIOECONOMIC DISPARITIES AND RACISM

Soon, a spirited discussion took place in our planning meetings on health and social disparities and racism in connection with citizenship. Ashley Clayton, project director for the collaborative, sent around an essay by Paul Farmer[16] on a new trend in medicine to deal not only with patients' clinical symptoms but their socioeconomic conditions and personal situations, since many symptoms and medical conditions are caused or exacerbated by the dire social and economic realities that patients experience.[17] Chyrell then sent out an article on Caitlin Rosenthal's research on modern business management techniques that, Rosenthal contends, were pioneered by slave owners in the 1800s in the United States.[18] Allison then noted that we had not talked about race in relation to citizenship. Lively discussion ensued. Chyrell spoke at another meeting about the "weathering hypothesis" that the health of

African American women may begin to deteriorate in early adulthood due to the cumulative effects of socioeconomic disadvantage, leading to higher rates of low birth weight infants.[19] At another meeting still, Kimberly Guy spoke of the frustration of people who completed courses to become certified as peer workers and then could not find work because of previous criminal records. Changes in the pardon process could change this situation, she said. We added the pardons process to our agenda.

Citizenship could not solve all of these problems, we knew, not in the mid-size city of New Haven or even in the little world of the mental health center. Still, citizenship would be an empty vessel if we failed to include these issues in our thinking and planning. From a more positive angle, citizenship and its 5 Rs were relevant to efforts to address health and social disparities and racism. Shortly after these discussions and at the suggestion of Mary Dansinghani, chaplain at the center, her group, the Spiritual Roundtable, along with the Committee on Health Equity and Cultural Diversity, and the *Citizens Collaborative*, agreed to co-sponsor a conference devoted in part to "microaggressions." Derald Sue describes these, in regard to race, as "brief and commonplace daily verbal, behavioral, or environmental indignities, whether intentional or unintentional, that communicate hostile, derogatory, or negative racial slights and insults toward people of color."[20] The conference was a success, with many clinicians in attendance.

The *Citizens Collaborative*: Projects and Research

We started work groups to address elements that we saw as contributing to our overarching mission of taking citizenship to scale in mental health care. They were manual development for the Citizens Project, voter registration for clients, community building at the mental health center, community connections, financial health, and citizenship-oriented care. This chapter will take up manual development, voter registration, and community building at the mental health center. The next will take up community connections and financial health, and the next and last of the three will take up citizenship-oriented care itself, with some overlap with earlier topics.

MANUAL DEVELOPMENT

I posed a dilemma above on how trying to force the *Citizens Project* into the strictures of a manual risked trading the spirit of the project for the letter of it. Patricia, Chyrell, and Kimberly took the lead picking and choosing useful material from earlier and too-brief drafts of a manual, expanding it conceptually and adding much new material.[21] They managed to pull off a balancing act of letter and spirit— enough detail on the letter of things to explain what the project was and how it worked, and enough spirit to give you a sense of how students experienced it. What they wrote, in fact, was not a manual but a guide. A guide shows the way without demanding that your boots fit into the prints hers left on the ground. She describes the terrain along the way, recognizing that the weather and other local conditions will change the looks of it before long but that the trail will still take you where you want to go, or thereabouts.

The guide tells a story, too, and to a particular reader:

> *If you are reading this introduction, it means that you are interested in the "whys" and "how-tos" of getting a citizenship project started. This guide helps to explain what a citizenship project is and why one might be beneficial to people in recovery in your area. It also outlines some of the key elements you need to put into place to get your project going...*

The story locates the reader in a place. That it's not the reader's place doesn't matter—what matters is that it's not taking place in an airless room. The opening narrative includes the citizenship foundation story of Jim deciding he needed to move out of his new apartment and go back to sleeping under the highway bridge:

> *Citizenship as we approach it...began with Jim, a man who was homeless and receiving services from the New Haven mental health outreach team in the mid-1990s...*

There's a passage about the 5 Rs and how they, and a sense of belonging, come together to define and embody citizenship.

The details and strategies the authors begin to introduce make of this guide a story in a particular setting that, paradoxically perhaps, allows the reader to create his own project mentally and visually while reading it. The details—when a landlord can and cannot come into your apartment and when he can and cannot bar you from entering it, the ins and outs and backstage wisdom of how the pardons process in Connecticut works for people with criminal histories—leave room for the reader to breathe rather than being smothered by them. And there are tips about how gestures, expressions, and personal and social space are the vessels that shape the words you speak to your listeners, and other pointers on the nuances of citizenship.

A hybrid thing such as a citizenship project, standing somewhere between program and "naturally occurring" community, can't be taught through the conventional form of a manual, but it need not defy description, either. The secondary effect of writing the guide was to set the stage for a new cohort that was to start soon, and start together as a group rather than trickle in through rolling enrollment. The course itself had been modified as well, laid out in the guide with more conscious attention to the relationship between class topic and the main R it addresses. Here is the list by order of presentation, with some topics involving two or more classes, and not including the four speeches that serve as the segue to the valued role projects:

Relationships: Intimate and Interpersonal	*Relationships*
Grief and loss	*Relationships*
Spirituality	*Resources*
Communication skills	*Relationships*
Negotiating the Criminal Justice System	*Responsibilities*
The Pardon Process	*Responsibilities*
Housing options	*Resources*
Vocational	*Roles*
Educational	*Roles*
HIV	*Responsibilities*
Advocacy/ADA	*Rights*
Healthy alternatives	*Resources*
Family matters	*Roles*
Citizens movement	*Rights*
Self-awareness	*Responsibilities*
Person-centered care in mental health	*Roles*
Culture	*Relationships*
Stigma and microagressions	*Rights*
Financial health	*Responsibilities*

You may have noticed, glancing at this list, that many of its items touch on more than one R. You might have substituted a different R for one or more topics. Indeed, it's the purpose and content of the lesson that determines which R it lands on most emphatically.

The manual also describes in detail the hiring, training, and work of peer mentors and the process and elements of creating and delivering valued role projects. The next step, after some fine tuning as we looked back and forth between the guide as a support for positive changes in the *Citizens Project* and put it into practice with a new class, was to work with DMHAS to support the development of new citizenship projects in other sites in Connecticut.

VOTER REGISTRATION

People with disabilities have lower rates of voter registration and voter turnout and higher rates of unemployment and poverty than the general population.[22] Disparities such as these contributed to support for passage of the Voting Rights Act of 1993, a corrective to limitations of the 1965 Voting Rights Act, aimed at eliminating discrimination against racial minorities. The 1993 Act was, in part, a response to loopholes used to get around the intent of the 1965 Act. It also held special importance for marginalized groups such as people with mental illnesses, as it charged state and local government agencies that serve people with disabilities to help them register to vote when they registered as clients.[23] Even with changes in the law, though, low voter registration has persisted among this group. Current estimates are that less than sixty percent of Americans with cognitive difficulties are registered to vote, the lowest among all disabled populations.[24]

In late spring 2012, Michael Sernyak asked me to form and chair an ad hoc committee to conduct a client voter registration campaign. I recruited Tomas Reyes, an administrator and former President of the New Haven Board of Aldermen, and Lucile Bruce, communications director for the center. Soon we had a committee of about fifteen clinicians, peers staff, case managers, administrators and researchers, along with collective enthusiasm for our mission. Two principles guided our work. First, voting was a right for people with mental illnesses as for all other citizens, and was a "gateway act" to other civic participation. Second, our activities would be non-partisan.

The story of our voter registration efforts, which began before the *Citizens Collaborative* was funded but later joined forces with it, can be told in two stages. The first is the 2012 Voter Registration Campaign. The second is infrastructure-related activities that followed the election.

2012 Voter Registration Campaign

Voter registration was not new to the mental health center, but earlier efforts had been narrower in scope and mostly led by an ambitious clinician or case manager or two. Now we had a committee, a charge from the CEO, and a Presidential election and open US Senate seat, both contests that appeared likely, early in the campaign season, to be closer than they turned out to be. Over several months we researched the voter registration process, including absentee voting and reinstatement of voter rights for people with felony convictions, and made initial plans for civic education activities at the center linked with voter registration. Along the way we identified a barrier to voter registration and other citizenship participation for CMHC clients, and had a disappointment that took the wind out of our sails temporarily.

The barrier was that an unknown but large number of CMHC clients did not have photo I.D. cards. In Connecticut you do not need a photo I.D. to vote. Instead, you can cast a provisional ballot that will then be checked against local voting records. In trying to support people who were marginalized in the political process, however, voting in a different manner than everyone else you're standing in line with is, at best, a fallback plan, even setting aside the fact that not all polling site staff are aware of this option. In any case, having a photo I.D. is something you need for more than voting, and the lack of one interferes with any number of practical interactions and transactions. Symbolically, not having a photo I.D. is a negative marker of full membership in society. In trying to solve the photo I.D. problem, however, we learned that getting one comes close to being a Catch-22, since having a photo I.D. of one form is the easiest and quickest way to get a photo I.D. of another. An original birth certificate is the mother of all forms of identification and of access to others, but helping people get one, as clinicians and case managers knew, could be arduous and time-consuming. The team psychiatrist who spoke above spoke on this topic:

> *It's difficult for people that have no I.D.s ... And the whole issue of get-*
> *ting someone an identification is, oh my gosh, especially after 9/11, it's just*
> *harder and harder. So they have to have a birth certificate and another form*
> *of I.D. just to get the nondriving driver's license at the motor vehicle depart-*
> *ment, that then enables them to get their checks cashed. For some people that*
> *can take months and months. You have to write to where they were born and*
> *try to get the birth certificate and then if you don't have any other I.D. [in*
> *order to get it] ...*

Given the challenge of pulling together a first-class voter registration campaign, we agreed to deal with photo I.D. problems individually and take up the collective problem of this form of marginalization after the election.

We also talked about civic education activities associated with voting, includ-ing in-center events such as Saturday matinee movies on civic and political themes, posters and videos in the lobby and waiting areas on voting and citizenship, visits to City Hall, and others. Most of these, too, we agreed, would have to wait until after voter registration was over. There was one exception, though. We thought the hotly contested campaign between Linda McMahon and Chris Murphy, the Republican and Democratic candidates to fill Senator Joseph Lieberman's seat in Connecticut, offered a perfect opportunity to sponsor a debate in New Haven on the candidates' mental health agendas. We would hold the event outside the center but encourage clients to come with their questions. We sent our request to DMHAS through the center's leadership.

The answer was no, out of an abundance of caution that, while the event would involve both candidates and be conducted in a non-partisan fashion, it could be interpreted as having elements of partisanship in a heavily Democratic city such as New Haven. We were disappointed, although the caution was understandable for a state funded program, which must do more than is absolutely needed to avoid any possible appearance of partisanship or the condoning of it. Yet where does the possible appearance of political partisanship end and and responsibility to encourage citizenship participation and citizenship capabilities of people who are excluded begin? This is a tension felt at all levels, not only by those the street level of conducting voter registration and related activities. One possibility is to work with center leadership and DMHAS administrators on developing guidelines for safely negotiating the Scylla of partisanship on one shore and the Charybdis of duty toward politically marginalized persons on the opposite shore. Less broadly and mythically speaking, when one way is blocked, the barrier, intuitively, may seem to apply to everything associated with the barrier. But if, working with administrators and policy makers, we could dissect the elements associated with civic education of various sorts, determine which were innocuous, which questionable, and why, and what steps might be taken to negotiate passage for some proposed activities and not others, we might be able to come up with a guide for planning and assessing the permissibility of such activities.

The campaign was a success in spite of its challenges. Peer staff worked the lobby and waiting areas of the center to register new and current clients. A case manager on one of the inpatient units talked up voter registration and helped many patients register. Committee members worked the crowd on farmer's market days in the center's parking lot. A satellite clinic conducted its own successful campaign a few miles away. In the end, a respectable number—at least 65 clients—registered to vote, and we had raised awareness of the importance of the topic at the center and among its clients.

Voter Registration: Infrastructure Development

We reassembled after a break. We agreed that the most compelling task we faced was to work toward voter registration being part of the work of the mental health center. Voter registration campaigns were important, but they were icing on the cake. Asking people if they were registered to vote when they came in looking for mental health care, helping them register if they needed it, and reaching current clients with the same question and offer of help was the cake itself, and that we did not have, not yet. It was unclear what the center's response to the 1993 Voting Rights Act had been at the time, but it did become clear from canvassing other mental health centers that ours was not alone in lacking a voter registration infrastructure, even though campaigns were conducted more informally at some centers. Since DMHAS had gone so far as to make a film in 1994 that encouraged its agencies and clients to put the law into practice, I think the most likely explanation for out being Johnny Come Lately pioneers is that centers, administrators, and staff intended to institute procedures to help incoming clients register to vote, but that the logistics for doing this got lost in the press of keeping up with day-to-day clinical work and its normal crises.

We asked to be recognized as an ongoing, rather than ad hoc, committee of the mental health center, and were. With the current Mayor of New Haven leaving after two decades in office, we decided to conduct another voter registration campaign, even if not on the scale of the first.

It floundered. There was no energy for it, and people started dropping off the committee. Tomas Reyes, a co-founder of the committee, left to become Chief of Staff for the Mayor-elect, State Senator Toni Harp. The *Citizens Collaborative* was getting started and I was putting most of my energy into it. Lucile and I talked about the possibility of having the Voter Registration Committee become a project of the *Collaborative* while maintaining its status as a committee of the mental health center. We broached the idea to both groups, had a joint meeting to discuss it, and all agreed to the semimerger.

While this process was going on, we were working with Peggy Bailey on building voter registration into the clinical intake process for new clients. After that we would come up with a comparable process for already-enrolled clients. Soon, we hoped to link broader civic activities for clients to the *Collaborative's* planned community-connection efforts in New Haven. Billy Bromage, a recruit to the Voter

Registration Committee from the *Collaborative*, was talking about educating public officials about the needs and the status, as constituents who vote, of people with mental illnesses.

In early interviews we conducted with clients who had been nominated by their peers and clinicians as making good progress in building community connections for themselves, a few noted their interest in voting and helping others get registered. They also spoke of the responsibility of knowing who you're voting for, and why. Here are comments from three nominated clients:

> *This year I was able to go out and help people enroll to register to vote . . . And just letting people know there's plenty of candidates. Don't just vote because you are told to vote. But if you vote, at least know who you're voting for and what they're about. Don't vote because, "Oh, they got this much money." What do they do for the community? That's what we're looking at. What do they do for your community? . . . Voting's a right. I have the right to speak up.*

> *I can't tell people who they need to vote for. I can empower people [to] do more study, have an interaction with that person [who is running for office]. And the most is, "What are you going to do for me?" What is going to be benefit where I can have faith again in my neighborhood? Where I can . . . like love and live happily ever in my neighborhood? "What can you offer me? I don't care if you have been in the neighborhood all your life. What can you offer me as a leader in this community?"*

> *Citizenship means a lot to me. My belief system, it ties in with my sense of self as a citizen. I try to make my actions consistent with my beliefs. I go through the motions with heart. I vote and I work the polls. I tell people what's on my mind, my take on the news, which may be different from someone else's take on the news.*

The last speaker, 21 years old, had been talking about his sense of responsibility to succeed in college and then in a professional career. His answer to one of the "reverse" questions we asked people, about the meaning of each of the 5 Rs in their lives—in this case, whether or not there were *responsibilities* he wished he *didn't* have—brought me up short reading the transcript. "The right to vote," he said. Not encouraging. But he continued:

> *Which sounds weird, but I feel like there are some decisions I don't want to make, that I don't want to make a mistake and choose the wrong person and could affect everyone in a whole broader respect.*

If that's not a form of civic consciousness, even if, ultimately, a wrongheaded one, then I don't know what would be.

The challenge that voter registration poses for mental health centers is linked with the challenge of supporting people's engagement in the 5 Rs of citizenship in the context of the demanding work of clinical care. As persons with mental illnesses have been, and continue to be, denied full membership in society, supporting their citizenship must factor in the lack of knowledge, for many, about the details and requirements of voter registration, the apathy or cynicism of some, who know they are not seen as an important voting bloc, and the demanding work of clinicians and mental health workers who are thinking, first, about keeping their clients alive and reasonably healthy in the context of poverty and mental illness in America. This is ongoing work for the Voter Registration Committee and the *Citizens Collaborative*, with support that goes deeper now for having started the work. It is not so hard, I think, to imagine a time when voter registration is just "what is done" at public mental health centers and clinics, assuming such entities survive, and when staff and clients, as well as the public, look back, scratching their heads, when they hear of a time when it was not.

COMMUNITY BUILDING AT THE MENTAL HEALTH CENTER

Michael Sernyak scans the horizon for new ideas. He became interested in the idea of mental health center staff and client involvement in discretionary spending as a means of community building and collective participation when he came across the Web site for the Participatory Budgeting Project in Washington, DC. Its Web site describes its mission and approach:

> *Our mission is to empower people to decide together how to spend public money. We create and support participatory budgeting processes that deepen democracy, build stronger communities, and make public budgets more equitable and effective.*
>
> *Our approach: Building on decades of experience around the world, we understand participatory budgeting (PB) as a democratic process in which local people directly decide how to spend part of a public budget.*[25]

The roots of the project were a collaboration between North American activists and academics. The first public instance of participatory budgeting in the United States coming out of this collaboration occurred in Chicago in 2009, when residents of the 49th ward voted on the use of over a million dollars of public funds that, in the past, had been doled out by the alderman. The Participatory Budget Project aims to "transform democracy" by fostering citizen involvement in government decision making, paying special attention to marginalized in the work of democracy people by poverty, race, and other forms of exclusion.

Michael asked me to coordinate a community building contest at the mental health center. He saw the contest as a way of building greater staff and client investment and participation in the life and operation of the mental health center, including developing annual performance improvement goals for the center. He had a thousand dollars to spend, he said. What could we do with it? I liked the idea of the modest sum of a thousand dollars, which in short order became two, as an impetus for broader change. I turned to Lucile Bruce, Billy Bromage, and Ashley Clayton, who did most of the heavy lifting, and thinking.[26] We formed a committee and began to work on contest guidelines and rules and the voting process for a mental health center with hundreds of employees and thousands of patients at the main building and a number of satellite clinics. We, by which I mean they, created an information packet, a submission form and ballots, held informational and proposal writing sessions for clients and staff, counted ballots, reported results, linked winners to the mental health center foundation that was funding the projects, and monitored the winners' progress in completing their projects and launching them with a celebration open to all at the center.

We defined community building as supporting one or more of the goals of enhancing the experience of clients and staff as a community, fostering a positive work environment, or bringing people together to meet, talk to each other, and celebrate. We encouraged proposals that were creative, collective, unique, and inclusive of all members of the mental health center. We required that all proposals come from at least two people. No solo projects. We encouraged entries designed by staff and clients together. We noted that there would be at least one winner, but possibly two or more, to divvy up a $2000 contest budget. We advertised electronically and with posters at the mental health center and its satellite clinics, and set a submissions window of two weeks, aiming for a balance between enough time to get a decent number of applications and a short enough period to maintain interest.

I thought we'd get two or three submissions for our first go-around. We got 13. Three were disqualified for lacking a two-person planning team and other reasons. We wrote brief descriptions summarizing the remaining 10 projects for voters and created a ballot. Voting was on the honor system. We put ballot boxes in several gathering places around the mental health center and at its satellites. I thought we'd get about 50 ballots. We got almost 700. I thought the satellite clinics would likely remain aloof for this first contest, and require coaxing to join in over the next round or two. The first-place winner was a satellite clinic that turned its waiting room into a polling station for two weeks and got more than 400 votes for its project, a mural to be created by clients and staff. The second place winner, for a barbecue grill for the mental health center's courtyard, got many of the remaining votes.

I've gone into some detail here to give a taste of how time consuming a modest community building effort at a large mental health center, or a similar setting, can be. In fact, the description fails to do justice to the effort. A better taste of this is in order. The following are a few of the ideas, discussions, spirited arguments, and considerations we had, with their imperfect resolutions:

¤ What should we do to get people involved in the selection process itself? A community building contest should include community- and consensus-building on what such a contest should be, what values it should reflect, and how fairly it represents a wide range of interests and groups, some more vocal and empowered than others. We wanted broad involvement from clients and inpatients, and from different sectors of the staff—clinical, maintenance, administration, public safety, and others. Yet we had limited time to foster such a process, and limited resources. In the end we opted for a smaller planning group, one that included peer staff, some of whom were also patients, and two or three other staff groups.

¤ The process should be fun. And funny. What would "community" be without it? We could have a town hall meeting with *American Idol*-like presentations of, and pitches for, the different proposals, the more inventive, bold, absurd, shy, moving, or generally attention-grabbing or seductive the better. See above for limitations of time and energy as well as competing demands. We went straight to a vote.

¤ Who could participate? Did involvement in the planning process preclude submission of a proposal? Yet some of the people who could throw off great ideas with a flick of the wrist were sitting on the planning committee. We decided, of course, that planning committee members could not vote.

¤ What about proposals involving projects that would take place outside the mental health center? After all, one of Dr. Sernyak's goals, and ours as a citizenship collaborative, was to reach out to the New Haven community. And then, again, look across the street from us. There was a major cancer center. We decided that proposals could include projects that took place outside the mental health center as long as they made a convincing case for how they built community at the center, too. In the event, we did not receive any.

¤ What about the voting process itself? How could we ensure the one person one vote rule? How did we know that there would be no ballot stuffing? The resolution to this dilemma was that we couldn't ensure any such thing, not with limited resources and time, and what kind of community-building message would a closely supervised vote on such a project as this be, in any case? The honors system was the way to go.

¤ How to maintain the link between a modest, though staff-intensive, contest and the ambitious leadership goal of democratic involvement at a community mental health center that is trying to support a "life in the community" for its clients, and which also happens to be a medical inpatient and outpatient hospital? This is partly a matter of experimentation, and of modesty about the contribution such an activity can make. But modesty, and sense of humor, notwithstanding, the connection between a community building contest and the larger goal of client and staff investment in the mission of the mental health center was at the heart of this project. Staying with the process and seeing how it could change and be shaped over time seemed to be the best response, for the moment, to the question.

Post contest, we were planning for the next one. We reported back to Dr. Sernyak on the questions and considerations above, and others. Community building contests, we concluded, while being enjoyable, must be linked to larger goals. Empowering people with a vote was a step in the right direction, but the choices must be meaningful and connected to broader change, or people would become disengaged. How could we use the contest to support a culture of engagement and participation at the mental health center for both staff and clients? The question, not the answer to it, which we didn't have, was the guide. A practical recommendation we gave was to build incrementally on our first project, requiring more participants for each proposal, including a town hall meeting before voting, and speeding up the process between award, completion, and celebration of the project. The first contest worked. We could build on that, while continuing to work on tightening and clarifying the link between discrete, small-scale community building projects and the larger aim of greater staff and client involvement in the direction of the mental health center.

7

Taking Citizenship to Scale

THE *CITIZENS COLLABORATIVE* II

We've long seen "community connections" as a core part of any citizenship project worth the name, and the same certainly applies to citizenship-oriented care. Financial health is newer on the mental health scene, but has taken up residence as well, and with the Citizens Collaborative. Much has happened with both.

Community Connections and Citizenship-Oriented Care: *Project Connect*

Billy Bromage, a young man, is an old-time social worker–community organizer, and I mean that as a compliment. About a year before the *Citizens Collaborative* was funded, some online research he was doing led him to *Project Friendship* in Prince George, British Columbia.[1] *Project Friendship* began about twenty years ago, drawing on the work of John McKnight, a sociologist known for community building work that focuses on the assets, rather than deficits, of troubled communities.[2] What struck Billy about *Project Friendship* was the simplicity of its approach to community inclusion for people who were socially marginalized by their disabilities. Rather than trying to connect them to generic community activities, *Project Friendship* staff ask people what their passions and interests are and then connect them with community members who have similar passions and interests. From there, if all goes well, people meet others with like interests and continue to branch out as they wish and as their individual capacities make possible for them.

Prince George is a small city, about 60% the size of New Haven, in another country—Canada—on the other side of the continent, with different demographics, community resources, and cultures. *Project Connect*, the name Billy chose, could and should not be a replica of *Project Friendship*, he knew. Still, the basic idea made sense to him as well as to Chyrell and me. When funding for the *Citizens Collaborative* came through, *Project Connect* became the *Collaborative*'s community arm, and later was largely absorbed into it as the community action group's learning and ambitions expanded.[3]

Project Connect's work begins by helping people identify their interests and deciding how they want to pursue them. Participants draw a map of their community as they see it. Staff—Billy or a peer life coach—talk with them about the map and how to use it to connect to their interests and vice versa, then work with them to find and make contact with people or organizations, eventually stepping back to allow the connection to flourish on its own. Here are a few case vignettes on the street-level work of the project, drawn from Billy's notes.

Oliver, in his fifties, wanted to join a book club. His peer life coach found a group that was reading bestsellers, but Oliver wanted something more intellectually challenging than that. After some fruitless searching, Billy called a friend of a friend, the director of a private library in New Haven. As luck would have it, the library director had been trying to get a book club started for some time, without success. Oliver's interest led to a meeting with the director. Then Oliver went with his peer life coach to the club for a first meeting of the club. No one there knew that he was the catalyst for it. A month later at a picnic in his neighborhood, Billy overheard two people praising the book club.

Peter, also in his fifties, has a broadcasting license and experience operating a ham radio. His peer life coach, Steve Olsen, has a basic knowledge of radios. The two talked about Peter's joining a local amateur radio club. Since then, Steve's contact with Peter has been through e-mail and an occasional phone call. After doing some research online, Peter decided to join a club in a town near New Haven. He and Billy made a plan to attend two different meetings. In each case, Peter cancelled. The plan stands, yet to be fulfilled.

Sandra, in her forties, lives in a rest home in New Haven. She has limited mobility due to severe nerve damage in her legs. She enjoys crafts and wanted to join a needlepoint group. Billy called the Director of Elderly Services for New Haven and found there was no such group, but the senior center in Sandra's neighborhood was looking for a volunteer to teach crafts. Sandra said she would try, even though it wasn't what she'd had in mind. She and Billy met with the site coordinator, the group was convened, and it worked, with Sandra teaching seniors a number of craft projects in addition to needlepoint. She told Billy the group kept her so busy that she had to use only her cane there, since her walker slowed her down. Sandra called the senior center one day to let them know she wouldn't be able to attend a holiday party because her transportation service had forgot to schedule her ride. The site coordinator said she had to be there, that she was part of the family, and sent a van to bring her to the party.

Alonso, in his forties, likes biking and wanted to meet other bikers in the New Haven area. *Project Connect* staff found a ride that the Parks & Recreation Department was sponsoring, but it was cancelled due to a thunderstorm. Billy stopped by a bike shop and heard about a weekly ride on Sundays. He told Alonso, but later heard that he didn't attend because he was confused about the meeting place for the riders. Billy realized that Alonso understood directions by landmarks rather than street names and so had not understood Billy's directions. Perhaps he was embarrassed to say so. Billy made a plan to meet Alonso at the social club and ride with him to the meeting place. Alfonso overslept, but he attends the Sunday ride now and is looking into others he's heard about from the other bicyclists. He's also looking for help from *Project Connect* again, this time to find a cooking class so he can improve the variety of his menu at home.

Marc, in his late forties, is an artist who attends many cultural events in New Haven with people from a social club. He approached *Project Connect* because he had fond memories of kayaking with his father as a boy, and wanted to take it up again. Staff contacted the Parks & Recreation Department and learned that kayaking would begin a few months later, in early summer. Billy suggested to Marc that he keep in touch with them about when the schedule would be posted. Marc called, but didn't hear back. *Project Connect* staff called, too. Eventually Marc got the schedule, only to learn that he would have to take a training course that cost $60 in order to participate. Marc didn't have that kind of money, and at that point *Project Connect* didn't either, so Marc put his plan on hold.

Dante, in his twenties, was already engaged in many activities and made frequent trips to New York City, but still wanted to get involved with *Project Connect*, although he wasn't sure what it was he wanted to do. In drawing his participatory map, Dante realized he wanted to join a running group. His peer coach helped him connect with one. He runs a few times a week now with the group and socializes with several of its members.

Simple is not always simple, as we've learned with Project Connect. The notion of connecting a person to another person or group with similar interests presupposes that such a connection exists when, in fact, it may have to be created, as occurred in the case of Oliver and his book club. A person may want to pursue a new social outlet but, as with Peter and the ham radio club or Alfonso and his bike riding group, may not be ready to take the plunge at first. Unexpected developments can prove to be positive ones, though, as with Sandra and her craft group. Community connection project may also help people build on the strengths of their strong social networks as opposed to starting from scratch, as with Dante.

Connecting people with specialized interests and high standards to community partners can be difficult, and may risk burning the latter. Joseph was fascinated with the idea of stock trading. Through *Project Connect* he made contact with Ed, an amateur trader, who told him about his experience and lessons learned from trading, gave him several books on the topic, and offered to have him over to his office to experience on-the-ground trading. Joseph's peer coach left the three-way meeting thinking that a solid connection had been made. Joseph called him a few days later, though, to say he thought Ed had not been "successful enough." Ed, who also thought that he and Joseph had made a good connection, was disappointed and perturbed. Project staff thanked him for the generosity of his time. Some time later and through a friend, a peer coach found another possible connection for Joseph, at his request. Joseph said he would follow up on his own.

Participants' mental or physical health can make it difficult for them to follow through with connections. Linda, who suffered from serious depression, wasn't able to get to an interview for a volunteer position she wanted. She's doing better now, and is working with her peer coach on another possibility. Andrea, who was having an increasingly hard time getting around because of physical limitations, was unable to start a volunteer position that her peer coach had helped her find. She, too, is looking at other options, this time in her neighborhood.

Let me offer a few points here. One, illustrated by Billy's account of his work with participants, is the importance of what Kim Hopper calls "committed work." Committed work involves going above the call and hours of duty to make improbable service transactions work. It may also involve violating or adopting a loose interpretation of agency protocol when going by the book won't get the job done. Such work, which generally happens at the margins of institutional care, happens in the moment and when no one else is available or willing to step up, runs the risk of violating its own standard of unstinting dedication to the welfare of its clients by letting more traditional care off the hook of *its* obligations.[4] Committed work, at least in the first sense, has been a characteristic of staff work on *Project Connect.* The project is still too new to run afoul of its second sense.

In the spirit of Lezley's caution against cultural miscommunication, by which touching someone on the shoulder might start a war, let me say that I don't think outreach and peer workers and people like Patty, Lezley, and Billy care more about their clients than clinicians and case managers in mental health centers do about theirs. The "kinds" of people who are drawn to the kind of work this trio is doing may be quite similar to the kinds of people who do other person-to-person work with people who are socially excluded by homelessness, criminal history, mental illness, dire poverty, or combinations of them. And work in or outside mental health centers will include those both more and less passionate and idealistic about the welfare of their clients. The committed work I'm talking about here, though, is the sort that often finds itself at the margins of what a work day, and work elements such as staff safety and client–staff boundaries, are understood or defined to be. It skirts or redefines those understandings and definitions of what work is and where it stops. The structure of the situation is different in mental health centers, where procedural requirements and organizational-bureaucratic presence are stronger, no matter the vibrancy and creativity of a given center. Redefining and transgressing boundaries happen there as well, but they define the work less boldly than they do at the margins, as in mental health outreach work.

A second point about *Project Connect* is that a reader might wonder why so much of the initial legwork and contacts were made by staff rather than having staff encourage and support the participant in making the contact. Such early contacts do happen, but the range and depth of participant interests and skills may partly obscure the difficulty many people have in taking the first step outside their social zones restricted by their social circumstances. Participants' experience in having made successful contact with staff support may encourage them to make next-step contacts on their own. Joseph, with his interest in stock trading, appears to be ready to make the next contact in his search for a mentor. If he does, and *Project Connect* staff learn of it, his previous decision not to go with Ed the stock trader, while awkwardly performed, may look like the style of a man who knows what he wants and has learned that he can't turn the work of doing it over to anyone else even if, as here, he still needs help in identifying possible connections. Even so, making the first move socially will be difficult for some people.

And not so far from the norm as it may appear at first. Many if not most of us have taken advantage of such help. They're called social networks, and they involve strategic help that, at times, a colleague or friend takes on your behalf because doing so increases your chances of success with the connection being made or the tip given. You don't have to be mentally ill to need help moving forward. Factor in the opportunities to ask for things we want, encouraged by forms, structures, and moments for inclusion that many of us have, and the chasm between where the excluded person stands and where his first step must land may look wider to the observer than it did at first. Here is the psychiatrist who spoke about the sense of being blamed that clinicians experience with the introduction of new approaches such as recovery or citizenship:

> *It's so hard to get people engaged in communities. And I'm trying to think of successful engagements. What is saddest to me is that for so many of our people there is not a community. I mean either they don't know what to do or know how to do it or they've been isolated for such a long time. So in a funny way, [the mental health center] has become a community to people... I mean I know there is... what's the project that Billy Bromage is involved with?*

"Project Connect."

> *Project Connect, and I think that has potential, that sounds wonderful. But when we think of [the clients on my treatment team], they don't even know what they want to connect with, really... We all try to sit with people and expand their world just a little bit and it's really hard... I just had a patient whose mother paid one of the workers at Dunkin' Donuts $20 every once in a while to feed her son when he came in so at least he'd have somewhere to go have donuts.*

A final point here is that these vignettes do not address the issues of discrimination and stigma that impede the social network building and flourishing of people with mental illnesses. This is a topic of study and action for the *Citizens Collaborative* as it tries to build bridges to the larger New Haven community.

COMMUNITY CONNECTIONS AND CITIZENSHIP-ORIENTED CARE:
THE CCC COMMUNITY ACTION GROUP

Billy and Patty became co-leaders of an action group to develop community connections for the *Collaborative*. Billy talked about the use of social networks, both face-to-face and electronic, for connecting mental health center clients to people and organizations outside the mental health sphere. This would involve training, for those who needed it, in the use of electronic media, thus increasing their social capital to boot. A similar approach had become the main source of connection-making prospects for *Project Connect* staff. The action group was also working with Steve Olsen, a peer life coach, and Rebecca Miller, the director of peer support services at the mental health center, on a community resources bulletin board for clients and staff. Billy is also thinking about working with a local networking site used by activists and nonprofit organizations to create a shared electronic clearinghouse for information about community resources, low-cost activities, and other programs. He wrote of the benefits that might come from joining in common cause with others:

> *From a community organizing perspective, there is definitely a benefit to maximizing the breadth of the working group that would plan a site like this. There would be shared interest in getting the work done and everyone would have less work on their own shoulders. A lot of organizations would benefit from a site that aggregates information in a user-friendly way... Beyond mental health service providers and people in recovery, groups that come to mind are schools, Boys & Girls Clubs, health centers, the City of New Haven, people trying to get the word out about their events, community activists, faith communities, people seeking various kinds of assistance, etc. I think pulling together representatives from these organizations to discuss the concept would be fairly simple. [But] is the* Citizens Collaborative *in the business... of pulling together or taking part in coalitions like this to address community issues?*[5]

As with some other ideas generated in the hot kitchen of the *Citizens Collaborative*, this idea runs ahead of our resources at the moment, but given the right shuffling of them it might work, under the *Collaborative's* direction or with other organizations.

The community action group has served, in part, as a second- as well as first-stage think tank, assessing and making recommendations on ideas that come up in *Collaborative* team meetings. One such idea involved walking tours of New Haven for team members, clients, clinicians, and others at the mental health center. I suggested this one, thinking it would serve the joint purpose of exercise, a strong interest and push the mental health is making for its clients and staff, and of getting to know the city and making contact with community members and leaders. Bridgett Williamson, a peer mentor who lives in an area that is home to many of the center's clients, offered to lead a tour of her neighborhood. The community group, of which Bridgett is a member, took up the idea and considered the possible downside of it. One was the possible perception of a do-gooding delegation from the mental health center elephant-in-the-room-of-the-neighborhood coming to have a look at where the poor people live. Also, they said, we needed to spend more time thinking about what we could bring to New Haven and its neighborhoods in addition to what they could do for mental health center clients. What was, and would be, our relationship to community members? And what would the follow up to a visit or tour be? As Billy wrote:

> *A one-off thing doesn't work. The whole point is to get to know who is in the community. What can we offer? What are we trying to learn? ... There have been conversations about how best to educate or inform clinicians and staff about New Haven outside of Park Street [where the mental health center is located] and its immediate surroundings. [There was a proposal] to take tours of various neighborhoods, maybe led by community leaders from that neighborhood. Several members of the community action group felt that sort of activity might not be the most effective. It doesn't provide the community leaders with anything substantive in return for their time, and it offers only one person's or organization's perspective about life in the neighborhood.*[6]

The way to go, the group proposed, was to "give back" to neighborhood leaders and residents by offering to help them with things that were important to them, such as neighborhood cleanups and community garden work days. As for gaining a broader understanding of the ways and means of community life in a New Haven neighborhood, working side by side with residents would give *Collaborative* members new perspectives on life in these neighborhoods and, perhaps, opportunities for clients to engage in the associational life of these small-scale communities.

Mary Ohmer writes that citizenship participation can help residents of neighborhoods to develop trust and shared expectations and norms for community life. Residents' identification with their neighborhood can decrease their isolation and empower them to become involved in local organizations. Community-based social work practices, she writes, can support citizenship participation, contributing to residents' self and collective efficacy.[7] The work of the community action group seems consistent with this approach.

The group came to consensus on an overarching approach and strategy. First, we would recruit clinicians, then grass roots community leaders, to the group to learn from their perspectives and, we hoped, get their buy-in. Second, the group would undertake a pilot intervention with one neighborhood partner, most likely the West River Neighborhood Association, given that group's well-established community activities and openness to people from outside the neighborhood. This association sponsored once-a-month Saturday morning neighborhood cleanups followed by work in a community garden. The action group suggested that we propose to help them with that. By doing so, we would meet residents, make a small contribution to the well-being of the neighborhood, and help to create a collective psychological space of openness for the participation of mental health center clients living in or near the neighborhood.

Stacy Spell, president of the neighborhood association, endorsed the idea, and plans were made to start with monthly events for four months with a process and outcome evaluation of the project. We would continue to work with the neighborhood in some form after that, but, if things had gone well with West River, also look to develop projects with other neighborhoods. One of our evaluation questions would be not only how the project did, but how to sustain it and others like it.

A Community Focus Group

The community action group conducted the first of what will be a series of focus groups with community members to get their ideas on how to connect clients of the mental health center with people, activities, and organizations outside the mental health center. This focus group would take place in the sober context of clients' and the community's socioeconomic situations, discrimination and stigma, and a lack of sufficient valued roles in society to be given out to marginalized persons.[8] The process for selecting community members was identical to those for choosing clinicians and community members. We were looking for leaders or well-connected folk in the community who would be able to give us advice on community connection-making as a key element of citizenship-oriented care. The action group itself chose some prospective focus group members, and took nominations from other New Haven residents.

Our selection method presumably ruled out people who might be hostile to our citizenship goals for mental health center clients, but we expected to hear some of those voices through "citizenship lunches" in which *Collaborative* members would have informal discussions with people who might, or might not, be friendly to our citizenship approach. Note that our decision to conduct focus groups with civic-minded people in New Haven contained an unarticulated assumption—that they would, naturally, welcome people with mental illnesses as "new" community members.

With last-minute cancellations, only four people attended the first focus group, but they had a lot to say. Paul, a novelist in his late thirties, also writes a well-known blog on cultural issues in the U.S. He is married with three young children and is active in his neighborhood and synagogue. Laura, in her early seventies, had a career working in mental health settings and still works part-time. A widow and mother, she is also a community activist with special interests in food, community gardening, and the environment. James, in his mid forties, is a social activitist with strong associations with faith organizations in New Haven. He lives with his wife in a diverse and socially liberal, neighborhood of New Haven. Ellen, in her late forties, is a community organizer at a state university in New Haven and lives in a communal apartment with her husband and four biological and adopted children.

She is involved with various community activities that reach out to people with mental illnesses.

The focus group lasted more than two hours. Questions, which required little follow-up help or prompting from the focus group leaders, included:

What does it take to connect people to their community?

Would making these connections be the same for people with mental health issues or other challenges, or different?

What do you think a person needs in order to connect to their community?

The session can be divided roughly into two parts—how people make connections in the community, and how people with mental illnesses make connections in the community.

The first question, "What does it take to connect people to their community?" elicited a response about *invitation*. Paul, the novelist, spoke of the importance of the invitation that comes from the person, already established in a relationship, group, or activity, who wants to welcome and include another:

It very often takes saying to someone, "Will you come on Saturday?" or, "Would you come to my house for dinner?" or, "I hear you have children. Why don't you come to my backyard [with them so they can] play with my children some afternoon?" Not that people won't respond to a flyer or a Facebook post or a poster, but when you say to someone, "Would you come?" and give them a specific time, make it a real invitation, "Would you come Sunday afternoon? We'd love to have you at the house of worship, at my backyard, at meetings at the farmer's market to say hello," or whatever, then it feels very real. You get a higher response, you get more people saying yes... So there's really no substitute, actually.

This idea makes sense and seems to offer a way in for some of the folk we want to help who are not well-connected socially. But who gets the invitation, and where?

The question of "who" involves social fit, the look and feel of it that the person who is considering whether or not to offer an invitation to another determines with a glance, before knowing the full answer to the question of his or her social fitness. The "where" involves opportunities that come with place—residing in the same neighborhood, the likelihood that people with certain social characteristics will set foot in certain areas, and so forth. Paul makes this point about the geography of connection:

One of the things that can stand in the way of connection is just geography... making sure [people are] not geographically isolated, physically isolated, as well, that they see other human faces. Why do they always put elderly housing 200 acres off of a main thoroughfare? It's like, God forbid they can still walk, there's not any place to walk.

Making the invitation, and accepting it, involve risk. Your offer might be rejected. The recipient has had the experience of being rejected before, a little bit or a lot.

If a lot, she will have learned ways—that will signal she's not interested in receiving an offer—not making eye contact, the determination of her stride to get her somewhere else, or other strategies that may nor may not be intertwined with the prompts of psychiatric symptoms. This is James, the social activist:

> *I think allowing ourselves to be vulnerable, exposed... can turn into a true community, in the sense that we all have our issues, we all have our things, we all have our pluses and our minuses.*

Yet there are different kinds and levels of risk depending on the quality of choices you've had and the consequences you may experience from losing or winning your bet—momentary embarrassment or personal devastation at having your offer rebuffed when offered, or not given at all when hoping for one.

James, as he says, holds high standards for what qualify as social connection and community:

> *There's two words, connect and community, and I think those can be defined very differently... I have probably a high standard for both, that maybe sometimes is a downfall for me, because I believe in real connectedness and real community. And there are a lot of barriers to true connectedness of community, a lot of things in society that seem to fight that nowadays... I think people can gather in places, people can come together, and act on a superficial level.*

Jane Jacobs, writing on the death and life of much larger cities and on neighborhoods with mixed residential and commercial uses, likely would have disagreed with James' standards and his implied definition of "real community." In her study of New York City, it was exactly the limitations, mutually observed, on one's social relations with the grocer, the family across the block, the group of runners you can mark the coming of spring by, and the freedom to keep one's private life private that make possible and partly fuel the energy, vibrancy, and safety of the small community of your neighborhood.[9] Your neighbor across the street will call the police or shout out at the intruder trying to pick your lock at midnight without your having to invite here over for dinner in return. This latter version of community and neighborhood life would seem to work better for some of the folk we work with who struggle with building close personal relationships. And for everyone else, Jacobs might add. Yet times have changed. Jacobs wrote of neighborhoods 50 years and another world ago. Mutual disconnection among neighbors and community members may have strayed farther from the benefits of "weak ties"[10] than Jacobs would have been comfortable with, and so, she might have more sympathy with James' lament now than she did in her own times.

Laura, the gardener with a background in mental health work, talks about the importance of having interests in common with others, although other elements emerge in her observations as well:

> *Where I've had the most success around this kind of thing [facilitating connections] is where people share common interests... I've had a lot of*

success over the last few years around gardening, on Whitney Avenue. I'm a part of the people that have been gardening there, and we have a very cool spot, because people stop by . . . and they start talking to us and they ask us about how they get to be a part of the garden . . . So I got to know June, who gardens at Thomas More and [through her] I joined the land trust. And I thought, this is a way that I can go into neighborhoods that I wouldn't ordinarily go into . . . I share an interest with the folks in the Hill and Newhallville and other parts of the city that, I wouldn't otherwise have a reason to go in their backyard . . . In the six or seven years that I've been doing this . . . I have met tons of amazing people that I probably wouldn't have met otherwise.

Two thoughts came up for me here. One is that Laura has the will, the wit, and the experience to go with her personality to help people with mental illnesses gain entrée to community life. Another is that the social skills that go with her natural curiosity and ability to mix and match with people probably vibrates at only a slightly higher pitch than what it takes the average person to "make it" in his or her work and social life. Some *Citizens Project* students and mental health center clients have pretty good pitch, and some do not. There's a question as to how much of this can be learned with the right combination of coaching and support. Some of it certainly can be, maybe enough for most. After all, it's not about having everything in place, but enough to get by with.

Years ago my colleague Larry Davidson, when asked if he had seen *Brokeback Mountain*, said that he had and that he and his wife had argued over the meaning of it. She talked about its social significance. He thought the movie was saying, "We're all f—d up and we're doing the best we can." I like that, because then the question becomes not whether you either have or lack what it takes to get by, but "How good does the best you've got have to be in order to get by?" And I might add that, often, we're not ready to go "out there," but we have to anyway, and so we try to go out with the best we've got, including what we've been able to do with the help we've been able to get from others over time, adding new tools, shortcuts, faking it until we're making it, and muddling through until then. And it's still hard.

Laura spoke of how working together and developing relationships run along parallel tracks, with the first providing the occasion for the second:

The group of us have worked every week together in the garden, and you're pulling weeds together, and doing things like that. I feel like what was just bringing people together to do something has grown into very important relationships. There's a number of people that are struggling with pretty significant depression that work in the garden, and they've come to trust other people, and I mean, there'll be days where you're working in the garden and somebody's crying at the same time.

After providing the occasion for meeting, the work is there, a foundation, something to do. What people talk about may have little or nothing to do with the work at any given time. This is Laura again:

> *Well, actually, it's very interesting…usually you don't talk about what you're doing at all… At the end you go back and look, and you see what you're working on, but the conversation that goes on during that, it's just like if you're sitting shelling beans, you know, you're not talking about shelling beans, you're talking about whatever.*

For Ellen the community organizer, the power of community comes from people "having equal standing," with all on board needed to make the group work:

> *And that whole personalizing, and the grass roots, that's it, like you've just made a connection there. People just walk away, and they'll come back, and [then] they'll start taking people to job interviews, take them on, you know, [or] "Come do this with us, we need you." I don't want to take on your task, too, you know. And so it's saying, "I'm owning my stuff, you own your stuff, and we can work together."*

Laura agreed with this "way things happen" looseness because the structure comes with the activity, which is enough without a lot of the what she sees as the stifling rules that govern other community gardens:

> *And so the way we run our garden is, if you can come, good, and if you can't, you can't, and we miss you when you're not there, and let us know what's going on. There's two people in our garden that are really depressed sometimes… But they come in there, and they pick out some vegetables, and it works.*

Paul, referring to Laura's description, thought there was something about size, too, critical mass, that helped to make such activities and community building happen in a context of people being together and able to spell each other when needed:

> *You just said there are certain people that come, it allows a little more organic thing, because people can pick up for other people's deficiencies somehow… So people can come at a certain time, if they need to be here and cry, they can be there and cry, and other people are going to be there to work. So there's something to me, about a critical mass of the numbers… There is that thing where people can pick up for each other… Stuff just kind of gets done, so that's the beautiful thing, I think.*

In the mid-1990s, musing on the work of the outreach team as it reached its maturity, I thought, "We'd really be flying if it weren't for people having to wait for Ted to catch up with every single new piece of learning we acquire." Now, it's true that sometimes people don't have what it takes for the work. If so, it's likely they'll be extruded by outreach workers who are at one and the same time the down and dirtiest of all mental health staff in their work and the most aristocratic in their expectations of each other's having the "right stuff."[11] Correcting myself later on about Ted, though, I had come to see that another important element is the uniqueness of the team. You make adjustments, you try to fix things, but if you try to make it perfect it becomes something else, and not necessarily something better, because compensating for others' flaws is part of the dynamic that drives the work and constitutes the "itness" of it. The same can be true in groups and small communities, I think, and such settings as Laura describes, with the right amount of support and anonymity, can provide niches for people who add to what the group becomes and is. Here's Ellen:

> The idea is that we bring good people together...and no matter how disabled someone is by what's going on with them, there's something they can contribute to that community. And if what you do is water the plants, but somebody else can help prepare the meal or plan the meal, [then] every single person within the community has something that they can do that they can contribute. And you figure out, so that everybody has a job, I mean, it's really important, there's nobody that gets to not have a job. And then the idea being...you're a part of that, you're making the whole thing happen...you have a role that has an impact on everyone else.

If this is beginning to sound a little too idealistic, then we're ready for the second part of the focus group, on how people with mental illnesses can connect with community. Ellen's comment, in fact, came in that second part and in the context of tension between James and Paul, on one hand, with their concerns about how to include these folk, and Laura and Ellen, on the other, whose comments suggested that the question of how to include people with mental illness compact with the question of how to include anyone. Paul gave the first response to the focus group leader's question about community inclusion for people with mental illnesses:

> Well, if they present as scary, it's going to be hugely different, right? Someone mentally...it depends on how they present, right? I've lived near mentally ill people. My parents live two houses down from a group home in Springfield...But they're, you know, none of them is actively schizophrenic. They don't present as scary. No one worries about their children around them. You know, I think it could be very difficult to connect if you moved onto my street, and you seemed in some way out of control, potentially violent, hearing things. I don't know. I just...when I think of some of the mentally ill people I see in downtown New Haven, if they're talking to people who aren't there and things like that, I'd worry about my children around them. So that would make it very, very different from someone who was depressed, or on the autism spectrum, or I mean...[i]f they seemed unpredictable in some way, I think that would change everything.

Ellen responded by noting that very few people with mental illnesses are dangerous or violent. She added, "I just think our world is turning into a place where people are so frightened of people dealing with various disorders that they [the people who are frightened] behave a little strangely."

James had a different concern—how difficult it can be, and how much energy it can take, to deal with people with mental illnesses:

> *In my experience, mentally ill people, they take a lot of time and energy, they take a lot of effort to try to connect to ... So the community has to decide for itself, that some people are going to take some extra effort. And unfortunately, communities don't always decide that ... I think people who are mentally ill, it's harder to connect, sometimes, from experience. But a lot of times, it's the community, as well, not willing to want to put in the time and energy to do that.*

"Do you think that's any different for other disabilities, like physical disabilities?"

> *[Yes,] I think it is ... If it was somebody who was in a wheelchair or something like that ... I can kind of deal with that. But if it's somebody that's ... [Let's just say] this has been a long day, and it takes a lot of emotional energy, I guess, to deal with that. In some ways, it's more exhausting, than, I would say, than other kind of more physical kind of things. It's kind of easier to get your head around, you can build a ramp, you can do whatever, these kind of pragmatic ways. Mental health, it's exhausting to kind of get your head around. You can't really, in my experience you can't really fix it. It's not like, it's not a quick fix type of thing, and that makes it very difficult.*
>
> *Laura: But I also think that that's ... the fact that you can't fix the situation, to wrap your head around it, you don't challenge yourself.*

In this latter part of the focus group, after Paul's comments about the "dangerousness" of people with psychotic mental illnesses, Paul and James raised questions about how, or if, people with mental illnesses fit into different community settings. Intentionally or not, their comments tended to characterize people with mental illnesses as a special group, set apart, needing to be "dealt with." As in James's comments, it seems, from some of their comments, that they see these persons as a group whose belonging in a given community is not assumed but must, instead, be assessed and decided upon that community. Laura and Ellen, on the other hand, spoke of the importance of inclusion and, while not denying that some people with mental illnesses could pose behavioral challenges, suggested that there were always people in groups who could do a better job than others of connecting with these folk and thus help all to connect and "make it together" in something like the same messy way that people make it together, with peaks and valleys, in most neighborhoods with diverse populations and different struggles.

Then the discussion took a an odd turn. Paul, after noting his understanding that the challenges experienced by people with developmental disabilities have different cognitive and behavioral difficulties or challenges than those of people with mental illnesses, told a lengthy story about inclusion in his synagogue of people with developmental disabilities from a group home in his neighborhood. The story centered around a particular congregant, described as a good and decent man, who worked hard, looked to his time in the synagogue as a place to seek peace, and had a trouble dealing with some of the group home residents due to their odd behavior.

Two things stood out in this long section of the focus group. The first is that the people from the group home seemed to be proxies for people with mental illnesses, as the discussion flowed from and often mirrored earlier discussions about the latter. The second is that the dilemma of inclusion that Paul posed for the other focus group participants in his use of the synagogue example focused almost entirely on how to support the congregant who was disturbed by the people from the group home. Heated words were exchanged.

The focus group was instructive and bracing. The four participants were intelligent and civic-minded and shared positive ideas and experiences of community building that will help the *Citizens Collaborative* plan its community outreach and connection making. The focus group also provided a cautionary note for us. I noted our, or at least my, unspoken assumption that the community leaders we identified would support the community inclusion of people with mental illnesses. This was certainly true of Laura and Ellen, both of whom had extensive experience working with this group. I wouldn't say it was untrue of James and Paul, but the invitation that James proposed as the first principle of community inclusion came with qualifications for him and for Paul when the discussion shifted from generic community-connecting to the relevance of that process for people with mental illnesses. We had not spent a great deal of thinking about discrimination and stigma up to this point. We needed to spend more.

Financial Health

Two years before the start of the *Citizens Collaborative*, Marc Rosen, a psychiatrist and leading researcher on money management and representative payees for persons with mental illness, asked me to work with him and his team on conducting "qualitative" research in the context of his larger "quantitative" studies.[12] Marc wanted to have some in-depth interviews done with study participants on their experience with money and external control of one's money. I was struck by how, with rare exceptions,[13,14] recovery folk weren't talking about money and money management folk weren't talking about recovery. I thought I knew why from the recovery end. Money management usually involves coercion, so recovery folk tend to be uncomfortable with it. I could only guess at two possible reasons money management researchers don't seem to talk about recovery much. One involves their relative lack of exposure to, or reservations about, it. Another is a sense that many recovery folk disapprove of their work.[15]

And yet the two are not incompatible. As Douglas Noordsy and his colleagues suggest, it is exactly a recovery approach that can keep involuntary or coercive approaches from becoming police interventions. Recovery within such interventions involves coping with external limitations while developing one's capabilities and the involuntary intervention as a challenge to be met and overcome.[16] For this argument to be most successful, I think, it should include attention to *entry, process*, and *exit* in regard to involuntary interventions, whether of conservatorship, money management, or outpatient commitment to mental health treatment, including coerced medication. These processes, it seems to me, to apply to work with people living under these bounded conditions whether or not you disagree with the use of one or more of the particular constraints in question.

Entry involves inclusion in the decision-making process of the person whose autonomy may be restricted, and a commitment to reasoning with, and listening to her counter-reasoning. If the process is honest—"We think you need someone else to handle your money for you right now, and we want to tell you why, and let you have your say, too" the person may at least feel that she *has* had a say, even if she lost the argument, or at the very least that she was forewarned. This, by the way, is not to suggest that such a process never happens now between clients and clinicians, psychiatrists, or others.

The client's feelings and thoughts about *entry* may be affected by advance discussion of *process* and *exit* during the entry stage as well as later on. Using money management of some form as the example, *process* includes training in handling her own finances that could be provided to the person during the involuntary intervention. *Exit* is the plan, discussed initially during the entry process and revised as needed during the intervention, for her "release," or staged release, from the intervention. Here I should note that a limiting factor in financial education under money management or representative payeeship is funding for money managers or representative payees to provide such extra support to their clients, as well as the training they may need for doing so.

In a qualitative inquiry we conducted as part of Marc's larger study of experimental financial counseling intervention, we found that core recovery themes such as self-direction and responsibility came up spontaneously and without interviewer prompts in client discussions of money management. Money management interventions, we came to think, should incorporate people's recovery-related motivations to acquire financial management skills as a means of eventually taking back responsibility for their finances, and money management staff should be trained to support their clients' recovery-related motivations and goals. We also thought the field of social recovery should attend to the issue of money in a way it generally does not at present. Finally, we argued that both money management- and recovery-based approaches should consider the use of asset building approaches such as subsidized savings to help move their clients out of poverty.[17] I don't exclude citizenship from this critique and these recommendations.

The next boost for our attention to money and finances came with the arrival of an anthropologist, Annie Harper, via the private nonprofit foundation associated with the mental health center. Kyle Pedersen, the foundation's director, hired

Annie to conduct an organizational study of the center's finance-related work and programs for clients and make recommendations for improving them. She found that most clients have some form of state or federal income support, that less than half are employed, many are homeless, and some are living in supported housing. Almost all of them struggle to meet basic expenses and spend much of their energy and time on coping strategies. She also found that while the mental health center offers a range of financial services from benefits counseling to direct money management services, there is high demand and limited slots for these programs. Annie's report concluded with a set of recommendations including incorporating discussion of financial matters into clinical care. This is a controversial topic, since some clinicians feel that money can poison clinical work and is best attended to elsewhere. She also proposed financial education services for clients with follow-up for opening bank accounts, consolidating or eliminating debt, and saving money.[18]

Annie then delved into the research and scholarly literature on financial health on the interconnections between poverty and mental illness.[19] There is disagreement on whether or not the cause of this interconnection is that people with mental illnesses are more likely to fall into poverty, or that poverty causes or aggravates mental illness such as depression and anxiety[20] and increased symptoms of psychosis and schizophrenia[21] or both. Being poor also appears to be a key factor in persistent physical health problems of people with mental illnesses.[22] Inadequate income my result in a struggle to meet basic needs, falling into debt, or both, and struggles such as these are strongly associated with mental illness.[23,24]

Many people who are poor don't have checking and savings accounts or access to ATMs, credit and debit cards, let alone mortgages, pension plans, stocks and shares, or the financial advisors, accountants, and stockbrokers associated with these.[25] Financial elements that are particularly relevant to mental illness are the in-and-out flow of people's money and the ability to turn financial resources into the resources needed to live. The latter can be called "financial capability," a combination of knowledge and skills and access to tools and services to transform financial resources into access to food, shelter, clothing, transportation, health, and social relationships. People who don't have bank accounts lack the ability to store, save, and get to their money cheaply or build up credit. Often, they have to rely on costly check-cashers, payday loans, and pawnshops.[26–28]

The difficulty some people with mental illnesses have in managing their money may lead their family members, providers of care, or others to take control of their finances, based on a doctor's assessment. People with mental illness who have a payee are less likely than others to be homeless or hospitalized and more likely to reduce their substance use and keep to their treatment plans, and these things appear to have a positive effect on their mental health.[29] Reliable payees are hard to find, though, and people who do have them may resent their loss of control over their money. In addition, payeeship usually does not include financial education or co-payment of bills to support people in developing financial skills that can lead to their reclaiming control over their money.[30]

A few programs to help people with mental illnesses improve their financial capability and build assets have shown some promising results for increasing their financial security, well-being, and overall functioning,[31-33] but the mental health field is only beginning to incorporate financial health approaches, including those from the fields of microfinance and asset building. One lesson learned from these fields is that financial supports and education need to be timely and connected with next steps, such as access to the financial tools and services that foster sustained financial capabilities.[34] Another is that asset building is unlikely to succeed unless basic income security is already in place.[35] Then, too, financial skills and capabilities tend to be more effective when they're part of people's efforts to build stronger social networks and achieve socially valued roles.[36]

Annie gathered information on financial tools and services in the New Haven area, including mainstream bank services, nonbank financial services such as check-cashers, non–financial institutions such as rent-a-centers or layaway options, unofficial lenders, nonprofit services such as financial literacy classes, financial counseling, tax preparation services, and savings support such as individual development accounts. She also made contacts nationally to connect the mental health center to new developments in the growing field of "financial health." After joining the *Citizens Collaborative,* she led a research project involving focus groups on money and finances with clients and clinicians at the mental health center, to gain a better understanding of what supports will help people do better with what money they have, and move toward having more of it.

We conducted six focus groups with a total of 39 clients who reported having money problems, being in debt, or having trouble opening a bank account. Of those who provided the information, more than 80% had incomes of less $1,000 a month and more than two-thirds received SSI or SSDI. Just under half said that they were never able to save money, and just under half again reported being in debt or in arrears on bills. Half had bank accounts and fourth had a payee or a similar arrangements for another's control of their finances.

Focus group questions for clients were:

How do you manage your money now, and how does that work for you?
Are there parts of dealing with your money that are easier or harder for you?
Are there people you talk to about your finances?
What do you think would help you to manage your money better?

We also conducted five focus groups with a total of 55 clinicians and other direct care staff. Focus group questions for them were:

Do clients bring up problems related to their finances?
What are the most common financial problems you hear about?
Are you able to effectively respond when your clients bring up these issues? [If "yes,"] what resources are available to you for this?

*Do you have any suggestions as to what other resources might be useful to help
your clients with these issues?*

We encouraged clients and clinicians to bring up whatever else came to mind on
the topic.

We had the focus groups transcribed. Several of us read and coded them, then
met and came to consensus on themes. I'll briefly review five here based on Annie's
summary of them: the intensity of poverty, coping strategies, mental health, poverty and stigma, seeking formal help and using formal financial services, and disincentives to work.

THE INTENSITY OF POVERTY

Poverty has many faces for clients. They include stretching your money to get
through the month, inability to afford anything other than bare essentials, and the
pain of any additional expenses that might come along. Here are comments from
two clients:

> *I take care of a family of six . . . I can't even afford toilet paper. By the time we pay
> the bills we don't have anything. It's hard.*
>
> *The co-pays and the over-the-counter things like vitamins, antioxidants, vita-
> min D, calcium, that I have to get and can't afford all the time, so I have gaps
> where I can't take [buy] them.*

Even clients who work make low wages and struggle financially. "I have two
part-time jobs and I still can't pay the rent," said one. Some had creditors for child
support or student loans. Many had their wages garnished. The first speaker in the
following comments on his reluctance to work for this reason; the second on struggling to make payments on her student loans:

> *I owe so much child support that if I work they'll take 30%. I'll be lucky if
> I get $2 an hour. By the time I'm done, I'm going to have worked 40 hours a
> week for $75.*
>
> *[With accrued interest, my student debt has] gone up from $2,300 to over $6,000.
> They harass me all the time to pay . . . I used to be in deferment because I didn't
> make enough money to pay them, but now that I'm working I'm worried they'll
> tax my check.*

Clinicians talked about how poverty affects their clients' states of mind, limiting the
types of relationships they are able to develop or their ability to seek work:

> *[My client] says to me, "How can I even think about going out on a date when I
> don't own a car or can't afford a taxi? Who will want to date me?"*
>
> *[My client's] eager to look for work, but she can't come up with the $10 to
> sign up for a clothing closet [store] where she can get interview and work clothes.*

They also talked about their clients' vulnerability to "deals" such as cable TV that is free for three months and then costs a bundle, or rent-a-centers that sell furniture and electronics for low monthly payments but for an overall high total price.

Since most clients don't have cars, they shop at corner stores where the food is unhealthy and expensive. And utility bills are a constant burden for many:

> *[My client] had her utilities cut off. When she got them put back on she had a light bill of $2,300 and gas bill of $1,800. She gets $629 a month, pays $30 for rent, then there's phone, light, gas, insurance, cell phone...She has food stamps. She supplements them with one bag of food a month from food pantries.*

COPING STRATEGIES

People are resourceful in navigating the world of poverty. They have careful and precise shopping strategies and do cost-benefit analyses of various financial decisions. "We go grocery shopping with a list, coupons, a budget, and we only get stuff on special," said one. "We stick to our plan." The first speaker in the following spoke of her budgeting principles, and the second about avoiding impulse spending and other bad financial decisions:

> *You need to make a budget to suit your lifestyle, what you want to buy—write it all down. It doesn't matter how much money you make, you just have to live within your means.*

> *When you see something that you want and you don't have the money for it, drugs or anything, it is self-discipline, you say to yourself..."I'm not gonna get this...I'll wait till next month," or "I can't get it because I'm an alcoholic or an addict."*

People also depend on food stamps and food pantries. Sometimes they exchange food stamps for cash to gain more flexibility in what they buy and where they buy it, especially when they don't have any money to supplement the food stamps. And there are opportunities in the informal economy—collecting and cashing in redeemable bottles and cans, rolling cigarettes to sell, selling your body...Many people spoke of the importance of family, friends, and others for financial help. Some of these arrangements worked well for people, and some not so well. Here are two examples:

> *I would borrow money from [my friend] all the time, $200 to $300 at a time. I would pay her back. She gave me advice to put aside $10 every month.*

> *I usually get loans from people downstairs from where I live. But I have to pay them more or they want me to do some hard work for them. If I go to the grocery store for them they will give me a dollar to bring all their stuff in. [And] he usually wants $5 to $10 extra [for each loan].*

Some people don't pay their utility bills, vacating the premises before their utilities are shut off or when they are about to be evicted for nonpayment of rent, or closing a utility account unpaid and opening a new one under their children or other relatives' names. Clinicians are well aware of their clients' poverty, and their means of coping with it. They frequently expressed admiration at people's resourcefulness. "I'm constantly amazed at how [our clients] live on so little money," said one. "I don't know how they do it." She continued:

> *It requires vast amounts of energy and effort for these folks to get their check, make sure it's safe, and even the folks that have conservators and arrange to get the money from the conservator and they spend, oh my gosh, hours and hours calling up the conservator's office for more money ... people have so little and so much of their time is really spent trying to secure the money and then figure out how best to use it. And I think because we do have a lot of substance abusers it's often like just more money, you know, they just want more money.*

MENTAL HEALTH, POVERTY, AND STIGMA

People run out of money, sometimes for simply lacking enough of it, sometimes because of cognitive problems or being taken advantage of, and sometimes because of struggles with impulse control or addiction. Addiction is the worst, clients and clinicians agree, especially when people get a lump sum of money:

> *It's the nightlife, going out, booze. I like to drink. There goes a lot of my money. If I cut out my three vices—smoking, drinking and gambling—I would probably have two or three hundred dollars a month. I am a risk taker. How do I cut this out? I do all this stuff when I get paid and by the third day I'm broke. I'm suffering for the rest of the month.*

Others spend the money early in the month on what seem to be frivolous purchases so that they don't have cash on hand to buy drugs. A clinician said of one of her clients:

> *Money is a trigger. It triggers her impulses. When she gets it ... she spends it right away so that she isn't tempted to use it on drugs. But more times than not she ends up relapsing [anyway].*

Often, though, difficulties with budgeting are related more generally to poverty and appear to have little to do with mental illness. Some clinicians see part of the problem as having to do with the fact that, poor or not and mentally ill or not on top of that, their clients—marginalized, stigmatized, rejected—are still members of our consumer society. One said:

> *I have a client who is really concerned with what it means to be a poor person in the world, and how people interact with her as a poor person. Clients want the same things that we do.*

Client focus group participants talked about wanting to feel like normal people by buying what they *want*, not just what they *need*:

You are suffering for three weeks because you had no money and then you get new money so you spend it to get yourself some joy."

When the paycheck comes in at the beginning of the month, the first thing I do is get a latte for $6, and then sometimes I get another one...I may be poor, but I can have one meal a month...like oysters, or I might buy a steak to cook at home.

Added to these desires to have a little luxury in their lives is the fact that many suspect things will never change for them, so why not splurge now and then?

An individual interview with a client who handles her finances well, paying her utilities and rent at the beginning of the month then dealing with everything else, deserves an extended look on the topics of coping with finances and on what constitutes a necessity, what a luxury. Kathy is 53 years old. She worked at one time and is thinking about part-time work, the most she can manage physically while also keeping within the income limits for SSI, which she receives due to her psychiatric disability and a stroke she had 11 years ago. Kathy also has bad arthritis. She lives in an apartment with a partner who does odd jobs now and then but otherwise is unemployed. She has three children and four grandchildren.

Kathy rescues dogs from being put down:

Money, there's just not enough of it. Just trying to balance everything...[After paying her utilities and rent:] And also my dogs get their food. I get a big bag of it. And Booger, my 7-year-old, he is on medication that costs me 100 bucks a month for his hip dysplasia, arthritis. So that comes right off the top, their care...I had vetting [taking a dog to the vet] last month. It was $200 just for blood work. I had to have his yearly exam, his blood work 'cause he's on these anti-inflammatories that can cause damage to the kidneys...The struggle is just, I don't make enough [and] so I've had to accept that I just can't work full time...There's just not enough. There's just not enough money...I was on a money management program at one time, and she said to me, "You don't have enough coming in for what you've got going on." Some people would say that having my animals is a luxury and I should get rid of them, or not that they would say that to me 'cause I would clock them...But the payoff that I get from it, it takes care of my mental and physical health. You can't put a price on that...[And then] the unexpected, like one time one got sick and they had to do an x-ray. His stomach had bloat and he couldn't move. So we took him to the emergency vet. That's 65 bucks to walk in the door. And then the x-ray is another 200 bucks. And then it's like okay, so now I'm short on...but it's a life. You can't...it's like, "All right, I'll sit in the dark. I'm not going to let a life suffer."...And now my computer is on the way out. My friends live in it, you know what I mean? 'Cause I do connections, so talking to people online or just kind of checking in...

And I do Facebook too. But it's an animal rescue thing and that's part of my community and my connection and what makes me feel good...don't go to movies and stuff like that, or vacations obviously...Also, too, I think even if you are struggling, you still have to do something nice for yourself. When I was working and getting regular paychecks, every Friday I would get myself a bouquet of grocery store flowers...for the table. And then you see that and you're like, "OK, I would work for those. I deserve something."...Or when the weather's warm I'll buy some flowers for in the yard or something like that...It could be a dollar store thing, but you need to treat yourself, too. And not feel guilty about it. But it's a tricky thing. It's a real fine line. But, you know what? My spirit needed it.

I've talked to people who are homeless who have to take their dog to the vet, and have had a quick, gut-level impulse to say, "You've got nothing for yourself, how can you take care of a dog?" But I've reconsidered, understanding what that connection means to them. Having nothing but a little love is not a justification for giving up the love, even if it costs money you don't have, and maybe means sitting in the dark.

SEEKING FORMAL HELP AND USING FORMAL FINANCIAL SERVICES

Some clinicians and other direct care staff offer ad hoc financial advice to their clients, but formal support is limited to conservator or representative payee mechanisms and only a small percentage of mental health center clients can have either of these at any given time. Some of those who do are happy with the arrangement. Here's a man who was:

About eight years ago I used to mess with drugs. They put me on a [limited allowance]. It was smart for them to do this, for them and for me...If I didn't have [a conservator] I would spend my check on the first day. I am happy with the way it is...If I don't get the money, I don't use drugs and I don't relapse.

Others, though, see control of their finances as an intolerable constraint on their autonomy and recovery. Many among this group understand why it happened to them, but that doesn't change their feeling disempowered and of being made to feel like less than a full-fledged adult:

With a conservator you really don't know what is going on with your money. I don't want to sit and argue with someone about my own money...It's like getting an allowance from your parents.

I understand trying to stop people from buying drugs and how that might be useful, but at the same time, I don't want anybody telling me what to do with my money.

As for the logistics of managing their money, some people operate only in cash, but most use some form of financial service such as a banking account, check-casher, or prepaid cards. The last allow people who don't have bank accounts to avoid using cash or overdrawing a checking account. This strategy is paid for, though, in high transaction fees. Many people can't open bank accounts due to having burned out too many banks or having been hit by with high overdraft fees, or don't open them in the first place for fear their creditors will garnish their accounts. But the downside of not having a bank account is the cost of cashing checks. Here's a clinician:

> *I had a client who got a $30 return from a co-pay, and Bank of America wanted to charge her $6 to cash it. Some people just say ok. They want the cash and can't get to another place. I had a client who paid $19 to have his SSI check cashed.*

Of those with bank accounts, some are happy with their services and tell stories of sympathetic and friendly bank tellers. Even many of these people, though, wish they had a place to put their money out of temptation's way:

> *I'd like an account where I would have to physically go to the bank to take the money out, something that I don't have direct access to but that I'm still in control of. That way I can't make so many immediate purchases. Online banking makes it harder for me to save money 'cause I just transfer money from savings to checking when I need it. It's so easy to find an excuse to move money. I wish I could put it in gold and just bury it.*

DISINCENTIVES TO WORK

The real and perceived disincentives to working embedded in the benefits system were a theme across all the focus groups. Both clients and clinicians spoke of the difficulty that people with mental illness face in procuring benefits, with lengthy and complicated application forms and corroboration of disabling illness from many different mental health providers. It's not uncommon for a first application to be denied. When this happens, people need to have the wherewithal to appeal the denial or reapply. Not surprisingly, those who succeed are reluctant to risk losing their benefits. People can work without losing benefits as long as they remain below a certain income cap, but information on such policies isn't widely available or well communicated, and fear of losing what you've got, along with a healthy mistrust of a complicated bureaucratic system, is a powerful disincentive to making any changes in your finances or health care benefits. It's better to stay where you are. The limited security that disability benefits provide may be preferable to trying, and maybe failing, to make it in the workforce.

Fear of losing benefits is often fueled by the asset limits imposed by the benefits system, which include bank account balances. This often discourages people from saving money and can lead them to spend it in ways that may appear irresponsible. Recipients also have to adhere to periodic redeterminations. Exceeding asset limits can lead their losing cash benefits or having a "spend-down" amount imposed on their medical benefits. And these can lead to disruptions in people's health care. Here's an example from one client:

> *I got my regular check from Social Security, and then they told me that unless I spent my money and kept my bank account under $2,000, they were going to*

> *take it away. [They] said to take it out of the bank and keep it at home. I live in a sober home. Yeah, right, I'm going to stuff $11,000 under my mattress? I had to go spend it. Then if I have an emergency I don't have any money saved up. They want you to blow all your money.*

That amount of money is unusual, but it may represent a back payment from a long application process for this person since benefits, once approved, are calculated from the original application date.

Both clients and clinicians were asked about supports that might help people become more financially capable and secure. Many in both groups said that as long as clients are afraid of losing their benefits they will be reluctant to take other steps that might help them become more financially secure. Incentives and protections exist, but it's hard to master the knowledge of them, and people don't trust that they'll work. Some clients talked about help they got from family members. Most were ambivalent about this kind of help, though. For some, it was humiliating, made them feel like children all over again.

Most clients wanted financial advice and education on budgeting and saving money rather than having it managed by someone else:

> *I feel the best way is to teach us to be as independent as possible. Giving you an allowance is not teaching you anything. Get someone to counsel you, help you work with a budget.*

Clinicians suggested that peer staff could be a valuable resource for one-on-one counseling with clients. Said one:

> *Finances are a sensitive topic, stressful. It might be easier to talk with someone who has been through the same situation themselves and who can recommend agencies that are helpful. It can be such an anxiety-provoking experience to talk about money. It can help to talk about it with someone who has been there.*

Clinicians are well aware of the poverty their clients endure. Many spoke of trying to help them with their finances, but whether they did or not, most also thought money and therapy should be kept separate. Both clients and clinicians also talked about the idea of community banks that would offer low- or no-fee accounts for clients, and the possibility of an on-site bank at the mental health center.

FINANCIAL HEALTH AND CITIZENSHIP

But why so much time on money in a book on citizenship? Consider three related themes that came out of this study. First, most problems that people have with money seem to be more connected to their poverty than to their mental illnesses. Some clients, particularly those with substance abuse problems, regularly spend to the point that they quickly run out of money, but even clients without such problems find it hard to get through the month. Many have so little money that they simply can't do that, or not legally. Others get by mathematically, but doing so month after month weighs heavy on the soul.

Second, many if not most of the clients we talked to work diligently and creatively to manage the little money they have. And third, they engage in these prodigious efforts in the context of the lack of meaningful choice on how to spend their money beyond bare survival, often with no hope that things will ever change or that they will have a chance to achieve their aspirations. They continue to invest vast amounts of energy into strategies to get by with very little, finding other sources of income, formal and informal, legal and illegal, when they can, planning carefully and practicing self-discipline, all in the midst of cultural norms of work, managing income to meet one's needs, and achieving one's dreams and goals based on self-sufficiency and hard work, the departure from which norm adds further stigma to that which they already face as people with mental illnesses And note that the other side of the coin of all this planning and self-discipline is, for people who are better off, the ability to splurge once in a while and still get through the month.

Following this study, Annie took the lead on a proposal for an intervention to develop and evaluate financial services and supports to help mental health center clients gain more secure incomes and use their money more effectively, even to build financial assets, little by little. Greater financial security, we argued, would make it possible for them to engage in more activities in their communities, and community participation would, in turn, support their financial health. Services would include training for direct-care staff in financial health principles and practices, peer-based support and counseling, incentive-based savings programs, favorable bank account arrangements, training from New Haven financial institutions, and integration of financial health with principles of citizenship and recovery.

The notion of citizenship-oriented care started with the gamble that putting a considerable amount of our energy, time, and resources into linking citizenship to clinical care would round out the citizenship approach after 15 or so years of operating pretty much independently of it. This notion, and what has come of it to this point, is the topic of the next chapter.

8

Taking Citizenship to Scale

THE *CITIZENS COLLABORATIVE* III

We started with three working principles for our work to arrive at citizenship-oriented care. First, we would not simply build on the *Citizens Project* as the most obvious and extensive example we had to go by and the one for which we had evidence to support its effectiveness. The *Citizens Project* was *the* example we had of a citizenship intervention, but that project took place outside the mental health center and, in part, drew its character from that fact. It also involved participants who, in addition to having mental illnesses, had criminal charges, which, we decided, would not be an inclusion criteria for the pilot projects we were looking to start at the mental health center, albeit not an exclusion criteria, either.

The *Citizens Project* would be one, no doubt the most important, source of information and example, then, but not the only one. Others would be our measure development research process and the measure itself as a potential treatment planning and tool. Others still would be our current projects of action, study, and learning including voter registration, *Project Connect* and other community outreach work, financial health study and the *Citizens Collaborative* itself as a reflexive speech community and planning group. We would also have the focus groups we conducted with clinical teams, individual interviews with clients and clinicians, and our "citizenship lunches."

The second of our three working principles was that citizenship-oriented care would be centered in individual treatment teams. This meant that while most of the attention and time given to specifically citizenship-related, as opposed to more purely clinically related issues, might largely be the province of peer staff and case managers, citizenship-oriented care would have to be a shared concept and set of values on the treatment teams that piloted it. The third principle, complementing the second, was that building strong connections to community resources and opportunities was an essential part of citizenship-oriented care and that our community work and resources must be linked directly to clinical care, not simply be available to clinical teams as "another resource out there." With this, it occurred to us that, on the basis of the joint community outreach and clinical components we were putting in place, the *Citizens Collaborative* had the potential to link the two main paths to citizenship for people with mental illness—the community's responsibility to offer it, as with *Citizens*, and individual support for "making it," as with the *Citizens Project*—that we had originally conceived of as the two main paths to full citizenship for people living at the margins of society.

Citizenship-Oriented Care Focus Groups

With a 12-item version of our measure of citizenship in hand for use in settings where all 46 items would be unwieldy and time consuming, we conducted seven focus groups with a total of more than 90 clinicians and team psychiatrists, case managers, peer staff, and rehabilitation specialists. After giving participants a brief explanation of the citizenship framework and our interest in adapting it for use on clinical teams, we handed out copies of the instrument, which read like this:

> *Thinking about your life in general right now, please read each statement and rate it on a scale of 1 to 5, from 1 for "not at all/never" to 5 for "a lot/all the time," or in-between for "sometimes," depending on how much you feel the statement applies to you:*

1. You have responsibilities to others.
2. You have knowledge about your community (e.g., knowledge about current events, policies, services, social events, and so on).
3. Your personal choices are respected.
4. You have or would have access to jobs.
5. You are connected to others.
6. You are a part of something greater than yourself.
7. You have the freedom of worship.
8. You have the right to protect yourself and others.
9. You have been or would be given second chances.
10. You take care of family, friends, children, or pets.
11. You are free from discrimination.
12. You feel safe in your community.

When everyone had read the statements, we asked them what they thought of them and whether or not the items were relevant to their clinical work with clients. Discussion was lively. "Clinicians" in the following refers to all direct care staff who participated in the focus groups.[1]

SUMMARY OF THEMES

A dual theme, most markedly on one treatment team, was the tension between clinicians' desire to make the measure accessible to clients and their tendency to underestimate clients' abilities to comprehend and respond to the items on the brief measure. Clinicians noted that many of the items were not concrete. Some saw this as making the instrument irrelevant to their clients, especially those with limited cognitive abilities or symptoms that disrupted their capacity for abstract reflection:

> *I am thinking about the schizophrenic population or persons who have problems with cognition and limited education. You would exclude [those] people from being able to respond.*

Clinicians in one focus group made suggestions for rephrasing some items to make them more accessible to their clients. None, however, noted the irony that it was people with mental illnesses, recruited largely from the mental health center, who helped to generate the items that they thought their clients wouldn't understand. This caveat does not necessarily negate the point about the abstraction that some noted about some of the items, since an item called out in a focus group might look and read differently on the page and in another format. But it should give one pause.

There was a general sense among clinicians that the domains captured the challenges that clients faced. They agreed with the importance of connectedness and social inclusion. Said one:

> *That's pretty intrinsic. You could probably throw out many of these and ask that one question about being connected to others.*

Clinicians said their clients' social connectedness often came in unexpected forms, from the solidarity of people living in a homeless encampment in town to the fidelity of immigrants, legal and not, keeping in close contact with their families living abroad. Addiction, clinicians said, interfered with many of their clients' social connectedness. Another was avoiding public places and encounters because of the stigma attached to mental illness.

Clinicians like the idea of a "second chance," but often saw it as an illusory thing for their clients, given the larger community's resistance to offering it. Having a felony conviction, they said, made finding a job, hard enough for anyone given the state of the economy at the time, far more difficult. Having been evicted from housing in the past made finding scarce housing even more of a challenge. The sort of discrimination that clinicians found most relevant to their clients' lives, clinicians said, didn't involve people's attitudes about their psychiatric symptoms, but potential employers' or property owners' wariness due to lack of tenure in jobs and housing.

Some clinicians thought their ability to promote their clients' citizenship was limited, especially for the most seriously disabled and disadvantaged among them. They talked about a tension between helping them meet their basic needs and promoting their overall psychological and social well-being. Many seemed to regard these goals as separate concerns. At least one clinician, though, suggested that helping clients meet their basic needs might put them on the path of achieving personal and social well-being. Most were frustrated that so many of the barriers their clients faced were "beyond the scope of the clinician and the patient." Community attitudes, stark poverty, and the limitations of mental health care assured that this was, and would be, so. "These are big political issues," said one.

Clinicians said some of their clients became too comfortable in the mental health system. They wanted to empower and teach them to advocate for themselves, but knew that social structures and the general public rarely supported such efforts. What were people going be empowered *for*, given the social, psychological, and economic challenges they faced? Even when client goals were relevant to some of the times covered in the brief instrument, and vice versa, some clinicians worried that including them in treatment plans might raise people's hopes now only to dash them later. One clinician of the brief instrument:

> *It's pretty broad and encompasses a lot . . . It looks like it would need a team working on this together. It's impossible for one person to do.*

This is exactly right.

Safety was a prominent theme. Clinicians said it was difficult for their clients to feel as though they were part of something bigger or spend their time giving back to others when they didn't feel safe in their own neighborhoods. For people with histories of trauma, lack of a sense of safety in their homes and neighborhoods, likely fueled and exacerbated at the outset by trauma, struck again the chord of those experiences, re-traumatizing them. And in any case, what does it mean to be a full member of one's community when that community is fragmented by poverty, substance abuse, and violence? In the aftermath of the school shootings in Newtown, clinicians also reported that their clients were wary of being identified as having a mental illness and being targeted as a threat to the public. This, in turn, put them in an untenable position in their neighborhoods, where they feared that, if they ever had to defend themselves, they would be seen as the aggressor because of their psychiatric histories. All of these concerns and others seemed to lead clinicians to feel, sometimes, as though they were simply "trying to keep people alive." This rendered dim their view of the prospects of offering meaningful support to their clients' efforts to master the 5 Rs of citizenship.

A few clinicians noted that treatment planning already incorporated some of the items in the brief measure. Others, though, said the measure highlighted elements of their clients' lives that were overlooked in most clinical work:

> *[The measure] hits on dimensions we don't usually explore. Like being treated with dignity and respect.*

The emphasis in the brief instrument on responsibilities and caring for others resonated strongly with them. They agreed that "the people that tend to do the best are the people who have found a way to give back." They also acknowledged that this truth could be more fully incorporated into their work:

I try and talk a lot with my clients about how they're making a difference [and]
giving back. Having it right here makes you think about it because you don't do
it with everyone.

Being "a part of something greater than yourself" was another item that surprised
some clinicians. Most responded positively to the idea, although many were skepti-
cal about their clients' ability to achieve such a lofty goal.

Clinicians distinguished the citizenship model readily from a recovery-based
framework. Citizenship was something with which anyone could identify, regardless of whether or not they saw themselves as being in recovery from mental illness
or addiction. "You can not want to be 'in recovery' and still want to be a citizen,"
said one. Despite the recovery model's emphasis on personal empowerment, citizenship seemed to some to capture more of a subjective sense of being treated with
dignity and respect than current person-centered treatment plans.

Clinicians talked about the importance of work for their clients, and the barriers they faced in trying to get any. Then again, not all jobs that were available to
clients were necessarily worth the taking, they said. "Sometimes working isn't the
best if you do a menial job," observed one. "It has to be something they value."
Only about 10% of clients at the mental health center are working. Often the jobs
that people do find pay little and have no prestige. The role of worker is far from
an equally valued role across a continuum from low-skilled and poorly paid to
highly-skilled and well paid. Clients may feel more stigmatized in a low prestige job
that has no connection with their interests, strengths, or talents, some clinicians felt,
than when they're not working at all. Clients are also concerned about how much
they can work and still maintain their benefits. Finally, as one clinician noted, some
clients saw work as falling outside the scope of individual therapy and impinging
on other uses they had for their sessions:

I had a client talk about voices and nightmares and not sleeping. "And oh, by the
way, I have a job interview later this week!" And that was helping her get through.

Clinicians talked about their own frustration of balancing their clients' needs
and interests with their own therapeutic goals as clinicians, along with administrative requirements and psychiatric assessments, all to take place in a 30- to 60-minute
session. They were especially concerned about their responsibility to assess their
clients' potential for harming themselves or others. How could they encourage their
clients to take more risks and reach out to people outside the mental health system when they, the clinicians, feared that doing so might exacerbate their clients'
symptoms and put them at risk of a psychiatric crisis? They talked about feeling
responsible when something "goes wrong" with a client, even when that person's
actions or setback falls outside of any what a clinician can be expected to be able
to predict based a brief risk assessment as part of each session. Thus there seemed
to be a sort of vicious circle of risk assessment that cut into any sustained focus
on clients' citizenship, and lack of citizenship work that, in its absence, tended to

highlight clients' fragility and need for risk assessment. Risk assessment was necessary and required in any case but was always imperfect, suggesting the need for a more extensive risk assessment.

One clinician commented on how the system of care encouraged and ensured such fears:

> *There are plenty of people without mental illness who make terrible decisions and destroy their lives. But somehow, when they're in this system it becomes different.*

Unfortunately, concern over risk to clients could keep clients stuck in another way, through the sedating effect of medication that might decrease their risk of a psychiatric crisis at the price of sapping any energy they might have for engaging in social activities. The system of care, then, including institutional accreditation and professional standards, narrows the discretion that clinicians can exercise. It also narrows the choices of people receiving mental health care, which can become, in effect, a school for educating clients about their lack of choice and diminished horizons.

Choice, as one clinician observed implicitly, is latent as well as active. It involves the knowledge that you can do a certain thing even if you chose not to:

> *I overheard a conversation the other day about someone who hadn't been out to eat for nine years. And it just made me think. I don't even like eating out, but I have the choice.*

This comment about lack of choice refers to clients' poverty, but it can also stand as a formula for the production of ever-narrowing psychological and practical choice for clients in which clinicians feel complicit. Such insights as these from the focus groups, with some interpretation here, risk giving short shrift distorting to the good that care can do. Yet they offer a portrait of a clinical staff that is aware of the limitations of its work, and, for most of its members, looking for ways to break out of it for, and with, their clients.

We conducted a focus group with a treatment team that worked with people in housing programs run by local nonprofit agencies, expecting that it might be a prime candidate for piloting citizenship-oriented treatment. This, of all teams at the mental health center, we thought, would have a natural connection to community and social inclusion, and to citizenship. It might be too easy for a pilot, though! In fact, although the clinicians and housing specialists on the team were interested in and supportive of the citizenship approach, housing agency program rules such as no smoking, no drinking, no living with partners, and others, restricted choice in important ways. One response to such a concern might be that our most significant and long-term citizenship intervention involved groups of people who were mostly still on probation, and thus working on their citizenship under conditions of significant constraint. So why not with people living under residential constraints?[2] The idea of pursuing greater autonomy in the context of restrictions on choice has come up before in this book. Still, the question of whether or not the residential teams were *of* the community as well as *in* it made piloting a citizenship intervention on the housing team loom, prospectively, as a challenging enterprise.

Clinicians both posed problems and were resources for our plan to develop citizenship-oriented mental health care. The problems they posed involved, for some, a sense of powerlessness to change things for their clients, and their under-estimation of their clients' potential to achieve full community membership and social inclusion. Some, assessing the citizenship goals and preferences reflected in the brief version of the citizenship measure, reverted to the example of their most severely disabled clients to suggest the naiveté of the citizenship idea. The resources they offered were, for many, their deeply held wishes and hopes for better lives for their clients. They were resources, too, in their overall interest in and support for the citizenship approach, and a modest arsenal of citizenship-supportive services they could draw upon. We had little feeling, in conducting the focus groups, of a "Here comes another researcher trying to make his bones off our backs" sentiment among clinicians. Instead, they gave us an honest and bracing look at their street-level work. Those few who seemed to be constructing a barricade against our intrusion with the examples of their most citizenship-defying clients did us a favor, in a way. There's something to evaluating your idea or intervention, in part, by who it threatens to send to the back of the bus. What level of citizenship, after all, should people be required to achieve in a democratic society? Should it not be their own level, and not that which their helpers or researchers would like to see them achieve?

Client and Clinician Interviews

We had planned to interview clients and clinicians in general at the outset. Given our *Collaborative* discussions, however, about taking a positive approach to citizenship work that, presumably, was already happening at the mental health center, we decided to ask for nominations of clients who were making citizenship progress and of clinicians who supported their clients' citizenship goals. We distributed flyers and forms for both. Both clients and clinicians could nominate in each category.

For clients, we asked for nominations of those whom the nominator saw as meeting three criteria from a list that included items such as showing a sense of responsibility toward others, having a connection to others in the community, knowing about events, activities, or issues going on in New Haven, supporting and encouraging others, knowing about their rights and pursuing personal goals even in the face of stigma and discrimination, and managing their finances well in spite of having a low income. For clinicians, nomination criteria included helping clients connect with community resources, working with them to meet their community-related goals, educating them about their rights, supporting them in taking on more responsibilities such as work, caring for friends, and others, and helping them deal with their finances. Nominators for both categories were a mix of clients and clinicians.

The interviews with clients were similar to those with *Citizens Project* clients, with questions about the 5 Rs, including those both present or missing and both welcome or unwelcome in their lives; their current and future goals; and what they regarded their community to be. Interviews with clinicians were similar to those with clients except that, in addition to asking about the 5 Rs and community in their own lives, we asked them to talk about the 5 Rs and community prospects of their clients.

CLIENT INTERVIEWS

Of the first several client interviews we've conducted, I'll profile two. Bill is 48 years old, African American, and as one would hope from the nomination process, quite involved with community activities, including advocacy. He has been homeless and has a history of drug addition and treatment. He lives with his sister, who helps him handle his disability income, but hopes to move into his own HUD-subsidized apartment at some point. Kathy, who spoke in the last chapter about money and taking care of her dogs, is 53 years old, white, and was a student of both the *Citizens Project* and the *Leadership Project*. She has been in prison twice for drug-related offenses. She had a stroke 11 years ago and receives visiting nurse help at home. Bill and Kathy, especially Bill, are perhaps more engaged in advocacy-related activities than most, although not all, members of the larger group of clients interviewed. Yet both also have long histories of serious psychiatric disorders and substance use and both receive disability income.

Bill

Bill is tall, a bit overweight. Given his looks and his advocacy experience you might expect a bigger or deeper voice. His is soft, but he has a presence that makes you want to filter out extraneous sounds to hear him better, rather than ask him to speak up.[3] With Bill, roles, resources, relationships, and community seem to mix and meld with each other, and advocacy seems to be his defining role and most prominent social activity:

> *Nowadays I'm more into advocating, helping out in the community ... And myself, I love helping people, especially in the community ... I love to get into politics to better a neighborhood ... I like helping others who have mental illness, to let them know that it's not over because we have mental illness.*

Bill's advocacy experience and sense of mission to help others with mental illnesses have roots in his own hard times, including years of homelessness and drug use. This stretch of his life started after his mother threw him out for coming home drunk, then getting into cocaine, and then into crack. He ended up in New York at one point:

> *I was homeless [and] someone helped me up ... This was a guy at this homeless shelter called the Redeemer in New York. It was a Christian shelter ... [This guy]*

encouraged me. "You don't have to be homeless. You know there's hope for you."
And he encouraged me that "You don't have to live like this, you can get back on
your feet. You can go back to school. You can be whoever you want to be, but you
got to want to change your life."

The theme of a moment when someone, who comes to be seen as a role model, mentor, or messenger, offers or says something to you at the right time and in the right place, appears across several interviews with clients. The lesson can hit home before you are ready to act on it, though. Bill came back to Connecticut, but he was still using:

I hit rock bottom where I was outside and my mom got in her car and she came
out where I was at, this abandoned building and asked me, do I want to go home?
I said, yeah. I said, listen, I'm tired, I want to go home. I'm tired of living out here
like this, going from soup kitchen to soup kitchen, wearing my same clothes for
five days, and beard growing, and I wasn't taking care of my eyesight...

Bill's experience with role models long preceded his encounter with the counselor at the *Redeemer* in New York City. It went back to his early childhood, and to his mother again:

My mother taught me how to help people. She told me, "You treat people the way
they want to be treated." You know my thing is, you see somebody hungry, help
them, feed them, encourage them to better themselves... And my mother raised
six children all by herself and she taught us well how to help people, be there for
people.

The theme of educating himself about others' experience by observing and talking to them and then taking action runs strong in Bill's story:

I went to different soup kitchens... to see how people survived... And [you] sit
there and you meet someone—"Hey, how you doing?" And [they say,] "Oh, I'm
okay. I'm blessed. I'm here in the soup kitchen." And I say, "Well, where you go
after you leave here?" And some would say, "Well, I may go to the shelter or
I may sleep outside, you know." And back in '94 I decided to start this group up
among myself and we called ourselves the Homeless Survivors... We slept out-
side for at least a week, just to see how people survived... I went underneath the
bridge just to see where people were staying, how they stayed warm. And just to
see people sleeping underneath the bridges reminded me how I could be if I was
stuck outside.

His role as advocate followed from his education:

My role was to go around and I was enrolling people to sign up for beds. Go to
the evening soup kitchens, to pick up their toiletries, like toothpaste, toilet paper,
vitamins, we were enrolling them to get them checked out for tuberculosis, HIV,
you know, we were like really being the outreach social worker...

The theme of being responsible first and foremost to and for yourself appears in the narratives of those like Bill as well as those far less socially engaged than he. Bill spoke on this:

It's important to me to take care of my health . . . In '04 I came down with diabetes and [it became necessary] for me to go to the doctor, for me to eat right, and for me to take care of my outside, and also to be more responsible for how I spend my money, be more responsible how I take care of my clothing . . . And I even tell people, if you don't take care of [yourself], own up to your responsibility, nobody will. You know what I mean? It was my responsibility to get myself clean and sober. It's my responsibility now to take care of me . . . It's my responsibility to get up every morning, brush my teeth, wash my face . . . And it's my responsibility to survive out here, you know, and I tell people, you don't have to try to do this by yourself. It's your responsibility to get help.

Let me note here that when we talk about the 5 Rs, it's easy to fall into the snare of describing them almost as things, objects, of social life. That is, we can end up reifying the 5 Rs as though people can pick them up at the citizenship store and hang them from their belts. That probably comes from talking about them for too long. This is less of a problem for people like Patty who do the work every day and have constant reminders that the 5 Rs have to stick people deep, come alive inside them, before they can use them well as tools. The oft-used AA and NA adage, "Fake it 'til you make it" would seem to contradict this, but I don't see that adage as meaning that, by acting the part, you will eventually you become the character you are portraying. I see it as meaning that you can act in ways you want or see yourself as needing to without necessarily experiencing, at first or often, a jolt of accomplishment, the high that comes from knowing what you're doing works, and you just nailed it. "Fake it 'til you make it" is an invaluable mnemonic for active and reflective living. Bill, though, seems to have reached a point where heart, will, and action are working together in him:

Just having that desire, the willingness, the open-mindedness and willingness . . . it's all about here in the heart, you know, to work in a community, you've got to have the mind and the heart and the desire to do so. If you don't have that then you can't help nobody . . . Helping a young person, helping an elderly person—"Listen, this ain't the end of the world. We're lost, but we can rise up again." I don't know how many more years I'm gonna be around, but while I'm here I just want to be able to make someone happy, or even just continue helping folks in the community. You know what I mean?

As already noted, Bill's ideas about rights and his advocacy related to them come out of personal experience:

Suffering from mental illness, I was told that I wasn't able to do nothing. And then if I was in a mental health facility, your rights are violated, your rights are being taken away. At the same time I tell people, "You're having to be in a facility, you have the right to make a phone call, you have the right to voice your opinion [about] the way that the place is going, or you're being mistreated."

"What kind of rights did you feel were taken away when you were in a mental health facility?"

My religion rights . . . They would tell me I would have to shorten my praying that I used to do and that's not right, telling me that I have to lower my standards of praying. And I tell anybody, if you happen to be in a facility you have rights to make a phone call . . . But there's a lot of people who don't know their rights, and I'm able to advocate for them and even call protection advocacy to ask them to come down and explain to people about their rights.

Bill has the zeal of an advocate. The community for his advocacy work is "people in recovery, people on boards of directors, people who like to pull together and to sit down and brainstorm something":

That's a community. Working together to come up with some type of plan. My thing is to connect and collaborate with people. Get them the information, getting them the resource. We need to open up more programs and at the same time, educate the community about what's available for them.

Kathy

Kathy's stroke of more than a decade ago wouldn't be obvious from sitting and talking with her if you didn't know. If you did, you might notice a slight drooping of her mouth on the right side and wonder if that really was the shadow of a slur in her voice trailing off at the end of some of her longer sentences, or wonder if you imagined it, knowing about her stroke. You'd be more likely to notice a hanging down slackness of her right arm if she got up to get you some coffee at her apartment.

Kathy's mental health and addiction problems started early:

I was 12. And then back in '87, I had a major bottom. I had gone into prison, came out, went into a program, stayed for like six years. And that's when they discovered that I had depression, but then later on we found out that it's bipolar and PTSD.

Kathy was homeless in the 1990s before she began to turn her life around. It started with a moment reminiscent of Bill's at the *Redeemer*:

There was this one woman. She gave me . . . I had nothing. I was staying in a shelter. I had three kids. [They] were all over the place back and forth with [relatives and others] . . . And she gave me a bus token. And that bus token, to this day, we're talking probably 16 years ago, I still remember the impact that she gave me that, and it was like I had a choice to do something, that I didn't have to stay stuck. It was just really symbolic and that she trusted me with that, that I didn't have to explain what I was going to use it for or anything.

This was a small act of kindness. The importance of such little things for Kathy as the giver now as well as receiver came up several times in her interview and in others of nominated clients. Such small acts and the practical help they bring in moments of dire need become acts of kindness rather than of charity when the giver offers them freely to a fellow human being of equal worth and dignity, not one who must demonstrate by her gratitude and reformed behavior that she was worthy of it.[4]

The homeless outreach team also made contact with Kathy and helped her get into housing and outpatient treatment at the mental health center. "I've had some really, really great women treaters," she said. "I really have to say that I wouldn't be where I am without them because they believed in me when I didn't believe in me, and didn't give up on me." In the early 2000s, Katy was a student in the *Leadership* and then the *Citizens Project*, a peer mentor, and also a member of a student-run project, called the *Citizens Council*, that was a first try at a next-step for students after the *Citizens Project*. The *Council* was to be convened and run by former students and others who would foster their own and others' community inclusion as well as engage in public education and advocacy. The project was a modest success, with strong support from Patty, and no funding available to keep it going after the first year. Still, Kathy remembered it fondly.

For Kathy, as for many other clients we interviewed, family members are her primary relationships. She has three children and four grandchildren, gets along well with all, and helps to take care of the grandchildren. She had to earn back her children's trust after years of homelessness, drugs, and two stints in prison:

> *I'll tell you, when I was homeless my relationship was not good with the kids. Even for a couple years after I cleaned up and everything 'cause they didn't trust me. So it took time.*

"How did you navigate that from having such strained relationships with them?"

> *It just took time. You know, trust. They saw that I was keeping my word. They liked being with me... And they like me... They're proud of me and stuff, and that feels really good.*

Like Bill, Kathy knew she had to take care of herself if she was going to be of any use to others:

> *My biggest responsibility is to myself—I've got to be true to me. My biggest responsibility is to just keep doing what I'm doing. 'Cause somebody else might get help from it, too. And usually, and actually a lot of times they do... Community connections.*

Kathy's community, somewhat like that of Nicholas with his geese but shared with others we've interviewed, includes animals and nature, living things:

> I have a house full of rescue animals...And I love being outside. I like to walk a while, you know, walk the dogs and stuff and go to the park. And I'm really into birding and planting and flowers and that kind of stuff...Being outside, being around nature and doing my birding, just watching them, I just feel really connected, especially the hawks and the birds of prey. Turkey vultures, believe it or not, are spiritual to me. They remove all the junk in a spiritual way. It's like, "Oh, I see a turkey vulture"...I know you mentioned about citizenship. And that's the first word that comes to my mind when I hear that [word citizenship], is "connected."

These passions of Kathy's are not a substitute for human relationships. She has those with her family members, we know. But her love of dogs connects her with other people as well:

> I do have a neighbor that lives up the street whom I've just gotten really friendly with, a young girl and her husband, another dog person. The animal rescue community...Next door they've got a dog...So we do a lot of dog talking. And coincidentally, he and his wife are both in recovery.

Kathy lives in a poor section of town—she calls it the ghetto—but feels safe in it, partly because it's a quiet little dead-end street, but mostly, it seems, because of the social connections she's made. Kathy would agree with Jane Jacobs on the idea of having neighbors you don't have to be best friends with, but with whom you can exchange bus tokens or just pass the time of day. She spoke of others she knew in the neighborhood:

> And then the new gal up the street, her and her husband, and I've met her mom and find out that she's in recovery for three years. And then, you know, there's the people across the street, the house across the street and we speak, you know, kind of hello. Nothing deep or anything like that. But just friendly and it's...you feel safe.

The mental health center and her clinicians are part of her community, true of others in some of the interviews we've done. Kathy's and others' comments about the center as a community for them did not suggest that they saw it as a "consolation community" for people with nowhere else to go but of being a place, and a group of people, with which and whom they had a personal connection. Whether such connections and sense of community with a mental health facility help or hinder people's efforts to build community with others, or whether those with more varied communities also can build a positive sense of community with their clinicians and centers are, as we say, questions for further study. We can say that Kathy and others we've interviewed show an ability to make strong personal connections with their professional providers of treatment and that those professionals appear to have a way of connecting with their clients as people. How well the latter's connection making works for clients who are less socially adept and inclined is another question for further study.

Kathy describes herself as a caretaker, and something more:

You know, helping out with my grandchildren when their parents are working. I have a role as a caretaker with my animals...and I guess [also] a responsibility within myself that if somebody reaches out for help, that I'm there. I think there are some people that I know that they know that they can call and I'll be there, and that feels good. Because I wasn't like real trustworthy, I didn't keep my word and stuff like that before. That connection, you know, just being there. So it's with the kids, with the animals, with the rescue, with people in recovery. Maybe that somebody else is struggling.

Kathy might seem almost too gentle to take on the role of advocate, but she has done so for her animals, and when needed, for herself and others. She talks about her activities with the *Citizens Project*:

It was kind of like making a difference and being a voice in the homeless community...I spoke up at the capitol. I served on that board [a Leadership Project internship] for maybe four years. And there were classes that teach you public speaking and just legislative process and all that kind of great stuff.

She said that citizenship, and also AA, gave her a voice. Her interviewer asked her about her rights:

I feel that I have the right to be treated with respect. I don't have to accept being talked down to. I don't have to accept that your word is like gold. And it comes [to] the same thing [with] my medical doctor. If I'm not feeling that I'm getting the care, then they got a boss. Same way with food stamps. They almost cut my food stamps one time. So the worker didn't want to work it, so I called my state rep. And I e-mailed like, I don't know, the governor. Yeah, I wasn't having it because it was an unfair situation. That next day, I had my food stamps.

Bill, Kathy, and others were nominated as people who were making progress in their social and community lives. We didn't provide for or demand from the nominators a precise standard for "a life in the community," but relationships and connectedness may be the strongest elements across these interviews. Advocacy and self-advocacy is a theme, too. "Community" is a meaningful term for all the interviewees and a primary one for many across their varying definitions and descriptions of it. Material resources are scant for all, though, and represent a major challenge for large-scale citizenship interventions.

CLINICIAN INTERVIEWS

Clinicians at the mental health center generally are psychiatric social workers. Psychology interns, residents in psychiatry, and others also have individual caseloads and lead or co-lead therapy groups. Psychiatrists, medical authorities on the teams, prescribe medications and, depending on the team and caseloads, may see clients for individual care. Wendy, a clinician, and Suzanne, a psychiatrist, were nominated for their work with clients on expanding their social and community lives.

Wendy

Wendy, in her mid-thirties, is a clinician in the acute services department, where people are first seen when they come in looking for help. Asked about the 5 Rs in her own life, she talked about wanting to adopt a child, or at least sponsor one through Big Brothers Big Sisters. Wendy describes herself as living a privileged life. She and her husband care "a lot about what happens politically within New Haven," she says, "and with the way services are delivered or with the way certain populations are treated." She knows that having a car and being able to drive to a grocery store that sells decent food distinguishes her from her clients who walk or take the bus and do their shopping at neighborhood stores with low quality food and high prices. Wendy was an Peace Corps volunteer before becoming a social worker. She believes in women's rights, the right to make as much money as men make, her right to own a home, and animal rights. She belongs to multiple communities—the professional social work community, the Latino community as she's half Latina, the white community since "that's how most people recognize me," the greater New Haven community, and the community of women.

Wendy talked about her clients' difficulty "breaking out of the mental health community." "They feel stigmatized," she said, "and that makes them hesitant to really partake in things. Or they don't know about opportunities outside of, for instance, going to [the local social club] or coming here." Safe affordable housing is a major barrier, too, along with lack of money, and people to help them manage what little money they have. People's treatment plans do include social, recreational, and leisure activities, she said:

> And I do try to encourage people to think about how to do more in their downtime and not think that going to appointments is a full day . . .

As for employment, it's difficult, she says, to know how to encourage people who seem to be ready to work. when they're afraid of it or of losing their benefits or both. She thinks work can raise people's sense of self worth, but there aren't many jobs to be had and the ones her clients can get don't pay much. Stigma is another barrier, and it's not something her clients are just imagining:

> It's important to validate that, because that does exist and people are marginalized, and so I think it's important to not pretend that [other] people aren't maybe making faces or not being so welcoming . . . It's important to validate that that's their experience. And then I just try to, you know, go at the person's pace, but still encourage them doing a little bit more outside of their comfort zone.

Wendy sees this comfort zone as a difficulty for many of her clients, ever more so as the time they've logged in the mental health system piles up. For this longer-term client group, even grasping the concept of a recovery-oriented, person-centered treatment plan, let alone contributing to the elements of such a plan, is a difficult step:

> *A lot of people still don't completely grasp that it's their treatment plan and the goals are their goals and whatever they actually want to accomplish is up to them ... [It's about] changing the way people think or how they view themselves, not just thinking of themselves as a mental health patient ...*

Perhaps the most formidable barrier to citizenship-oriented care, even working prospectively with clinicians like Wendy who were nominated for their community orientation, is a focus on simply keeping their clients alive that, perhaps, makes citizenship look like a luxury for their clients. Wendy says it better:

> *The biggest challenge is all of the other major issues that we are helping people with, before you can even think about citizenship as being on the table, because there's housing and food and shelter and psychiatric crises and medical issues. So many of our people come not with just a couple of those things, those issues, but like five or six and so we can't always get to [citizenship], or that gets put on the back burner as far as, "What do you want to do besides worry about where you're going to sleep tonight and if you're going to have food at the end of the month?" Certainly more permanent supportive housing is needed. More money management access is needed. Less red tape to get people connected to various services ... To get people a bed at the Columbus House Shelter now you need to fill out a referral and get them put on a list ... And [some agencies] discharge people for not showing up for appointments and so forth. [As for subsidized housing], these things are closed, for years sometimes, and then open very briefly and you have to catch them and they have a lottery to get picked, like for Section 8 housing.*

I've heard similar comments to these from outreach workers when the word "recovery" comes up, as though the "not getting it" crowd has just walked in the door with cupcakes for their clients when they, the outreach workers, are trying to figure out how they'll persuade those very clients to come into the shelter on a Friday afternoon in January and the temperature dropping. The recovery and citizenship folk might say, first, that there are always too many problems that stand in the way of recovery and citizenship to do anything to promote either, so you have to go ahead and start, anyway. Second, attending to the principles of recovery and citizenship are not inconsistent with the goal of keeping people alive, although sometimes, it's true, you need to bring people in from the cold first, and talk recovery later.

Neither group is wrong, except when they're convinced they are right. Wendy alluded to this tension in regard to people who arrive at the mental health center in crisis:

> *There's probably room to ask more specifically about those kinds of things ... other than like their demographics and medical issues and whatnot ... And then if we do admit people, there isn't really a question about citizenship or rights [in the intake forms]. I mean we ask about people's ... if they're responsible for any children,*

and in the suicide assessment we ask about what kind of protective factors make them want to live. Whether they feel responsibility for children or pets or whether spirituality helps them, but it's connected to suicidal thoughts, not broadly, like, "Is this something that's missing in your life?"

Wendy also talked about new resources at the center, including a full-time case-worker from the Department of Social Services to help people with determinations of eligibility and applications for state assistance of various forms. Clinicians also had contacts for energy assistance and other services with a local community action agency. Money management help, however, either voluntary or involuntary, was in short supply:

The concept of savings . . . So many people I think just are used to living paycheck to paycheck—you know—social security check every month and being broke after the first week, versus seeing how they can stretch it out, seeing how they can go to like a certain grocery store to get better prices, versus another. Just being more thoughtful with their purchases, I think education around that would be good and expanding the money management program . . .

This statement appears to contradict Wendy's comments on awareness of her privileged status in being able to drive to where the better, and cheaper, food can be bought. But perhaps this was a statement more of frustration than of judgment.

Suzanne

Suzanne, a team psychiatrist from whom we heard in the last chapter, has been at the center for about 15 years. Her first responsibilities, she says, are to her family— her son, her husband, and her elderly parents. "In terms of citizenship," she says, these responsibilities anchor her in "a large community of my colleagues at work, because I feel responsible not just to my employer but to the people I work with." She experiences these responsibilities as positive ones, but also as draining at times. Her rights are political rights, free speech, "rights to my body, rights to be happy, rights for security, I suppose . . ."

Suzanne commented on a sense of powerlessness of clinical staff that mirrors the disempowerment of their clients:

There are rights within the organization that employees don't always have. I think it's not as empowering a place as it could be . . . There's this myth that everything is a medical model, but I don't so much see that, not that I want things to be a medical model, but it's really . . . a sort of top-down sort of place so that I think it kind of mirrors what we sometimes do or don't do with, I call them patients because I'm a doctor . . . Things don't start from on the ground in the community where people really know what they're doing, but come from on high.

Her possible hypothesis-in-the-making that client empowerment requires greater staff empowerment would seem to support the *Collaborative*'s view of citizenship work as organizational and systems work as well as individual client work.

Suzanne has a gift for looking at things from different angles, eschewing simple answers to the big problems that underfunded and overworked agencies and staff and their marginalized clients face. "We have the role to take care of people and yet to empower them," she says, capturing in a sentence a world of contradiction and challenge in the age of recovery in public mental health care. Then, too, living in a neighborhood where "people look out for each other, people know each other," and knowing of the social capital that such conditions represent and continue to produce for her and her family, she has complicated feelings about home visits to her clients:

> *We'll often do home visits with two people partly because the neighborhoods are not so safe and partly because people bring different things to the relationship . . . I feel like it's such a privilege to be able to do home visits . . . I've been doing home visits for probably 30 years. But as I've been doing them more and more, I also see the down side and the risk, [and] that can be judgmental because . . . people don't bathe or don't take care of their house, but I think the really important thing is to be able to talk to people about it and express that. And then other team members can often say, "Well, wait a minute, they live in a different way that you do." . . . But also to respect how people might not want you that close into their space . . . And to try to be careful to, each step through the door, "I'm here, is it okay?" "Where should I sit?" Giving the person as much power as possible because, here you are! And the really sad thing is that we so often come to their house to put them in the hospital.*

Asked, asked about the R of resources, she alluded to her awareness of the links among money, the relational resources of friends, and personal and social resources of things to do, compared with those of her patients:

> *The other resource is of things to do, just ways to fill time . . . when I see poverty, the day stretches out ahead of [my clients] and what are they going to do? Well, they'll watch a little TV. They'll fall asleep. They'll sit in a chair, [and this] is so tied in to their lack of relationships, I think.*

The work of mental health care is multifaceted, as Suzanne describes it, from the "clinical side where our goal is to help people stay out of the hospital and be as well as they can be," to "the skill building component where they are coupled with people that are hired as skill builders," to helping people manage what little money they have. Suzanne understands the deprivation that fuels spending sprees that people can't afford:

> *I think when people have been so deprived, they get that money and they just want to spend it, period. It's really hard for people to think through, "OK, if I spend all this money today I won't have anything at the end of the week or the end of the month." But they think, "I will figure that out when it comes to that," I guess.*

Yet there is something more fundamental about spending sprees—it's likely that Suzanne understands this, and would have talked about it if the conversation had stayed on this topic—that is epitomized in Nancy's comments in the last chapter on buying flowers for the table. It's not just about wanting to spend a little money, to splurge, to do something nice, although it is about these things, in part. It's also about wanting to do something that normal people do, normal in this context meaning "what people do just as a part of being alive"—the luxurious necessities and necessary luxuries that can trump what will happen at the end of the month when the lights may go out.

Suzanne does talk about the money management program at the center as being too judgmental. She also wishes that clinical staff did not have to get in the middle between people and their money. And then...:

> There are times when there's nothing I can do...Everyone is pulled in different directions to give people things when we see people are struggling so. I think there's an impulse, well, let's figure out a way to buy them their medication if they can't afford it...But I mean we, really, our people are struggling.

People are struggling, too, when it comes to the issue of community outside the mental health center:

> You know, it's been so hard to get people engaged in communities. And I'm trying to think of successful engagements. What is saddest to me is that for so many of our people there is not a community. I mean either they don't know what to do or know how to do it or they've been isolated for such a long time...I wish we knew what would work to build community because I think we all know that's what people need.

These, and others not included here from Suzanne and others, are sobering words from an empathic clinician seen as having a special orientation toward supporting people's lives in the community at large. If there's consolation in them, it's that there is ample interest among this group in doing something else, or more than is being done now, to match community mental health treatment with "a life in the community" and the means to sustain it.

Citizenship Lunches

We were already conducting individual interviews on citizenship and financial health with clients, clinicians, community members, and *Citizens Project* graduates. "Citizenship lunches" was an experiment. The idea was to talk to people, mostly not associated with the mental health center, more informally on the topic of citizenship than we could in the other formats. *Citizens Collaborative* members would be given $25 to take people out to lunch. They would give or read to their lunch guests a brief introduction to citizenship and the 5 Rs and our use of them to support people with mental illnesses. At some point during the lunch they would ask two questions of their guests. The first was, "Does citizenship have anything to do with mental health care?" The second was, "How so?" or "Why not?" depending on the answer to the first question. Hosts could also ask their guests questions about the 5 Rs or other elements of citizenship if the flow of discussion allowed it. The hosts would write up a brief report on each lunch and submit it with their receipts. I encouraged CCC members to host people host people who might not be supportive of our citizenship work, as well as those they suspected would be. We needed to learn from hostile or cynical views as well as supportive ones.

We were all busy with other things, though. Every once in a while I'd ask Ashley Clayton, the project director, how the lunches were coming along. Slowly, she said. I'd almost forgot about them when she e-mailed me reports on the first three. The experiment was working, albeit mainly because team members went above and beyond the call of the paragraph or two worth of reflections we'd asked of them. One report took up four single-spaced pages. No doubt the strong reactions that hosts got from some of their guests helped to fuel the diligence they brought to their reports.[5]

Rachel is a primary care physician at a community health center in San Francisco whom one of the team members met with during a visit there. Melissa is a visiting nurse in New Haven who often cares for people with mental illnesses. Cecilia is a check casher in New Haven who sees people with mental illnesses when they come in with SSI or other checks.

RACHEL

Citizenship as we practice it in New Haven can't simply be replicated in another city or area of the country, or for that matter other countries that we're working with now, without attention to clientele, culture, socioeconomic, and service system elements. Even within a local ethnic group or culture, citizenship and its interrelationships will have different nuances or emphases. Patty has been telling me for a long time that *relationships* should be the first-named R, since all the others follow from it, and I've told her for a long time that I need to keep the order they're in now because that's how I remember them. Recently, though, I got a look, behind her *Citizens Project* experience, at why relationships are so central for her. "In the Native community," she said, "when we meet someone we ask them what tribe or nation they belong to and who are they related to, or who they know, not what they do." Think of the world view reflected in the different between the first sorts of question and the last.

Caveats such as these would, of course, also apply to recovery, social inclusion, capabilities, and other applied theories in different cultures and countries. The comments of Rachel, whose patients are all poor, homeless, and often have mental illnesses and addictions, reflect and give clues to a different service system in a community with different characteristics and, perhaps, some different values, or shades of them, from the one I've logged time in. On the last—values—her description of her patients' volunteer work as peer health educators may suggest that volunteering has a somewhat higher status in mental health circles in San Francisco than it does in New Haven. Rachel's patients who volunteer in soup kitchens and shelters seem to her to have a better quality of life and better health overall than those who do not. She notes that the causal direction of these activities—people doing better because they volunteer or people volunteer because they're doing better—is not established.

For Rachel, the 5 Rs are tied up with resources. She worries that the Affordable Care Act will create even greater health disparities between US citizens and undocumented migrants and immigrants than it does now. Decent and affordable housing, she said, is a form of health care, as people who are housed cost less to the state in mental or physical health care:

> The more attractive and livable the housing, the lower the move-out and mortality rates...New housing in San Francisco for homeless people has in-house nursing and social work. It connects people to community events and work and volunteering. And there are spaces in them for community building. Still, that means a "community within a community," not necessarily connection to the larger community.

Rachel seems to look at responsibilities and roles as one, with roles being defined by responsibilities and responsibilities usually involving valued roles. It is social workers, she said, who have the greatest impact on people getting involved in citizenship activities, and doctors and psychologists who help their patients get or stay healthy enough to participate in their communities. She talks about unsanitary conditions and poor upkeep of the building and "a certain level" of violence and drugs in the SROs, but also says said that "people seem to take care of each other and look out for each other." Some sub-groups, though, including gay and transgender folk, are marginalized even within already-marginalized communities. For these groups, some community groups and churches step into the gap, including *Glide*, a "spiritual movement" that describes itself as "a radically inclusive, just and loving community mobilized to alleviate suffering and break the cycles of poverty and marginalization."[6]

Outside of such oases, San Francisco has many free community events, but "it's very unusual to have homeless people attend," Rachel says, "because without treatment, healthcare, clean clothes, transportation, they're not 'socially solvent' and they feel stigmatized, even traumatized, interacting with the larger community." Socially solvent—a great phrase for citizenship work, and you won't find it on the Web. I looked. And stigma, including internalized stigma, is available everywhere—San Francisco, New Haven, you name it.

Melissa

Melissa is a visiting nurse who provides home care for people with mental illness or HIV or both. After reading the information sheet on *Citizenship* she said to her host:

> *Oh, this is funny, really. It's stupid. You are a group of people who say that people need to achieve greater independence, but really, I think it's just a way to cut spending. Even if you all don't have that goal in mind, that's what they'll do with it, they'll use it to justify spending cuts.*

Janet Weiss offered a similar critique of "systems integration" theory more than 30 years ago. Often, she wrote, services are integrated and unnecessary "duplication of services" is eliminated as a means of cutting costs.[7] Melissa added that she agreed with the idea of supporting the increased autonomy of "these people," but not across the board and not blindly.

> *We need to recognize that some of them can't go further. We can't constantly push the envelope—it leads to instability. I have a patient, Theresa. She's had lots of nurses and in the past they kept trying to get her to wear new clothes, to wear proper boots in winter, but she doesn't want it. I've been her nurse for two years and I don't care what boots she wears. I just need to make sure that she takes her HIV meds and that she is safely housed. That's all I worry about, and it works. She's taken a big step recently. Her abusive boyfriend is not allowed to come into her housing, and they stick with it. So even though she hangs out with him, she can get away when she needs to.*

Some of Melissa's cynicism appears to involve frustration not only with researchers who don't get it but with funding cuts and administrative structures that don't get, or don't want to get, how much onerous reporting, charting, and billing requirements cut into the care she gives:

> *It's all about funding cuts. Theresa is with the [mental health center's] ACT team, but now they have to focus on increasing autonomy because they've had their funding cuts. I've had my funding cut. I need to produce a 60-page dissertation every two weeks to justify why Theresa and my other clients need continued visiting nurse care... Theresa can't handle more autonomy. She's schizophrenic, and she is really really sick. She has constant auditory hallucinations. She needs to not be pushed. She's paranoid.*

Her lunch host asked Melissa about the 5 Rs as they applied to Theresa. Melissa touched directly on all but responsibilities, and indirectly on that in her reference to the local social club for people with mental illnesses:

> *Rights. Yes, of course she has rights. The main one is to safe, affordable, decent housing—and she gets that at [the housing program where she lives]. She also has the right to quality medical care... Roles. What does she do? She hangs out*

with her abusive boyfriend. She holds up a sign on the boulevard. She should go to [the local social club] but she doesn't ... She has three kids but they were all taken away the second they came out of her body ... Relationships—her boyfriend, me, her caseworker. Resources. She gets subsidized housing. She gets food stamps that she sells to her boyfriend's mother ... She spends the money on crack.

Another response would be sorrow and pity, in the deepest and most charitable sense of those words. Martha Lawless, a colleague who was project director for an evaluation of a SAMHSA-funded program for women with behavioral health disorders who were homeless became, in effect, a member of the intervention team. She spoke, with sorrow and pity, of intimate partner violence in some clients' lives, of their abuse, at times, of their own children, and the emotional, even traumatic, impact on project staff, including peer mentors with similar experiences to those of their clients.[8]

Melissa believes that Theresa gets very good care, citing especially her psychiatrist at the mental health center. As for her comments on people like Theresa who can't and shouldn't be pushed, she also saw other categories of clients who are too institutionalized to change, or too "entitled" to try.

There are some patients for whom it really doesn't work, but honestly, I see that they aren't playing along at all. They're so institutionalized. Or entitled. I hate that word because I know what people think about me when I use it, but it's true. They have never been givers, they don't know how to give back. They were born into poverty and mental illness, it's intergenerational, their families were worse than dysfunctional, they were sick. They don't know how to give. [To her host:] Do you try to help with that?

Drugs, Melissa thinks, are the biggest problem for people like Theresa, but consistency of care comes next. "Carers," she says, "need to be on time, and they need to stay in place over time so that the relationship gets built. These people have never had consistency, they don't know how to trust in social relationships." On this some of our interviewees, who talk about frequent changes in therapists, would agree with her. This is a problem in teaching hospitals like the mental health center, with July first as an annual day of dread for many clients.

Melissa's host asked her about her personal views on citizenship. She said:

Honestly, what does "being a citizen" mean to you? The question is stupid. It's smarmy. It's not a real question and it's not looking for a real answer. It's looking for a made-up answer. It's like asking someone, "Are you happy?" ... Honestly, I'm so jaded ... I have the right to walk down the street, work, quietly get on with it but hate it all at the same time. My work and my health care are screwing me up so bad, I'll tell you the truth, I've decided never to vote again. It's all bullshit ... The only possible good thing about the ACA is that it will fail and something better might come out of it ... What would make me vote again? If the changes actually affected me. They should use the tax money for public services

for me as well as for the poor and the rich. At the moment I feel more disempow-
ered that I did under Bush. It's even worse now. The health care, the foot dragging
on immigration, the damn wars and drones. Responsibilities? To work hard, do the
right thing, not suck on the system...Don't drop litter, be kind to my neighbors.
Mostly try to make sure my children aren't assholes! Roles? My work is really
important, but it is so undervalued. As time goes by I'm getting paid less to do
more. I am exhausted and overwhelmed. This job is killing me...The shit rolls
down to us. I want to go back to school to be a nurse practitioner, to work in one
place, not have to go around to people's homes. To get paid better. But I have to
finish my bachelor's. Who's got the time or money? [To her host:] Are you a case
manager for your patients?

I've quoted Melissa at some length here because she shares at least one thing with
Suzanne the psychiatrist, if to a different degree—a sense of powerlessness in her
work.

Cecilia

If you asked 10 people working in public mental health care to say the first thing
that came to mind about people who work in check-cashing stores, my bet is that
none would say "valued role" or anything like it, a few would say "predator." Check-
cashing stores and their staff are typically seen as gouging the people who can least
afford it, can barely squeeze by on the piddling sums they're getting even before being
gouged. Annie Harper has shown us a different picture of some check cashers, and a
complementary picture of respectable banks with high monthly fees and high overdraft fees for people with miniscule balances who don't quality for waived fees or
overdraft protection. It's not that check-cashing stores are run by princes, but they do
offer people a way to get cash quickly, do help people pay bills, for a fee, and sometimes more than that, as with Cecilia, whom Annie hosted for a citizenship lunch:

I see people with mental disabilities getting taken advantage of. I was in T-Mobile
once, and there was this guy buying a phone, he was saying that he only earned
$710 a month, and wondering if he could afford it, and he seemed really slow, and
the guy selling him was just thinking about his commission. He only gets that
commission on his check once, but the person buying the phone might be on the
way to spiraling into a world of debt...I see them come into the store [here]. I
always count their cash out so they can see, then put it in an envelope with the
right amount written on it, and I staple the receipt to it. I've told you that some
check cashers rip off the customers, so I make sure they know they can trust me.

Cecilia witnesses greed and desperation both, and sees both in the context of a
system many of us are caught up in:

It's not just people with mental illness who get taken advantage of. I was accused
last year of stealing $500 from an elderly lady. Luckily I was away the week she
said it was stolen...I know she had daughters who wanted her money all the

time...When they kept asking for money, she told them she didn't have it because the check casher had ripped her off...People always just want to get ahead, be like a person who can be in luxury. Even me...I always buy my kids stuff from Lands' End, LL Bean, Ralph Lauren, though I get it cheap...If I don't have these things, I feel like I don't measure up.

Cecilia's job is not secure. Five stores in the area have closed recently. She thinks the people she sees are better off with what they get from her than what they will get from the banks. "Unless you are good with money," she says, "you're better off without one. Overdraft fees can go over $100 for just one dollar over." She helps some of her customers with their bills, too:

I have a customer, she's old, I've got close to her. She pays her bills here. TV and phone all in one...I buy her toilet paper, Tide and stuff. She always asks me. She used to order her food from catalogues, ham and stuff, it was so expensive...Finally I persuaded her to get food stamps, but she still has to ask me for money. Her daughters don't help, they come and eat her food...And they do their laundry [there] so she runs out of detergent...And she pays all this money to her church she's been going to for 30 years. She should be getting help from them!

This elderly lady may or may not have a mental illness, but the same story could and does apply to people who do.

Cecilia understands her customers because she's gone through hard times herself, and she's not past them. Identification with others on the basis of personal experience may not be imperative, but it can help. It's a fundamental ingredient of peer work, too, but working in the mental health field these days it's easy to forget that "peers" come in many forms. They may also work at the margins of mental health care, as in check-cashing stores. Cecilia's description of getting by is not so far removed from the ones that mental health center clients have described in our interviews with them:

I pay $925 rent, $400 sitter, $150 light, $150 gas, then cell phone, bus pass. I used to have a car but don't anymore. I can't afford it...And I earn, after tax, $2000 a month. I can hardly make it. But that's where you hustle. Pampers for example. I write to them and tell them that one split, then they give you vouchers for free ones. I did the same with Tide detergent and got it free for a year. I would get someone to take me to Sam's Club so I could use the vouchers for the biggest container...

Cecilia has a bank account, but only for getting her tax return. "I'm not a citizen," she says. "I was born in Canada and came here when I was a baby." But that doesn't matter so much, she says. What matters here is the color of your skin, and money:

Look at me, I'm black. That's all that matters in this country when it comes to being a citizen. I'm a black person, and people look at you differently when you're black. For example, if I saw someone foreign—Pakistani like your husband, or Chinese—out there getting out of a limousine, wearing fancy clothes, I'd think to myself that they've done well for themselves. But if I saw a black man doing the same thing I'd be thinking he must have taken out a second mortgage to be able to afford it, that at home he's sleeping on thrift store sheets. He's gotta be putting up a front, it can't be for real... When my oldest daughter was growing up, I was living in the projects and I didn't want her playing with the project kids, so I put her in Audubon Music School and I signed her up for a country club. Now she has these Yale friends and I keep telling her to hang with them. She'll get ahead using those networks. Now I'm putting the younger two in French lessons. It's all about money. Steve Jobs said he did all he did to change the world, but you can be sure he left something behind for his kids, too. If there was one thing I could do for our customers that we can't do, I wish I could give them financial stability. That's what we can't give them.

Summing up the *Citizens Collaborative*

We had a better view of the terrain now based on the work reported in this chapter and the two preceding it. We had a strong creative team and a supportive administration. We had made some good contacts with clinicians and teams at the mental health center, with more to do and lots to prove. We had clinicians, peers, and administrators as well as researchers on our team. My insistence that we hold most, if not all, of our meetings at the mental health center proved to be on the mark. We gained more credibility from bumping into people in the halls at the center and being the source of spirited voices coming from Room 135 than would have been the case if we'd dropped in only as needed from our research headquarters on the other side of town. We also had the problem of riches—too many ideas, too many insights, all boldly urged, about what should fit under citizenship's umbrella—but this is a problem I'll take any day over a poverty of thought and nerve.

We had a bona fide *Citizens Project* manual after 12 years. We had linked voter registration with the collaborative's work. We had looked at the notion of connection-to-community from a few different angles and realized that the connection, and the contribution, would have to go both ways, from community to clients and from mental health center, staff, and clients to community. We had made a modest contribution to community building within the mental health center itself. And we had added the issue, and problem, of money and finances to the citizenship R of resources that people needed to make it as full-fledged community members.

We had started the *Citizens Collaborative* with three principles that helped to guide us through the early planning stages for citizenship-oriented care at a large urban mental health center as a pilot project for DMHAS. The first principle was that we would not be locked into the *Citizens Project* model, but would look at other sources for guidance, too, from measure development and our current research, and perhaps even back to *Citizens*, as we had now come full circle back to the charge of building connections to community resources for and with people with mental illnesses. The second was that bringing citizenship-oriented care into individual treatment would require that all team members, from psychiatrist and team leader to clinicians, case managers, peer mentors, and other specialists understand and buy into the principles of citizenship, regardless of who it was that spent how much time on street-level citizenship work. And the third was that the community connections, contacts, and resources we were developing in the New Haven community would be linked directly with, and be immediately available to, clinical teams, rather than being external services to which team members could refer their clients.

These three themes hold up, with the exception that we had moved back, a bit, toward the *Citizens Project* as the place from which to build and modify citizenship-oriented care. Still, the original principle of using that project as only one model of several made sense. We needed to be able to think away from it and its dominant presence as our chief exemplar of putting citizenship theory into practice. And we did, in fact, have other findings, tools, and research to bring to bear on our planning, all of which enriched our understanding of citizenship and mental health.

Coming on fast at the tail end of our first year as a collaborative, there were new developments in each of the topic areas—manual development, voter registration, community building at the mental health center, community connections, financial health, and citizenship-oriented care—of this and the last two chapters. These helped to push us into a planned transition from a relative focus on planning, brainstorming, research, and networking to a focus on action and tangible projects during the second year.

We shipped the *Citizens Project* manual off to DMHAS. It still needed some touchup and additional material, but it was far enough along for us to show to the Commissioner and Chief Financial Officer and others, and get their take on it. With revisions we would make based on their ideas, we hoped to get started with them on replicating the project in other sites across Connecticut.

The voter registration project had reached a milestone. We had a process, approved and about to be put in place, to ask people if they were registered to vote as they registered as patients, or clients. This was a long time in coming, but from what we could gather we'd be the first mental health center in the state to make voter registration a formal part, inscribed in its approved policies and procedures, of the work of providing public mental health care in our state. Soon, we'd be training the front door and peer staff in voter registration, and getting started. Doing the same for people already registered at the center would come next.

There were no major developments on the "community building at the mental health center" front, except to move ahead incrementally with what we were already doing, but my thinking about community had shifted a bit. "Naturally occurring" communities and organizational communities were different animals, but they had some common markings. And all of them, in their different ways, were hybrid communities in a transitional world. This is saying both too much and too little, and too late in the book, but the practical impact of this thinking, for me, has been to neutralize, which is not to say negate, the notion of community. "Community" is morally neutral. It involves people living or working together, or both. It can be weak or robust, supportive or constraining, rich or poor in affective and instrumental ways, and not always both or neither of each. And community can change, if most often, or in many ways even in a global world, like Issa's snail climbing Mt. Fuji, but slowly, slowly.

The community action group had been busy. A second community focus group was far more hope-inspiring than the first, so much so that its participants asked to become involved in our work. We decided to start an advisory group for the collaborative, with them as the founding members. It is worth noting, as regards their enthusiasm, that all had some connection to mental health work. Our outreach efforts with the West River Neighborhood Association was off to a good, if slow moving, start. There were more of us cleaning up the neighborhood on Saturday mornings than there were residents. If institutional and naturally occurring communities both tend to change slowly, the pace and nature of community change and community time are still qualitatively different than those of institutional change and time. The former has more of people in it, the latter of the clock. The former is an association that begins with living in the same place, the latter with being hired for work that is performed in a certain place. Still, if change happens slowly, it may take deeper root for being pushed hard. We needed to be in West River for the long haul, and the evidence of our worth be staying power, not fireworks. Finally, the community action group would be playing the lead role in developing new and ongoing valued role projects and opportunities that, we hoped, would include connections to paid work for people with mental illnesses.

On financial health, a proposal we wrote for a pilot financial health project at the mental health center was approved by DMHAS, adding to our repertoire and our funding. The project would be largely ethnographic and exploratory at the outset, but eventually would test different forms of financial supports for clients. Financial health continues its march toward the center of the citizenship agenda.

As for citizenship-oriented care pilot projects, we were looking in two different directions, and beginning to plan with the teams for each. One direction was work with young adults, many of whom had "aged out" of being clients of the state's Department of Children and Families. What would citizenship-oriented care look like for people who had barely had a chance to gain or lose their citizenship? The other was the assertive community treatment (ACT) team, working with older clients with more longstanding histories of serious mental illnesses who would challenge the citizenship approach in another way.[9] What would citizenship look like, and how much could it offer, to people who were assessed as being among the most "chronically ill" and of long-term clinical care, including home visits, of all of those receiving public mental health services?

Yet the newly-reconstituted ACT team after a brief state experiment to eliminate them, needed to go through its own growing pains. The timing might not be the best for the ACT or the citizenship team, tempting as it was for the latter to get in on the ground floor of things. Peggy Bailey, Director of Clinical Operations at the center and a former ACT team director, had another idea. What about placing *Citizens Collaborative* folk on several of the mental health center's treatment teams, without any particular time pressure for integrating citizenship-oriented care onto those teams? It would give the citizenship folk an object lesson in clinical care in process, and an opportunity to team members to hear about citizenship. From that process, a more organic way of bringing citizenship into mental health care might emerge. It was a good idea. To it, I proposed to add some specific help with community connections that *Citizens Collaborative* folk could offer to clinical team members for individual clients.

There was one aspect of our thinking about citizenship-oriented care that would apply to any pilot project we undertook. Citizenship-oriented care, we had come to think, with Patty's urging and insistence, could be integrated with the clinical work of teams without holding all, or even most, citizenship-related activities at the mental health center. This was obvious, of course, when it came to community activities or connection making, to helping people venture outside the narrow social and physical circles they occupied to other spaces and people in the community at large. It might also apply, though, to citizenship groups and meetings of various sorts. Why not meet at the public library, for example, or, for young adults, at a basketball court, rather than the mental health center?

Citizenship's beginning in the boundary encounters of Jim and Ed, his outreach worker, took place in the context of a mental health system of care, even if their meetings occurred at its farthest margins. These meetings, which provided the spark and impetus for the citizenship framework and approach, thus involved not only what citizenship looks like at the individual or small group level, but what citizenship can mean and might have to mean to have its own staying power at the level of mental health systems of care and their relationships to the communities in which they do their work. Would they be *of* those communities, or only *in* them?

9

A Model of Citizenship and Mental Health

Starting with homeless outreach and continuing with citizenship, I've made much in this book of an iterative learning-and-action process in which mastery of the task at hand and its application in practice set the stage for the next task by exposing the limits of what the current one can accomplish. We applied this process in outreach work, where we learned how to find people who were homeless, then how to identify those among them who might have a mental illness, then how to make contact and build trust slowly with the person not the patient, then how to start talking about help we had to offer, then how to negotiate with and persuade people to accept services such as mental health treatment and housing. This last step exposed a limit that mental health outreach could not master—how to help people become neighbors, community members, and citizens—due to the limitations of its charge and its expertise. Reaching the outer limits of mental health outreach, then, suggested the idea of a different kind of next step, that of supporting people's full citizenship as outlined by the 5 Rs. This iterative learning-and-action process has been slower and less concrete in our multistage application of the citizenship framework, but it's at work there, too, nonetheless.

I need to call on this process one more time to write about citizenship-oriented care writ large in communities and mental health "systems of care." I use quotes here not to indicate a term of art but to qualify the shorthand message of the term, since the very limits of what a system of care is, and where the system fades into associational life, are in play in trying to construct a model of citizenship and mental health. And I include under "citizenship-oriented care" the idea of "citizenship-oriented systems of care" because of a lesson learned from our *Citizens Collaborative* work. We've come to think that citizenship-oriented care in the most specific sense—integrating citizenship principles and supports on treatment teams—is unlikely to endure and thrive unless citizenship principles are persuasive to, and come to be reflected in, the workings and ways of mental health centers and their staff and clients. Citizenship will fail if it is something we do only for other people and not a set of values and assumptions shared and acted upon by all. It will also fail, though, if citizenship is the province of mental health systems of care and not of communities and society as a whole.

Citizenship as a framework for the social and community inclusion of people with mental illnesses is intended to help individuals, but it also involves interventions that take place in systems of care and local communities as a whole, and in the relationship between system and community. "Citizenship" is a fairly new concept in mental health care, but its vision and principles, as I noted earlier in the book, go back to the beginning of the community mental health movement in the 1960s with its dual goal of providing effective mental health care outside the hospital *and* supporting a "life in the community" for people with mental illnesses. And so, with the halting, sometimes incoherent, and poorly-funded introduction of community mental health centers to provide effective clinical care and the even more halting, incoherent, and poorly-funded attempts to support community living and membership for people discharged from state psychiatric hospitals, was the "treatment system and community living" character of public mental health set in motion as the deinstitutionalization era receded.

A model of citizenship and mental health could move in different directions toward its goal, but by any path it takes it will proceed with consideration of, in comparison, reaction, or as an alternative, complement, or corrective to, current models of community mental health care in the United States. Therefore, a full model of citizenship and mental health should show where it started out, how it might reach its goal, and the broad outlines of what it might look like for individuals, mental health care, and society. "Outline" is the operative term here, not "exhaustively describe." I propose to offer here an initial model of citizenship and mental health as a way of addressing the dual goal of effective community-based treatment and life in the community, with the caveat above about "problematizing" the idea of "system of care."

Three caveats and an explanation are in order. The first caveat is that the *model* of citizenship and mental health with which this chapter will end makes certain assumptions that only its being a model can excuse. The model assumes stability, or moderate progress, in areas such as housing, income support and employment, integration of mental health and primary care, and other domains. These are partial assumptions, since a model of citizenship and mental health might be expected to have a positive impact in some of these areas. But the model makes other assumptions, too, about issues that could enhance, weaken, bar, or open doors it, and over which it has little, if any, control. For example, as I noted in the preface, this book, and now the model, do not address the impact of the Affordable Care Act on public mental health care, including its impact on socially-oriented mental health approaches such as citizenship. The model does not address possible cuts or increases in funding for mental health care and social services. Nor does it address policy changes—for example, an increase in the use of outpatient commitment for persons people who are not engaged in treatment and are deemed at risk of harm to self or others—that could have an impact on the development of citizenship-oriented systems of care. The model also assumes local communities that remain at, or close to, their current level of stability or instability. Large assumptions, indeed.

The second caveat is that the two figures accompanying the text in this chapter—a "premodel" and model—freeze in time what is actually a process that takes place across it in both cases. In the "premodel" figure, my attempt to incorporate elements of a citizenship-oriented system of care in its relationship to community includes our work from mental health outreach up through the *Citizens Project*. In the "model" figure that follows, my attempt to incorporate system and community elements and relationships reflects both our current *Collaborative* work and extensions of the citizenship work into the future.

The third caveat has to do with particular limitations of a "model" in regard to citizenship and mental health, which I'll get to by way of returning to some other comments I made in the preface to this book, on the "generalizability" of the citizenship framework. There, I wrote about the potential limitations of the framework for mental health care in general, given that the theory and the work emerged from mental health work in the Northeast in a liberal city and state with a progressive state mental health authority. Thus, I wrote, the citizenship framework could not be assumed to be applicable, without modification, in other areas, regions, and urban or rural settings with varying cultural and socioeconomic elements in play. At the same time, I'll argue here that the citizenship framework is more specifically defined and has been more closely studied than most other socially-oriented approaches to mental health care, and that this study has supported its basic structure and premises while offering guidance for both replication and modification. On another note, the term "model" can be misleading, since it seems to fit the world of systems more than the messy world of associational life, while citizenship locates itself in both worlds and between the two.

The explanation I promised just above involves returning to the broad categories of "system" and "associational life." "Associational life" involves mainly direct, voluntary, and informal interactions and experiences that take place in, and partly constitute, the everyday life of neighborhoods and communities and of individuals, families, and groups that live and work in them. The "associational world" may include social organizations such as community centers, and religious organizations.[1] A related term, "lifeworld," involves personal and social life outside of "systems." "Systems" represent what Max Weber described as the "rationalization of the world"[2] through bureaucratic organization, logic, and hierarchies of order and authority employed in state, financial, banking, industry, human service, and other sectors.[3]

Increasing system encroachment on the various forms of associational life is a major theme in contemporary social theory. A reverse encroachment—in which the lifeworld penetrates the system—is rarely discussed, but is present in systems from the outset and asserts itself in various ways in organizational operation and life. David Schwartz writes about the underworld of non-regulated relationships and care in mental health organizations and systems.[4] As in other systems, this under-, or unofficial, world is peopled by the secretary who knows everybody and how to get the boss's ear, mid- and lower- level staff on the totem pole who talk outside during smoke breaks about what's really going down inside, research interviewers who double as counselors and referral sources for social services for research subjects, and many others. The dual clinical and social nature of public mental health care, while not an exact parallel to the system–underworld dichotomy, tends to ratchet up of the tension of that dichotomy, since mental health care involves a connection to a broader swath of people's lives than is the case in many other service systems.

Toward a Model of Citizenship-Oriented Systems of Care: Outreach and Citizenship Work

OUTREACH WORK

Outreach workers leave their offices to find, meet, and engage in transactions with people who are homeless and live outside the protections of society with the exception of various, mainly systems-connected, interventions to ameliorate their situations. This is an oversimplification of homelessness, as it implies that people stay homeless until outreach workers happen along, when in fact many people are homeless for longer or shorter periods of time, with alternating periods of being "barely housed" in rundown motels, staying with friends, or even in apartments. That said, long-term homelessness is generally associated with a higher percentage of persons with serious and chronic mental illnesses than among people who are episodically homeless.[5]

Outreach workers bring with them a wide range of services and supports including mental health treatment and housing. Outreach teams generally are more or less closely tied to their local mental health systems of care. In New Haven at the time of the ACCESS program, for example, the outreach team was a program of the mental health center. Eventually, most outreach teams' clients are referred to office-based clinicians and teams for ongoing mental health care. The mental health system of care can take many forms, but a common model is that of a state mental health authority that develops and promulgates policies and distributes funds for public mental health services, with local mental health authorities, or LMHAs, which negotiate contracts with and distribute funds to participating agencies, provide quality assurance based on negotiated services and outcomes, and coordinate care including referral to LMHA-member organizations for clinical, rehabilitative, housing, and other services and resources.

The ideal of integrated systems of care, or systems integration, which has been called the Holy Grail of social policy makers,[6] emerged from 1960s War on Poverty programs that came to be seen as inefficient, costly, and ineffective due to the lack of coordination of care among them. Systems integration in mental health care can be described as matching and coordinating services that are to be adequately funded and coordinated and that address the full range of social as well as clinical needs of people with mental illnesses. Starting in the late 1970s and never fully implemented due to funding cuts during the Reagan era, the "community supports system" approach to community mental health care aimed to correct the deficiencies of the community mental health center movement. As Howard Goldman and Joseph Morrissey wrote in the 1980s, previous attempts at mental health reform had redefined social problems of poverty, crime, deprivation of resources and opportunities, and racism as mental health problems. Community support systems, by contrast, would address the social challenges of people with chronic mental illness as *social*, not clinical, problems.[7] Community support systems would also provide effective mental health treatment within integrated systems of care.

Goldman and Morrissey's work was a foundational document for the federal Substance Abuse and Mental Health Services Administration's ACCESS program and its test of systems integration theory in work with people who were homeless with mental illnesses. An integrated system of care that addressed the social problems of people who were homeless and provided effective community based mental health care would, finally, give full due to the social problems of this group. The ACCESS approach, seeking its solutions systems of care, provided a vision and blueprint for what mental health systems of care could be, building on what was, by then, a 30-year experiment in shifting from institutional to community mental health care.

Homeless outreach, a microcosm of integrated systems of care based on the Goldman-Morrissey model, simultaneously demonstrates the advance of this approach and exposes its limits, which are the limits of all mental health systems of care, no matter their resources' richness and integration—their inability to offer their clients the status of neighbors, community members, and citizens, but only a bounded citizenship within integrated systems of care. Citizenship proposes that the 5 Rs of rights, responsibilities, roles, resources, and relationships, and a sense of belonging that is validated and reinforced by others, may be linked to integrated systems of care, but that people will find their sea legs as citizens outside of them, in their home communities and society at large. In addition, we identified two main pathways for achieving citizenship. In one, society opens its doors, often as a result of advocacy on the part of marginalized and excluded groups and their supporters, to those marginalized groups. In another, personal supports, skill- and community-membership building activities, along with a trial run of taking on a valued role in society, as in the *Citizens Project*, aim to help individuals make their way to full membership and participation in society.

INITIAL CITIZENSHIP EFFORTS: CITIZENS AND THE *CITIZENS PROJECT*

Citizenship started on a grand scale by taking on the first of the two pathways to citizenship. We may have erred in putting our money on a prospective community welcoming of people who were homeless than on more pointed advocacy efforts, although *Citizens* did have elements of both social activism and broad appeal to the New Haven community's democratic ideals. We certainly erred in our ambitions, since neither a social activism nor a community education and acceptance model had much chance of succeeding this early in the development of the citizenship model and with our limited funding. Still, *Citizens* gave us a test run at a community-level approach to community membership for persons with mental illnesses, especially those who were or had been homeless.

The *Citizens Project* took up the second, individual-level approach, with people receiving public mental health services who had criminal charges and who, mostly, had been or were currently homeless, or were at risk of it. The *Citizens Project* can be called a hybrid of social service program and community association. This makes it an apparent contradiction to our original argument that solutions to non- or second-class citizenship had to be found outside mental health systems of care. Those systems provided a false "solution" of bounded or program citizenship for people who were seen as too vulnerable and lacking the cognitive and social tools to compete in the marketplace of community and society where the real thing is bargained for. This contradiction inherent in the *Citizens Project* was modified, in the beginning, by its non-clinical nature and its focus not on clinical improvement but on full membership in society. It was further modified over time as the project became a mini-community within the larger community of New Haven.

PREMODEL OF CITIZENSHIP AND MENTAL HEALTH

The following "premodel" figure illustrates key elements in outreach work, mental health systems of care, and the *Citizens Project* in relation to mainstream society:

At the left hand side of the figure under the heading "Outside Society," outreach work signifies both itself and other systems-spanning approaches—jail diversion is one—for people socially excluded by homelessness, mental illness,

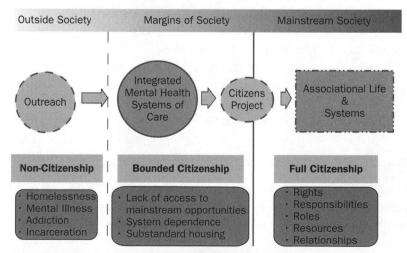

FIGURE 9.1 The Current Landscape of Citizenship and Metal Health.

addiction, and incarceration, and by poverty, lack of economic opportunities, and other deprivations. Outreach work provides multiple services to its clients, and is capable of helping them move across the border of society and into more or less integrated mental health systems of care. Such systems, which include housing, employment, disability entitlement, and other services and supports, occupy a marginal space in society and can provide, as above, only a bounded citizenship with lack of, or severely constrained, access to mainstream social and economic opportunities, dependence on mental health staff and other providers of care, and substandard or barely adequate housing in poor and often crime-ridden neighborhoods.

The *Citizens Project*, which can stand for other programs that share its principles and general approach, straddles the margins and mainstreams of society. Although participant are students in a time-limited program with inadequate follow-up resources, they are studying to take on valued social roles in mainstream society with its associational life and systems of health and social care, services, the law, finance, and more. The "margins of society" does not indicate middle-class or "median" worldviews, values, work, or housing, but access to the means to make a living or maintain oneself on an adequate income, to social interaction and opportunities with one's fellow citizens, and to freedom from exclusion based on discrimination, stigma, racism, or other excuses used to limit the rights and full access to society for all individuals and groups.

As occupants of the margins of society before making a successful transition to the mainstream of society, *Citizens Project* students need not be technically or legally excluded from mainstream opportunities to be excluded, in effect, from full participation due to severe poverty and other deprivations and barriers built into the structure of their lives and their social and economic surroundings. As citizenship students, their efforts are directed toward securing a strong connection to the 5 Rs, a sense of entitlement to the benefits of membership, and recognition of their status as citizens not only legally, but personally and socially. Retaining its funding and other links to public mental health care, however, the *Citizens Project* has one foot in the mental health system of care and the other in a mainstream world in which associational life and systems exist in dynamic tension with each other. The broken circle indicates the porous nature of the *Citizens Project*, with traffic between systems and associational life and between the margins and mainstream of society.

A MODEL OF CITIZENSHIP AND MENTAL HEALTH

Citizenship-oriented care writ large in mental health care and society is the next stage and logical step beyond the premodel figure above. The *Citizens Project* points in its general direction. The *Citizens Collaborative*, considered as part of the future of citizenship and mental health, has much work to do, but has reached the point of being able to suggest an outline, in figure and text, of that possible future.

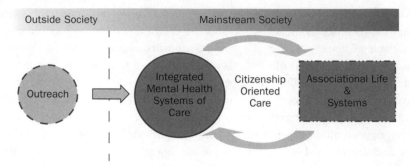

FIGURE 9.2 The Future Citizenship and Metal Health.

As in the premodel figure, Outreach, doing its work "Outside Society," stands for itself and other approaches for reaching out to people with mental illnesses, many of whom stand, with others, beyond the protections of society that others enjoy. The work of Outreach here essentially duplicates that of the premodel figure, with the important exception that, in this ideal-future model, outreach supports its clients' transition not only to integrated mental health systems of care but to associational life and other systems, all located in mainstream society. "Citizenship-oriented care," located in the figure between mental health systems and associational life and systems, is simultaneously reflected in the mental health system of care and mediates the interaction between mental health treatment and associational-systems domains as well as between individuals receiving mental health care and the associational-systems domain, in part through the medium of valued roles.

Arguably, another premodel figure could have been included after the first, showing the mental health system as having migrated from its "margins of society" location in the first figure, to a point where it has come to straddle the margins and mainstream domains, thus taking the place of outreach in the first premodel. But since the model I'm presenting here gives a "possible future" look at citizenship and mental health, and leaps over several previous iterations that would lead to it, filling in one more step to come before it would only suggest the need for another to come before or after that one.

In this ideal-model, stand-alone citizenship interventions may continue to exist and even expand, but the integrated mental health system of care has achieved, at a much larger scale, the porous character of the *Citizens Project* in the premodel figure. The broken line of the mental health system's circle indicates its hybrid system-community status due to its inculcation of citizenship practices and its increased links to, and collaboration with, community institutions, neighborhoods, resources and opportunities. This leap to hybrid status may not be quite as high or long as it seems, given that community mental health care is already a hybrid discipline within health care as a whole due to its involvement with the non-medical, social aspects of mental illness and mental health care. Links to other systems of care and to associational life of the community are shown as two-directional arrows, further suggesting the porousness of the integrated mental health systems of care. This transformed system, however, maintains intensive clinical interventions including inpatient beds, or alternatives to them, for people experiencing psychiatric crises, and continues to support the integration of mental health and primary care.

The hybrid community-system of this possible future mental health system of care, nimbler than its predecessor, will partially de-emphasize business complexity and bureaucratic procedures in favor of associational complexity and creativity. As Michael Sernyak said to me, "We have a hierarchical system here. Sometimes you need that, for medical crises, but most times you don't. Yet the hierarchy is still here, and it applies to everything we do." The movement toward differentiating the need for hierarchy in crisis from the need for more collaborative "loosely coupled" systems of care,[8] will be a slow one, but the potential for it to happen, as above, seems more likely in mental health systems of care, given the personal-social nature of mental illness and poverty, whether or not current system of care adequately addresses the dual nature of the challenges its clients face.

By now, though, the overworked case manager looking for help, and the social scientist or advocate examining the logic of the model, may have some burning questions. "But what about this thing called poverty? What about housing? What about work? Where's the link between citizenship and these things? And if it's not there, then what does citizenship and mental health amount to? Telling yourself that you're a citizen when you're just as shut out of things as before?" The answer is that we're trying to figure these things out as we go along. We have done the obvious— linked money and finances and the prospect of work to the *Citizens Collaborative*. We include health and social disparities and inequities in our work because a citizenship response must include them, even if our response is inadequate.

The work of people like Jim Mandiberg on self-sustaining social and economic enclaves of persons with mental illness, with the potential to pass back and forth flexibly between it and other communities of identity, is intriguing. Mandiberg argues that mental health systems of care conflate issues of illness and issues of inclusion. The mental health system, he writes, cannot support the social inclusion of its clients. The general public, on the other hand, lacks the commitment or interest in taking up this cause or welcoming this group. Socioeconomic subcommunities, he thinks, offer more promise than either.[9–10,11] While Mandiberg would not, I think, give a vote of confidence to the citizenship model I'm proposing here, his is the kind of against-the-grain approach that might find a place in a model such as this. Capabilities theory, as applied to the roles and well-being of people with mental illness, has enormous promise, including a possible pairing of financial health and capability approaches. Social recovery including peers as direct care staff, not to speak of researchers for generating and studying the problems of poverty and disability, can draw on enormous intellectual and human resources and conviction for collaborative ventures aimed at community membership and valued roles for people with mental illnesses. And social inclusion, with its cross-systems and cross-disability approach to mental health reform, has much to offer to a hybrid systems-community approach to mental health care as well.

At the policy level, Amber Wichowsky and Donald Moynihan have criticized the failure of governments and administrative agencies to encourage and monitor the adoption of citizenship outcomes. Administrative theory, they write, gives priority to cost achievement over citizenship values such as fairness, equity, and civic engagement. They argue for the capacity and the responsibility of governments to develop and encourage adoption, among funded agencies, of citizenship outcomes that address civic capacities, social reciprocity, and trust in addition to narrower program outcome measures. Policy feedback research, they note, has shown that social policies have an impact on social capital, sense of belonging, and sense of self-worth as a citizen. They also note the capacity of social policies to encourage political participation, using the example of Social Security leading to the increased political activities of seniors.[12]

Looking to in-depth, ethnographic sources of information with which to pursue new paths of system-community interaction and increased attention to social as well as clinical outcomes in mental health care, it is likely that many natural associations are already taking place between people with mental illnesses and fellow neighborhoods and community members without the help of planners and policy makers. Ethnographic and participatory research can help us understand the ways in which people with illnesses make, or don't make, contacts and connections with the postman, the grocer, the landlord, and others, leading to social relationships and resource opportunities that help them to be successful in their neighborhoods and communities.[13] Study of interactional rights and obligations derived from Erving Goffman's microanalysis of interaction order, as Paul Colomy and David Brown describe its adaptation to a citizenship context, can enrich our understanding of respect, regard, and dignity that reward or withhold citizenship rights and corresponding obligations at the day-to-day micro-interaction level in communities and associational life.[14]

As for the link between citizenship and mental illness and the criminal justice system, the citizenship framework and model may contribute to new collaborations between behavioral health systems and the courts and between professionals and community members and institutions, including new training for criminal and mental health professionals and the introduction of "forensic peer staff" into prerelease and re-entry programs.[15] Joint mental health and criminal justice efforts organized around the citizenship framework might, over time, contribute to a reduction in criminal justice costs through use of less costly interventions and putting money and resources back into communities in the form of increased productivity of currently disenfranchised persons with mental illnesses.[16] The citizenship model also provides a framework, and empirical evidence, for fostering new diversion and rehabilitation programs to give people opportunities to take on productive roles in society. The citizenship model and its core peer component can be adapted, too, for prerelease citizenship programs and re-entry planning and expanded community release efforts for people with mental illnesses being released from prison.

Scholars of mental health policy and practice in the United States have written of recurring historical cycles of mental health reform in which seemingly new models of care echo earlier ones with their missions of providing community versus hospital care, integrating medical and social aspects of care, and fostering the full community membership of its clients.[17] In one of our citizenship focus groups with a treatment team at the mental health center, a veteran psychiatrist said that such ideas and initiatives as citizenship promised, including the involvement of local community leaders, had been tried back in the 1960s with little success. Such reminders are bracing, and should be welcomed for use in honing the particularity of new approaches while drawing on what worked before and trying to avoid replicating what didn't.

This said, the cyclical model critique downplays new knowledge that puts the comparison of different eras and cycles into question. For all the failures of the past 50 years and the imperfections of its successes, there were no ACT teams in earlier eras of mental health reform, no supported housing or Housing First, no motivational interviewing, dual disorder treatment, or illness management and recovery programs. Social inclusion, recovery, capabilities, and citizenship have echoes but not mirror images in earlier approaches. Social work, particularly of the community organizing persuasion and with its grasp of the meaning of empowerment, builds on a grand tradition but has new tools to use in its effort to put the community back into community mental health care. Individual and collective trauma in communities, and resilience in the face of trauma,[18] can be a link between traditionally individual and individual-diagnosis–based mental health care and the mental suffering, and capacity to persist in the face of suffering, that co-exist in many communities and residents of those communities in the United States.

In addition to rigorous empirical research, one way to think about staying awake and attentive to the question of whether or not one's new approach is a dressed-up version of an earlier one, or that improves and goes beyond them, is to strike a middle path between forgetting the past on one hand and giving into it on the other, using such questions and historical processes and cycles reflexively and dialectically in citizenship-oriented planning processes that include all parties—people with lived experience of mental illness, caregivers, researchers, and policy makers. The components of such a process are fairly close to being in place in our own mental health care system and community, and the 20-year process of arriving at this junction need not be replicated over the same period of time in other settings. That's what theoretical frameworks, with flexible models based on street-level practice, are for.

10

CONCLUSION

I had just paid the cashier for coffee in the cafeteria of the mental health center and turned to find a table.

"MIIIIE-CULL!"

It was Angela, who taught me that homelessness depends on how you define it and what home means to you, also whether or not it's wise to "confess" to being homeless, especially to someone you've just met who has an audio recorder going. I hadn't seen her in more than 15 years, and damned if she really *didn't* look a day older. And at least she recognized me. Angela was doing well. Soon, she'd be moving out of the residential program she had been living in for years into her own apartment. It was good to see her, and to know she was happy to see me. I told her how much I'd learned from her when she got angry with me for asking her about being homeless.

"I was never homeless," she said.

I had thought for years about trying to get in touch with Jim, to thank him. We were a couple of months into the *Citizens Collaborative* and talking about ways to let people know what we were up to. Lucile Bruce reminded me that the communications director at DMHAS, the one who had made a short film 20 years ago about the 1993 Voting Rights Act, was still there. Maybe he'd be interested in doing a film on our work. I liked the idea, and wondered out loud about finding Jim and his outreach worker, Ed, to see if they'd agree to be in it. I contacted Debbie Fisk, the clinical director of the outreach back then, now running one of the mental health center's treatment teams. I asked what she knew of Jim and Ed's whereabouts.

She told me that Jim had been transferred to the ACT team years ago, when Debbie had been running at. He made a threatening statement about a state official that he had some circuitous connection with. Debbie was legally obligated to report it to the police, reluctantly since she didn't think Jim was going to act on his threat and knew that he'd be furious with her. As it turned out, a threat had been made against this official around the same time that Jim made his comment about him, and a suspicious package had been sent to the man's home. The bomb squad examined it. It was a fake bomblike contraption. The FBI grilled Jim and concluded that his angry statement was a coincidence and that he had nothing to do with either the other threat or the package and no intention of harming the official. "He refused to speak to any of us again," said Debbie.

And Ed? Debbie hadn't been in touch with him in years. She knew the same thing I did, that he'd finally been able get a state job, which paid a lot better than what he got working at the shelter when he'd been with the outreach team.

I still think about looking up Jim one day, but I doubt that I will. I don't think he'd be happy to see me.

I was in the middle of writing the chapters on the *Citizens Project*. I'd just interviewed a few of the recent graduates and had thought about Ned, who'd been a client of the outreach team and a student with one of the early *Citizens Project* cohorts. The last time I'd seen him was about 10 years ago, when he gave his piano recital at the social club as his valued role project. I'd always liked Ned, and wondered how he was doing. I asked Patty if she ever saw him and told her I'd like to interview him. A couple of days later she told me that Ned wanted to see me and was up for an interview. She gave me his cell phone and told me to call soon, because he bought minutes at the beginning of the month and ran out near the end until his next SSI check came in.

I called a couple of times. He must have run out of minutes. A week or so later Patty told me Ned had minutes again. By then, though, I was immersed in this book you're about to finish, and just couldn't do it. I asked Christa Morris, who was working with us on the way to medical school, if she could. She could.

Ned had been back in jail early in 2013 for a parole violation, he told her. When he got out in July he and his girlfriend split up. The relationship wasn't good for either of them. But splitting up with his girlfriend meant putting himself out on the street again, his third time homeless. Then in December his father died, and Ned, who'd been out of treatment for a while, became depressed and suicidal and started seeing his old therapist. But he didn't go back to drugs. He's been clean for eight years now, he told Christa.

Since December he'd been recovering, he said, and is hopeful about the future. He found a subsidized apartment. He hasn't been able to find work because of his criminal record. He spends a lot of time at the social club, at his church, and with clients at the mental health center that he's reconnected with. He's writing and singing again. He's always felt better when he's doing that. And most importantly he's trying to rebuild a relationship with his son, Nathan, who's 18 now. Ned got divorced from his wife after the first time he went into the psychiatric ward and missed out on most of Nathan's childhood, spending about 15 years in and out of prison, mostly for drug-related charges. At one point Ned's ex-wife told Nathan that he had died.

Ned wants to become more of a father to Nathan by opening up to him, telling him about his experiences. He has profound life lessons to teach his son, he says. He's also worried that his ex-wife is overprotective of him. He's been teaching Nathan to be more independent, to take the bus and develop some street smarts, but also to appreciate nature and stay close to his extended family. They meet about once a month to buy comic books at the store on Chapel Street, feed the birds on the Green, and go to church. His ex-wife is the biggest barrier between him and his son, he says. And money. He struggles to have enough left over after his rent and child support to take Nathan on a bus trip, buy him something, take him out to eat.

Ned talked about the *Citizens Project* and how much it meant to him and the experience of community he got from it. After he graduated, he got involved with outreach to people who were homeless, helping them figure out their social security paperwork or calling people who could help them. I wondered if he'd done that with Bill, whom we had interviewed recently as one of the mental health center clients nominated for making progress on his life in the community. "I used to go around and tell people about opportunities that they could have," said Ned. "It felt good. I found my own self-worth." He considers his fellow outpatients at the mental health center to be his family now. His own family has struggled with his illness, but patients at the center appreciate and understand and look after him.

Ned likes being out in nature. Often he takes walks before sunrise:

I like watching the sun rise at the end of the water and stuff like that. You know, the sun at the end, that's amazing. That's beautiful. I like watching and checking the formation of clouds sometimes. Sit back and just watch the sky change up a little bit. I'm an observer. I like watching the stars at night even though they stay in the same place. I'm a gazer. I got faith.

He wanted to tell Christa about a time when he was homeless and met up with his brother, a Jehovah's Witness:

I said, "Come and spend a day out with your brother in tent city." He was laughing, "Why you in tent city? Why you out here in the street homeless?" [I told him,] "I've been out on the street since I was 15 years old running away from home when you was a baby." He ain't know nothing about that. And he said [to me], "You could have been a superstar. You could play and you sing. You should have been up there in the spotlight. You should be on TV. You could have been." "Things happened," I told him. [Then I said,] "Why don't you try staying out with me for 24 hours, sleep on the green with me? Matter of fact, bring some money with you. Do what you want to do, but stay out on the street with me." You know what he said?

"What did he say?"

He couldn't do it. I said, "Why not?" He said, "Because somebody might rob me." I said, "Please, nobody's going to rob you. Where is your God? Where's your faith? What are you worried about?"... You got all this God and you can go home at the end of the day and close your door and lock your door and you can go and sleep. You got all these people that sleep out in the street on a daily basis. You can't do it for one day? I have places I still go out and go and sleep, and be fine.

"Yeah?"

I still go nap on the Green on a bench. I just sit up like this and nap and sometimes just lay my head on the metal part without a pillow and just nap there. And I'm comfortable still. I'm not spoiled like that. I don't ever want to get spoiled like him and do something like that.

"There's something valuable in being able to be out in the world."

I feel like that's priceless, to be able to do something like that. You can't take that from me. Only God gave me that blessing. You can't take that from me. That means something to me . . . I can have money in my pocket and still stop and go to sleep for an hour or two. Feed the birds . . . I was watching the little kids on the Green chasing the birds and stuff. I love watching kids play. I love that in snow or whatever. That's the joy I get out of Christmas and my birthday . . . watching kids play in the snow, the lights around town . . . Just being out there with nobody. I have no way to celebrate my birthday. My family doesn't come looking for me. I ate out of garbage cans to survive. I slept behind the school. I slept in trucks that were parked in somebody's yard and got out of there before they would come out. I've done stuff.

"But something came out of it from what I'm hearing you say."

I count blessings every day. I count blessings when I wake up. That's a blessing to me . . . I appreciate that. I'm seeing another day without a broken bone. I don't have no enemies. My enemies are my friends. My enemies that were my enemies to this day, they're not my enemy no more. They don't bother me. They don't move me. They're speaking to me.

These are inspiring words, good enough to end a book with. But this is a book about citizenship and mental health. So, two citizens, one privileged by usual standards and one not, meet to talk about life and citizenship. The citizen lacking in privilege teaches and inspires the one who has it. Or, you can find the 5 Rs of citizenship in Ned's words without looking too hard. His responsibility toward his son, the richness of his inner resources in contrast to the poverty of his outer resources . . . But finding the 5 Rs when you're looking for them can get a little too easy, a little too pat. Something else came up for me, though, the second time I read this part of the interview. "Flourishing," and what people need for it, came to mind. I gravitated, naturally, toward affective goods and instrumental goods, and the combination of the two, as the answer. I thought about part of the work of citizenship as helping people build skills and gain access to tools that can help them make it in society. But another part of the work, Ned made me think, is to give people a place for learning, yes, but one that also allows enough gaps in it teaching and process to nourish an inner flourishing and give it room to come out.

I don't know how much the *Citizens Project* helped Ned. He says it did. And inner flourishing or not, he continues to struggle. A week after interviewing him,

Christa got a phone call from him asking if there were any studies she was doing that he could get paid for. He'd just lost his housing. But that moment, or two hours, of Ned teaching his interviewer is still a cause for celebration, I think. To celebrate means to praise publicly or observe an occasion with ceremony or festivity. We honor what we celebrate. Between troubles and the facing of them, we also remind ourselves to celebrate, and are encouraged.

NOTES

Preface

1. Allison Ponce was the first among our research group to talk about the "aspirational" nature of citizenship. Aspiration may be implied in the 5 Rs of rights, responsibilities, roles, resources, and relationships of citizenship as we define it, but naming a quality changes its presence. A similar example is Chyrell Bellamy's pointing out the "rites of passage" elements of the *Citizens Project*. We were dimly aware of this idea—I even came across the term among the archives of one of our published articles—but did nothing with it until Chyrell brought Shadd Maruna's work on it to our attention. Maruna uses the concept in relation to prisoners being released to their communities after serving their sentences.

Chapter 1

1. Rowe M. *Crossing the border: Encounters between homeless people and outreach workers*. Berkeley, CA: University of California Press, 1999. Many passages in this chapter and others draw on material from this book, and the book's relevance can be assumed without further citation. I do cite my and my colleague's other publications on homelessness and outreach work, in their places.

2. Rowe M, Hoge MA, Fisk D. The bright yellow sneakers: A case example of assertive outreach with mentally ill homeless persons. *Continuum: Developments in Ambulatory Health Care*, 1996, 3 (4), 265–269. Here and throughout I've changed names, biographical details, and clinical information that might identify clients. I've also changed names for people—clients or not—whom I've not been able to find if I have any doubt about whether or not they'd want to be identified.

3. The text of *Crossing the Border* has Jim responding "Good" to my question about the food. I wrote the book considerably earlier in time, but the repeated "You asked the question, you already know the answer" seems more characteristic of Jim and is what I remember now, although my memory have have correct then and be faulty here.

4. The term, and the title of Edgar Allan Poe's eponymous story, refers to the urge to knowingly say or do the wrong thing at the wrong time, to one's own harm.

5. Sells D, Davidson L, Jewell C, Falzer P, Rowe M. The treatment relationship in peer-based and regular case management services for clients with severe mental illness. *Psychiatric Services*, 2006, 57 (8), 1179–1184.

6. Sells D, Black R, Davidson L, Rowe M. Beyond generic support: The incidence and impact of invalidation within peer-based and traditional treatment for clients with severe mental illness. *Psychiatric Services,* 2008, 59 (11), 1322–1327.

7. Rossi PH. *Down and out in America: The origins of homelessness.* Chicago: University of Chicago Press, 1989.

8. Rowe M, Hoge M, Fisk D. Critical issues in serving people who are homeless and mentally ill. *Administration and Policy in Mental Health*, 1996, 23 (6), 555–565.

9. Ibid.

10. Cohen NL & Tsemberis S. Emergency psychiatric interventions on the street. *New Directions for Mental Health Services*, 1991, 52, 3–16.

11. *Reaching out: A guide for service providers*. Washington, DC: Interagency Council on the Homeless, 1991.

12. Chafetz L. Why clinicians distance themselves from the homeless mentally ill. In RH Lamb, LL Bachrach, FI Kass, eds. *Treating the homeless mentally ill: A report of the task force on the homeless mentally ill.* Washington, DC: American Psychiatric Association, 1992, 95–107.

13. Cohen NL & Marcos LR. Outreach intervention models for the homeless mentally ill. In RH Lamb, LL Bachrach, FI Kass, eds. *Treating the homeless mentally ill: A report on the task force on the homeless mentally ill.* Washington, DC: American Psychiatric Association, 1992, 141–157.

14. Swayze FV. Clinical case management with the homeless mentally ill. In RH Lamb, LL Bachrach, FI Kass, eds. *Treating the homeless mentally ill: A report of the task force on the homeless mentally ill.* Washington, DC: American Psychiatric Association, 1992, 203–219.

15. Morse GA, Calsyn RJ, Miller J, Rosenberg P, West L, Gilliland J. Outreach to homeless mentally ill people: Conceptual and clinical considerations. *Community Mental Health Journal*, 1996, 32 (3), 261–274.

16. Randolph F. Improving service systems through systems integration: The ACCESS program. *American Rehabilitation,* 1995, 21, 36–38.

17. Randolph F, Blasinsky M, Leginski W, Parker LB, Goldman HH. Creating integrated service systems for homeless persons with mental illness: The ACCESS Program. *Psychiatric Services*, 1997, 48 (3), 369–371.

18. Agranoff R. Human service integration: Past and present challenges in public administration. *Public Administration Review*, 1991, 51, 533–542.

19. Randolph F, op cit.

20. MacBeth G. Collaboration can be elusive: Virginia's experience in developing an interagency system of care. *Administration and Policy in Mental Health*, 1993, 20, 259–281.

21. Buckley R & Bigelow DA. The multi-service network: Reaching the underserved multi-problem individual. *Community Mental Health Journal*, 1992, 28, 43–50.

22. Substance Abuse and Mental Health Services Administration. *Services integration: A twenty-year perspective*, 1991.

23. Weiss J. Substance versus symbol in administrative reform: The case of human services coordination. *Policy Analysis*, 1981, 7 (2), 21–45.

24. Warren RL, Rose S, Bergunder AF. *The structure of urban reform.* Lexington, MA: Lexington Books, 1974.

25. Warren RL. Comprehensive planning and coordination: Some functional aspects. *Social Problems*, 1973, 2 (3), 355–364.

26. See also Snow DA, Baker SG, Anderson L, Martin M. The myth of pervasive mental illness among the homeless. *Social Problems*, 1986, 33 (5), 407–423.

27. Jacobson N. *Dignity and health*. Nashville: Vanderbilt University Press, 2012.

28. Rowe, 1999, 107.

29. Goffman E. *Strategic interaction.* Philadelphia: University of Pennsylvania Press, 1969, 3.

30. http://store.samhsa.gov/shin/content/SMA04-3870/SMA04-3870.pdf.

31. http://www.prainc.com/soar/cms-assets/documents/74697-776854.homelessness-defs081512.pdf. See also http://homeless.samhsa.gov/ResourceFiles/0abwdb1u.pdf.

32. Erikson K. *A new species of trouble: Explorations in disaster, trauma, and community.* New York: Norton, 1994, 158.

33. Ibid, 159.

34. Hoffman RE. A social deafferentation hypothesis for induction of active schizophrenia. *Schizophrenia Bulletin,* 2007, 33 (5), 1066–1070. doi: 10.1093/schbul/sbm079.

Chapter 2

1. See Ware NC, Hopper K, Tugenberg T, Dickey B, Fisher D. Connectedness and citizenship: Redefining social integration. *Psychiatric Services,* 2007, 58 (4), 469–474.

2. Rowe M, Kloos B, Chinman M, Davidson L, Cross AB. Homelessness, mental illness and citizenship. *Social Policy and Administration* 2001, 35, 14–31. This article is the primary source for the material on *Citizens* in this chapter, not including the sections ion the book, *As I Sat on the Green,* and on the *Leadership Project.*

3. Author's interview with Lezley TwoBears, November 22, 2013. Unless otherwise noted, as in my stated memory of a conversation with Lezley, quotations from her in this chapter come from this interview.

4. "Moments" is a term I've adapted from a Norma Ware article on social inclusion and capacity building for people with mental illnesses: Ware NC, Hopper K, Tugenberg T, Dickey R, Fisher D. A theory of social inclusion as quality of life. *Psychiatric Services,* 2008, 59 (1), 27–33.

5. Baumgartner JN & Herman DB. Community integration of formerly homeless men and women with severe mental illness after hospital discharge. *Psychiatric Services,* 2012, *63* (5), 435–437.

6. Tsai J, Mares S, Rosenheck RA. Does housing chronically mentally ill adults lead to social integration? *Psychiatric Services,* 2012, *63* (5), 427–434.

7. Yanos PT, Stefanic A, Tsemberis S. Objective community integration of mental health consumers living in supported housing and of others in the community. *Psychiatric Services,* 2012, *63* (5), 438–444.

8. Heater D. *A brief history of citizenship.* New York: New York University Press, 2004.

9. Tocqueville AD. *Democracy in America: Volumes I & II.* H Reeve, trans. New York: Alfred E. Knopf, 1953, 1945.

10. Durkheim É. *Division of labor in society.* G Simpson, trans. London: Collier Macmillan, 1933.

11. Marshall TH. *Class, citizenship and social development.* Chicago: University of Chicago Press, 1964.

12. Janoski T. *Citizenship and civil society: A framework of rights and obligations in liberal, traditional, and social democratic regimes.* Cambridge, UK: Cambridge University Press, 1998.

13. Bellah RN, Madsen R, Sullivan WM, Swidler A, Tipton SM. *Habits of the heart: Individualism and commitment in American life*. Berkeley, CA: University of California Press, 1996.

14. Werbner P & Yuval-Davis N. Women and the new discourse of citizenship. In N Yuval-Davis & P Werbner, eds: *Women, citizenship and difference*. New York: Zed Books, 1999, 1–31.

15. Lister R. Dialectics of citizenship. *Hypatia*, 1997, 12 (4), 6–26. doi: 10.1111/j.1527-2001.1997.tb00296.x.

16. Duffy S. The citizenship theory of social justice: Exploring the meaning of personalisation for social workers. *Journal of Social Work Practice: Psychotherapeutic Approaches in Health, Welfare, and the Community*, 2010, 24 (3), 253–267. doi: 10.1080/02650533.2010.500118.

17. Goffman E. *Asylums: Essays on the social situation of mental patients and other inmates*. New York: Anchor Books, 1961.

18. Gambino MJ. *Mental health and ideals of citizenship: Patient care at St. Elizabeth's Hospital in Washington, D.C., 1903-1962*. Urbana, IL: University of Illinois, 2011.

19. Anderson ES. What is the point of equality? *Ethics*, 1999, 109, 287–337.

20. Mouffe C. *The return of the political*. London: Verso Press, 2005.

21. Honneth A. *The struggle for recognition: The moral grammar of social conflict*. J Anderson, trans. Cambridge, MA: MIT Press, 1995.

22. Rowe M & Pelletier J-F. Citizenship: A response to the marginalization of people with mental illnesses. *Journal of Forensic Psychology Practice*, 2012, 12 (4), 366–381. doi: 10.1080/15228932.2012.697423.

23. See McKnight JL. Regenerating community. *Social Policy,* 1987, Winter, 54–58 for his comments on associational life. This term is derived from de Tocqueville's "associationalism" involving voluntary contributions to community life and spirit, and the forming of associational bodies as defenses against increasing state domination of society.

24. Bourdieu P. Forms of capital. In JG Richardson, ed. *Handbook of theory and research for the sociology of education*. New York: Greenwood Press, 1983, 241–258.

25. Coleman JS: *Foundations of social theory*. Cambridge, MA: Belknap, 1990.

26. Portes A: Social capital: Its origins and applications in modern sociology. *Annual Review of Sociology*, 24, 1998, 1–24.

27. Hannum R, Myers-Parelli A, Schoenfeld P, Cameron C, Campbell H, Chrismer L. Promoting social integration among people with psychiatric disabilities. *Innovations & Research*, 1994, 3, 17–23.

28. Thoits PA. Multiple identities: Examining gender and marital status differences in distress. *American Sociological Review*, 1986, 51 (2), 259–272.

29. Hall S & Cheston R. Mental health and identity: The evaluation of a drop-in centre. *Journal of Community and Applied Social Psychology*, 2002, *12* (1), 30–43.

30. Stryker S & Burke PJ. The past, present, and future of an identity theory. *Social Psychology Quarterly*, 2000, 63 (4), 284–297.

31. Cast AD & Burke PJ. A theory of self-esteem. *Social Forces*, 2002, 80 (3), 1041–1068.

32. Deaux K & Martin D. Interpersonal networks and social categories: Specifying levels of context in identity processes. *Social Psychology Quarterly*, 2003, 66 (2), 101–117.

33. Davidson L, Mezzina R, Rowe M & Thompson K. "A life in the community": Italian mental health reform and recovery. *Journal of Mental Health*, 2010, 19 (5), 436–443.

34. Anthony WA. Recovery from mental illness: The guiding vision of mental health service systems in the 1990s. *Psychosocial Rehabilitation Journal*, 1993, 16, 11–23.

35. Davidson L & Roe D. Recovery from versus recovery in serious mental illness: One strategy for lessening confusion plaguing recovery. *Journal of Mental Health*, 2007, 16 (4), 459–470. doi: 10.1080/09n638230701482394.

36. Larry Davidson uses the "living outside" term in his book, *Living outside mental illness: Qualitative studies of recovery in schizophrenia*. New York: New York University Press, 2005.

37. *The President's New Freedom Commission on Mental Health. Achieving the promise: Transforming mental health care in America*. Rockville, MD: DHHS Pub. No. SMA-03-3832, 2003.

38. Davidson L, Tondora J, O'Connell M, Lawless M, Rowe M. *Transforming mental health care: A practical guide to recovery-oriented practice*. New York: Oxford University Press, 2008.

39. Weisser J, Morrow M, James B. *A critical exploration of social integration in the mental health recovery literature*. Vancouver, BC: Centre for the Study of Gender, Social Inequities, and Mental Health. (CCSM) http:www.socialinequities.ca, 2011.

40. Hopper K. The counter-reformation that failed? A commentary on the mixed legacy of supportive housing. *Psychiatric Services*, 2012, 63 (5), 461–463.

41. Edgley A, Stickley T, Wright N, Repper J. The politics of recovery in mental health: A left libertarian policy analysis. *Social Theory & Health*, 2012, 10 (2), 121–140. doi: 10.1057/sth.2012.1.

42. Turner-Crowson J & Wallcraft J. The recovery vision for mental health services and research: A British perspective. *Psychiatric Rehabilitation Journal*, 2002, 25, 245–254.

43. During the Civil Rights era of the 1950s and 1960s in the United States, African Americans, then "negroes" or, more derisively, "colored" people in segregated Southern states, were expected to sit at the back of the bus, with whites in the front.

44. Davidson L, Stayner DA, Nickou C, Styron TH, Rowe M, Chinman MJ. "Simply to be let in": Inclusion as a basis for recovery from mental illness. *Psychiatric Rehabilitation Journal*, 2001, 24, 375–388.

45. Silver H & Miller SM. Social exclusion: The European approach to social disadvantage. *Indicators*, 2003, 2 (2), 1–17.

46. Randolph, Improving service systems, op cit.

47. Hopper K. Rethinking social recovery in schizophrenia: What a capabilities approach might offer. *Social Science & Medicine*, 2007, 65, 868–879.

48. Jacobson, op cit, chapter 1.

49. Sen A. Well-being, agency and freedom: The Dewey lectures, 1984. *The Journal of Philosophy*, 1985, 82 (4), 169–221.

50. Hopper K. The counter-reformation that failed? A commentary on the mixed legacy of supportive housing. *Psychiatric Services*, 2012, 63 (5), 461–463.

51. Mattison A, Benedict P, TwoBears L. *As I sat on the green: Living without a home in New Haven*. New Haven, CT: Citizens Project/Columbus House, 2000, vi.

52. Rowe, *Crossing the border*, op cit.

53. Butterfoss FD, Goodman RM, Wandersman A. Community coalitions for prevention and health promotion. *Health Education Research,* 1993, 8 (3), 315–330.

54. Francisco VT, Paine AL, Fawcett SB. A methodology for monitoring and evaluating community health coalitions. *Health Education Research,* 1993, 8, 403–416.

55. Kloos B, Benedict P, TwoBears L, Rowe M. *Citizens process evaluation: Documenting the creation of a community-based organization.* New Haven, CT: Consultation Center, 1999.

56. Mattison A, Benedict PO, TwoBears L. *As I sat on the green: Living without a home in New Haven.* New Haven, CT: Columbus House, 2000, 4.

57. Ibid, 6.

58. Ibid, 6.

59. Ibid, 8.

60. Ibid, 9.

61. Ibid, 10.

62. Rowe M, Benedict P, Falzer P. Representation of the governed: Leadership building for people with behavioral health disorders who are homeless or were formerly homeless. *Psychiatric Rehabilitation Journal,* 2003, 26 (3), 240–248. This paper is the primary source for this section. Other sources are also cited.

63. Gutierrez LM. Beyond coping: An empowerment perspective on stressful life events. *Journal of Sociology and Social Welfare,* 1994, 21 (3), 201–219.

64. Snow DA & Anderson L. Identity work among the homeless. *American Journal of Sociology,* 1987, 97, 1337–1371.

65. Berger PL & Neuhaus RJ. *To empower people: The role of mediating structures in public policy.* Washington, DC: American Enterprise Institute for Public Policy, 1977.

66. Callahan S, Mayer N, Palmer K, Ferlazzo L. Rowing the boat with two oars. *NFG Reports,* 1998, 3 (5), 3

Chapter 3

1. Communication to the author from Madelon Baranoski to the author on January 13, 2014.

2. Hopper K, Jost J, Hay T, Welber S, Haugland G. Homelessness, severe mental illness and the institutional circuit. *Psychiatric Services,* 1997, 48 (5), 659–665.

3. Lamb HR & Weinberger L. The shift of psychiatric inpatient care from hospitals to jails and prisons. *Journal of the American Academy of Psychiatry and the Law,* 2005, 33 (4), 529–534.

4. Department of Justice. Mental health problems of prison and jail inmates. *Bureau of Justice Statistics Special Report,* 2006, NCJ 213600.

5. Baillargeon J, Binswanger IA, Penn JV, Williams BA, Murray OJ. Psychiatric disorders and repeat incarcerations: The revolving prison door. *American Journal of Psychiatry,* 2009, 166, 103–109.

6. Baillargeon J, Hoge SK, Penn JV. Addressing the challenge of community reentry among released inmates with serious mental Illness. *American Journal of Community Psychology,* 2010, 46, 361–375.

7. Hoge SK. Providing transition and outpatient services to the mentally ill released from correctional institutions. In RB Greifinger, ed. *Public health behind bars: From prisons to communities.* New York: Springer, 2007, 461–477

8. Roman C & Travis J. *Taking stock: Housing, homelessness, and prisoner reentry.* Washington, DC: Urban Institute, 2004.

9. McNeil DE, Binder RL, Robinson JC. Incarceration associated with homelessness, mental disorder, and co-occurring substance abuse. *Psychiatric Services*, 2005, 56, 840–846.

10. Hartwell S. Triple stigma: Persons with mental illnesses and substances abuse problems in the criminal justice system. *Criminal Justice Policy Review*, 2004, 15, 84–99.

11. Osher FC & Steadman HJ. Adapting evidence-based practices for persons with mental illness involved with the criminal justice system. *Psychiatric Services*, 2007, 58, 1472–1478.

12. Uggen C, Manza J, Thompson M. Citizenship, democracy, and the civic reintegration of criminal offenders. *Annals, American Academy of Political and Social Science*, 2006, 281–310.

13. Rowe M & Baranoski M. Mental illness, criminality, and citizenship. *Journal of the American Academy of Psychiatry and the Law*, 2000, 28 (3), 262 261.

14. Lamberti JS, Weisman R, Faden DI. Forensic assertive community treatment: Preventing incarceration of adults with severe mental illness. *Psychiatric Services*, 2004, 55 (11), 1285–1293. doi: 10.1176/appi.ps.55.11.1285.

15. Mueser K, Myer PS, Penn DL, Clany R, Clancy DM, Salyers MP. The illness management and recovery program: Rationale, development, and preliminary findings. *Schizophrenia Bulletin Suppl 1,* 2006, 32, S32–S43.

16. Burns T, Catty J, Baker T, Drake RE, Fioritti A, Knapp M, Lauber C, Rössler W, Tomov T, Busschbach J van, White S, Wiersma D. The effectiveness of supported employment for people with severe mental illness: A randomised controlled trial. *Lancet*, 2007, 370 (9593), 1146–1152.

17. Bellamy CD, Garvin C, MacFarlane P, Mowbray OP, Mowbray CT, Holter MC. An analysis of groups in consumer-centered programs. *American Journal of Psychiatric Rehabilitation,* 2006, 9 (3), 219–240.

18. Panas L, Yael C, Fournier E, McCarty D. Performance measures for outpatient substance abuse services: Group versus individual therapy. *Journal of Substance Abuse Treatment*, 2003, 25 (4), 271–278.

19. Taxman FS & Bouffard JA. Substance abuse counselors' treatment philosophy and the content of treatment services provided to offenders in drug court programs. *Journal of Substance Abuse Treatment*, 2003, 25 (2), 75–84.

20. Flores PJ. *Group therapy with addicted populations: An integration of twelve-step and psychodynamic theory, 2nd ed.* New York: The Haworth Press, 1997.

21. Fram DH. Group methods in the treatment of substance abusers. *Psychiatric Annals*, 1990, 20 (7), 385–388.

22. Vannicelli M. *Removing the roadblocks: Group psychotherapy with substance abusers and family members.* New York: Guilford Press, 1992.

23. Garvin CD. A task-centered group approach to work with the chronically mentally ill. *Social Work with Groups*, 1992, 15 (2/3), 67–80.

24. Kurtz LF. *Self-help and support groups: A handbook for practitioners.* Thousand Oaks, CA: Sage, 1997.

25. Garvin CD. *Contemporary group work.* Boston: Allyn and Bacon, 1997.

26. Connors GJ, Tonigan JS, Miller WR. A longitudinal model of intake symptomatology, AA participation and outcome: Retrospective study of the project MATCH outpatient and aftercare samples. *Journal of Studies on Alcohol*, 2001, 62, 817–825.

27. Humphreys K. Professional interventions that facilitate 12-step self-help group involvement. *Alcohol Research and Health*, 1999, 23, 93–98.

28. Humphreys K, Moos RH, Cohen C. Social and community resources and long-term recovery from treated and untreated alcoholism. *Journal of Studies on Alcohol*, 1997, 58(3), 231–239.

29. McKellar J, Stewart E, Humphreys K. Alcoholics Anonymous involvement and positive alcohol-related outcomes: Cause, consequence, or just a correlate? A prospective 2-year study of 2,319 alcohol-dependent men. *Journal of Consulting and Clinical Psychology*, 2003, 71, 302–308.

30. Moos RH & Moos BS. Sixteen-year changes and stable remission among treated and untreated individuals with alcohol use disorders. *Drug and Alcohol Dependence*, 2005, 80 (3), 337–347.

31. Moos RH & Moos BS. Participation in treatment and alcoholics anonymous: A 16-year follow-up of initially untreated individuals. *Journal of Clinical Psychology*, 2006, 62 (6), 735–750.

32. Noordsy D, Torrey W, Mueser K, Mead S, O'Keefe C, Fox L. Recovery from severe mental illness: An intrapersonal and functional outcome definition. *International Review of Psychiatry*, 2002, 14, 318–326.

33. Rowe, Citizenship, community, and recovery, op cit. This, and the next two references are among the papers that give the most detailed descriptions of *Citizens Project* components.

34. Rowe & Baranoski, 2011, op cit.

35. Rowe M & Pelletier J-F. Citizenship: A response to the marginalization of people with mental illnesses. *Journal of Forensic Psychology Practice*, 2012, 12 (4), 366–381. doi: 10.1080/15228932.2012.697423.

36. Snow and Anderson, Identity work, op cit.

37. Copeland ME. What is wellness recovery action plan® (WRAP®)? http://www.mentalhealthrecovery.com/wrap/. Accessed on January 5, 2014.

38. Davidson L, Chinman M, Sells D, Rowe M. Peer support among adults with serious mental illness: A report from the field. *Schizophrenia Bulletin*, 2006, 32 (3), 443–450.

39. Christens BD. Toward relational empowerment. *American Journal of Community Psychology*, 2012, 50 (1–2), 114–128. doi: 10.1007/s10464-011-9483-5.

40. Fisk D, Rowe M, Brooks R, Gildersleeve D. Integrating consumer staff into a homeless outreach project: Critical issues and strategies. *Psychiatric Rehabilitation Journal*, 2000, 23 (3), 244–252.

41. See also Rowe M. Alternatives to outpatient commitment. *Journal of the American Academy of Psychiatry and the Law*, 2013, 41 (3), 332–336, for information on outpatient commitment.

42. Barrett-Leonard GT. Dimensions of therapist response as causal factors in therapeutic change. *Psychological Monographs*, 1962, 76, 1–36.

43. Simmons J, Roberge L, Kendrick BS. The interpersonal relationship in clinical practice: The Barrett-Leonard Inventory as an assessment instrument. *Evaluation and the Health Professions*, 1995, 18, 103–112.

44. Sells, 2006, op cit.

45. Sells, 2008, op cit.

46. Davidson L & Rowe M. *Peer support within criminal justice settings: The role of forensic peer specialists*. National GAINS Center, 2007.

47. Maruna S. Reentry as a rite of passage. *Punishment and Society*, 20i1, 13, 3–28.

48. Rowe, op cit, 32.

49. This quote and others in this chapter are from a 2013 interview with Patty Benedict.

50. This quote is from a circa 1995 interview with Ned.

51. This quote is from a 2013 interview with Ned.

52. The following section on course topics and themes and students' connection to them is adapted from Stacy Brown's unpublished paper, "Student-teacher interviews."

53. This is another example of the absurdities that are inseparable at times, or of a piece with, the logic that gives bureaucracy its ability to take human service work to scale. The Salvation Army shelter did not qualify as an emergency shelter by HUD's algorithm, and thus Carlos, while staying there, did not meet HUD's eligibility requirements for permanent supported housing for people who are homeless, and had to become "more homeless" in order to achieve that status.

54. Wang C & Burris MA. Empowerment through Photo Novella: Portraits of participation. *Health Education & Behavior*, 1994, 21 (2), 171–186. doi: 10.1177/109019819402100204.

55. Rowe M, Bellamy C, Baranoski M, Wieland M, O'Connell M, Benedict P, Davidson, L, Buchanan J, Sells D. Reducing alcohol use, drug use and criminality among persons with severe mental illness. *Psychiatric Services*, 2007, 58 (7), 955–961. This and the Clayton et al. article following are sources for more detailed explanations of research procedures on the randomized controlled trial of the *Citizens Project*.

56. Clayton A, O'Connell M, Bellamy C, Benedict P, Rowe M. The citizenship project, part II: Impact of a citizenship intervention on clinical and community outcomes for persons with mental illness and criminal justice charges. *American Journal of Community Psychology*, 2012, 45 (2). doi: 10.1007/s10464-012-9549-z.

57. Teplin LA. Psychiatric and substance abuse disorders among male urban jail detainees. *American Journal of Public Health*, 1994, 84, 290–293.

58. Johnson SL, Sandrow D, Myer B, Winters R, Miller I, Solomon D, Keitner G. Increase in manic symptoms after life events in goal attainment. *Journal of Abnormal Psychology*, 2000, 109 (4), 721–727.

59. Myers J, Lindenthal J, Pepper M. Life events, social integration and psychiatric symptomology. *Journal of Health and Social Behavior*, 1975, 16 (4), 421–427.

60. Bolton JM, Robinson J. Sareen J. Self-medication of mood disorders with alcohol and drugs in the National Epidemiologic Survey on Alcohol and Related Conditions. *Journal of Affective Disorders*, 2009, 115 (3), 367–375

Chapter 4

1. Except for the interviews from which I quote individuals later in this chapter, student comments come from focus groups conducted periodically over the past 10 years. They were not audiotaped, but detailed notes were taken.

2. Significant parts of this chapter draw from, quote, or edit material from Patty Benedict's project notes or responses to my queries.

3. Swidler A. Culture in action: Symbols and strategies. *American Sociological Review*, 1986, 51, 273–286.

4. See Nisbet RA. *The quest for community: A study in the ethics of order & freedom*. New York: Oxford University Press, 1953.

5. Kim Hopper and Jim Baumohl may not actually use this term, but they say as much in talking about surplus populations of people who are homeless and do not have access

to valued roles in society in their article, Held in abeyance: Rethinking homelessness and advocacy. *American Behavioral Scientist*, 1994, 37 (4), 522–552. doi: 10.1177/00027642940 37004007.

6. Honneth, op cit.

7. Kant I. Grounding for the metaphysics of morals. In Michael Morgan, ed. *Classics of moral and political theory*. Indianapolis: Hackett, 1992, 991–1041.

8. Honneth, op cit.

9. See Yule G. 2006. *The study of language, third ed.* Cambridge, UK: Cambridge University Press, 2006.

10. Habermas J. *Legitimation crisis.* T McCarthy, trans. Boston: Beacon Press, 1973.

11. Outhwaite W. *The Habermas reader*. Cambridge, UK: Polity Press, 1996. Note: both Thomas McCarthy, translator of *Legitimation crisis*, and William Outhwaite, editor of *The Habermas reader*, give excellent introductions to Habermas' work that I have drawn on, as well as Habermas himself.

12. Maruna, op cit.

13. Maruna & LeBel, op cit.

14. Simon J. *Poor discipline: Parole and the social control of the underclass, 1890–1990.* Chicago: University of Chicago Press, 1993.

15. Cohen P & Cohen J. The clinician's illusion. *Archives of General Psychiatry*, 1984, 41 (12), 1178–1182. doi: 10.1001/archpsyc.1984.01790230064010.

16. Giddens A. *Modernity and self-identity: Self and society in the late modern age.* Stanford, CA: Stanford University Press, 1991, 26–27.

17. The full story that Nicholas told me is a good deal longer and more complex than what I've included. This abbreviated version shortchanges the nuances if the male power struggle that Nicholas described himself as having taken part in with the male geese, and the lessons he claims to have taught them. Still, I think this version captures the "community" aspect of his story that is also present in the longer version.

18. http://sakisan.hubpages.com/hub/What-is-K2-drug-Answered.

Chapter 5

1. Marshall, *Class, citizenship and social development*, op cit.

2. Bellah et al., op cit.

3. Most of the measure development text in this chapter is derived and edited from Rowe M, Clayton A, Benedict P, Bellamy C, Antunes K, Miller R, Pelletier J, Stern E, O'Connell MJ. Going to the source: Citzenship outcome measure development. *Psychiatric Services*, 2012, 63, 461–463.

4. Trochim WM & Kane M. Concept mapping: An introduction to structured conceptualization in health care. *International Journal for Quality in Health Care*, 2005, 17, 187–191.

5. *Diagnostic and statistical manual of mental disorders 4th ed., text revision.* Washington, DC: American Psychiatric Association, 2000.

6. Kessler RC, Berglund P, Demler O, Jin R, Merikangas KR, Walters EE. Lifetime prevalence and age-of-onset distributions of DSM-IV disorders in the National Comorbidity Survey Replication. *Archives of General Psychiatry*, 2005, 62, 593–602.

7. Stanton A & Revenson T. Adjustment to chronic disease: progress and promise in research, In Friedman HS & Silver RC. *Foundations of Health Psychology.* New York: Oxford University Press, 2006.

8. Pickett SA, Cook JA, Cohler BJ. Caregiving burden experienced by parents of offspring with severe mental illness: Impact of off-timedness. *Journal of Applied Social Sciences*, 1994, 18, 199–207.

9. Fine M, Torre ME, Boudin K, Bowen I, Judith C, Hylton D, Martinez M, Rivera M, Roberts RA, Smart P, Upegui D. Participatory action research: From within and beyond prison bars. In Camic J, Rhodes JE, Yardley L, eds. *Qualitative research in psychology: Expanding perspectives in methodology and design.* Washington, DC: American Psychological Association, 2003, 173–198.

10. Viswanathan M, Ammerman A, Eng E, Garlehner G, Lohr KN, Griffith D, Rhodes S, Samuel-Hodge C, Maty S, Lux L, Webb L, Sutton SF, Swinson T, Jackman A, Whitener L. *Community-based participatory research: Assessing the evidence.* AHRQ pub no 04-E022-2. Rockville, MD: Agency for Healthcare Research and Quality, 2004.

11. Wallerstein NB & Duran B. Using community-based participatory research to address health disparities. *Health Promotion Practice*, 2006, 7, 312–323.

12. *Concept System Software, Version 4.0.* Ithaca, NY: Concept Systems, Inc., 2007.

13. Davidson ML. *Multidimensional scaling.* New York: Wiley, 1983.

14. Everitt B. *Cluster analysis, 2nd ed.* New York: Halsted, 1980.

15. This sub-section is based on a paper under review: O'Connell MJ, Clayton A, Stern E, Bellamy C, Benedict P, Rowe M. Reliability and validity of a newly-developed measure of citizenship among persons with mental illness.

16. Streiner DL. Starting at the beginning: an introduction to coefficient alpha and internal consistency. *Journal of Personality Assessment*, 2003, 80, 99–103.

17. http://www.socialresearchmethods.net/kb/convdisc.php. Accessed February 22, 2014.

18. Lehman AF. A quality of life interview for the chronically mentally ill. *Evaluation and Program Planning*, 1988, 11, 51–62.

19. Hogan D & Owen D. Social capital, active citizenship and political equality in Australia. In I Winter, ed., *Social Capital and Public Policy in Australia.* Melbourne: Australian Institute of Family Studies, 2000, 74–103.

20. McMillan D & Chavis D. Sense of community: A definition and theory. *Journal of Community Psychology*, 1986, 14, 6–23.

21. Ridgway P. The recovery markers questionnaire. Unpublished.

22. SPSS, IBM. *SPSS Statistics Version 19.0.0.1;* 2010.

23. Freedman DA. *Statistical models: Theory and practice.* Cambridge, UK: Cambridge University Press, 2005, 23.

24. Hocking RR. The analysis and selection of variables in linear regression. *Biometrics*, 1976, 32.

25. This sub-section is based on an unpublished report written by Patricia Benedict and Erica Stern.

26. Portis EB. Citizenship and personal identity. *Polity*, 1986, 18 (3), 457–472.

27. This section draws heavily on Ponce AN, Clayton A, Noia J, Rowe M, O'Connell MO. Making meaning of citizenship: Mental illness, forensic involvement, and homelessness. *Journal of Forensic Psychology Practice*, 2012, 12 (4), 349–365. doi: 10.1080/15228932.2012.695660.

28. Ware et al., Social connectedness, op cit.

29. See Chiricos T, Barrick K, Bales W, Bontrager S. The labeling of convicted felons and its consequences for recidivism. *Criminology*, 2007, 45 (3), 547–581. doi: 10.1111/j.1745-9125.2007.00089.x.

30. Goffman, *Asylums*, op cit.

31. Stellar JE, Manzo VM, Kraus MW, Keltner D. Class and compassion: Socioeconomic factors predict responses to suffering. *Emotion*, 2012, 12 (3), 449–459. doi: 10.1037/a0026508

Chapter 6

1. Mueser, Illness management and recovery, op cit.

2. Rowe, op cit.

3. Ibid, 147.

4. Ibid, 147.

5. Wiseman J. *Stations of the lost: The treatment of Skid-Row alcoholics*. Englewood Cliffs, NJ: Prentice-Hall, 1970.

6. MacKay K. Compounding conditional citizenship: To what extent does Scottish & English mental health law increase or diminish citizenship? *British Journal of Social Work*, 2011, 41, 931–948. doi:10.1093/bjsw/bc010.

7. Schwartz DB. *Who cares? Rediscovering community*. Boulder, CO: Westview Press, 1999.

8. Davidson et al. *A practical guide*, op cit.

9. Whitley R, Strickler D, Drake RE. Recovery center for people with severe mental illness: A survey of programs. *Community Mental Health Journal*, 2012, 48, 547–556.

10. From Lucile Bruce's e-mail to me.

11. Honneth, op cit.

12. From Chyrell Bellamy's e-mail to me.

13. Allison Ponce made this comment in a *Citizens Collaborative* team meeting.

14. From another Chyrell Bellamy e-mail to me.

15. From Allison Ponce's e-mail to our study group on citizenship-oriented care.

16. Farmer P. Investigating the root causes of the global health crisis:Paul Farmer on TED book, *The upstream doctors*. http://blog.ted.com/2013/06/05/investigating-the-root-causes-of-the-global-health-crisis-paul-farmer-on-the-upstream-doctors/.

17. Manchanda R. *The upstream doctors: Medical innovators track sickness to its source*. New York: TED Books, 2013.

18. See Johnston K. The messy link between slave owners and modern management. http://hbswk.hbs.edu/item/7182.html.

19. Geronimus AT. The weathering hypothesis and the health of African-American women and infants: Evidence and speculations. *Ethnicity & Disease*, 1992, 2 (3), 207–221.

20. Sue DW, Capodilupo CM, Torino GC, Bucceri JM, Holder AMB, Nadal KL, Esquilin M. Racial microaggressions in everyday life: Implications for clinical practice. *American Psychologist*, 2007, 62 (4), 271–286.

21. Benedict P, Guy K, Bellamy PD with Rowe M, Baranoski M, Hunter-Gamble C, Herring Y, TwoBears L, Harper A, Crespo M, Antunes K. *Guide to implementing a citizenship project*, 2014.

22. Schur L, Shields T, Kruse D, Schriner K. Enabling democracy: Disability and voter turnout. *Political Research Quarterly*, 2002, 55 (1), 167–190. doi: 10.1177/10659129 0205500107.

23. Kelly PD. The power gap: Freedom, power and mental illness. *Social Science & Medicine*, 2006, 63 (8), 2118–2128.

24. *Voting and Registration in the Election of November 2012*—Detailed Tables. United States Census Bureau, 2012 http://www.census.gov/hhes/www/socdemo/voting/publications/p20/2012/tables.html.

25. http://www.participatorybudgeting.org/about-participatory-budgeting/what-is-pb/.

26. Most of the text that follows on our Community Building Project and its aftermath comes from documents—a report and a follow-up plan—written by Lucile, Ashley, Billy, and me.

Chapter 7

1. Rans SA & Green M. Project Friendship, Prince George, BC: Bridging the gap. In Rans SA & Mike Green (authors), Kretzmann JP & McKnight JL (co-directors). *Building community connections by engaging the gifts of people on welfare, people with disabilities, people with mental illness, older adults, young people*. Evanston, IL: School of Education and Social Policy, Northwestern University, 2005, 27–40.

2. Kretzmann & McKnight, op cit.

3. This section on *Project Connect* draws heavily from Billy's reports.

4. Hopper K. Redistribution and its discontents: On the prospects of committed work in public mental health and like settings. *Human Organization*, 2006, 65 (2), 218–226.

5. From Billy Bromage's e-mail to me.

6. From another Billy Bromage e-mail to me.

7. Ohmer ML. How theory and research inform citizen participation in poor communities: The ecological perspective and theories on self- and collective efficacy and sense of community. *Journal of Human Behavior in the Social Environment*, 2010, 20 (1), 1–19. doi: 10.1080/10911350093126999.

8. Hopper & Baumohl, op cit.

9. Jacobs J. *The death and life of great American cities*. New York: Vintage Books, 1961.

10. Granovetter MS. The strength of weak ties. *American Journal of Sociology*, 1973, 78 (6), 1360–1380. doi: 10.1086/225469.

11. Wolfe T. *The right stuff*. New York: Farrar, Strauss & Giroux, 1979.

12. I use quotation marks around qualitative and quantitative research in recognition of Jeff Draine's circa 2012 e-mail comments to me that we should abandon these terms, as they fail to give their due to the wide range of research methods available to us today in the social sciences. I agree, but don't know of good alternatives to these terms.

13. Elbogen E, Tiegreen J, Vaughan C, Bradford DW. Money management, mental health, and psychiatric disability: A recovery-oriented model for improving financial skills. *Psychiatric Rehabilitation Journal*, 2011, 34 (3), 223–231.

14. Elbogen E, Bradford D, Swartz M. A recovery-oriented money management intervention. *Psychiatric Services*, 2013, 64 (1), 99.

15. See this article for a similar phrasing of this argument, and relevant research: Rowe M, Serowik KL, Ablondi K, Wilber C, Rosen MI. Recovery and money management. *Psychiatric Rehabilitation Journal*, 2013, 36 (2), 116–118.

16. Noordsy et al., op cit.

17. Rowe, Serowik, et al., op cit.

18. Harper A. *Improving the financial health of Connecticut Mental Health Center (CMHC) clients: Consultancy report for the CMHC-Foundation*, 2012.

19. Much of the literature review and the study described in this section is derived and edited from a research paper: Harper A, Clayton A, Foss-Kelly L, Bailey M, Sernyak M, Rowe M. Financial health and mental health: Making the connections. Under review.

20. Hudson C. Socioeconomic status and mental illness: Tests of the social causation and selection hypotheses. *American Journal of Orthopsychiatry*, 2005, 75 (1), 3–18.

21. Burns JK & Esterhuizen T. Poverty, inequality and the treated incidence of first-episode psychosis: An ecology study from south Africa. *Social Psychiatry and Psychiatric Epidemiology*, 2008, 43, 331–335.

22. El-Mallakh P. Doing my best: Poverty and self-care among individuals with schizophrenia and diabetes mellitus. *Archives of Psychiatric Nursing*, 2007, 21 (1), 49–60.

23. Butterworth, op cit.

24. Jenkins R, Bhugra D, Bebbington P, Brugha T, Farrell M, Coid J, Fryers T, Weich S, Singleton N, Meltzer H. Debt, income and mental disorder in the general population. *Psychological Medicine*, 2008, 38, 1485–1493.

25. FDIC 2012, National survey of unbanked and underbanked households. https://www.fdic.gov/householdsurvey/2012_unbankedreport.pdf.

26. Barr M. *Financial services for low- and moderate-income households: Detroit area household financial services study.* Ann Arbor: Survey Research Center, University of Michigan, 2006.

27. Figar D. Institutionalist policies for financial inclusion. *Journal of Economic Issues*, 2013, XLVII (4), 873–893.

28. Servon L. The real reason the poor go without bank accounts. *The Atlantic Cities Place Matters*, 2013. http://www.theatlanticcities.com/jobs-and-economy/2013/09/why-poor-choose-go-without-bank-accounts/6783/.

29. Rosen M. The check effect reconsidered. *Addiction*, 2011, 106, 1071–1077.

30. Carpenter-Song E. Anthropological perspectives on money management: Considerations for the design and implementation of interventions for substance abuse. *The American Journal of Drug and Alcohol Abuse*, 2012, 38, 49–54. doi: 10.3109/00952990.2011.643980.

31. Swarbrick M. Asset-building, financial self-management service model: Piecing together consumer financial independence. *Journal of Psychosocial Nursing and Mental Health Services*, 2006, 44 (10), 22–26.

32. Burke-Miller JK, Swarbrick M, Carter TM, Jonikas JA, Zipple A, Fraser V, Cook JA. Promoting self-determination and financial security through innovative asset building approaches. *Psychiatric Rehabilitation Journal*, 2010, 34 (2), 104–112. doi: 10.2975/34.2.2010.104.112.

33. Cook JA & Mueser K. Economic security: An essential component of recovery. *Psychiatric Rehabilitation Journal*, 2013, 36 (1), 1–3. doi: 10.1037/h0094739.

34. Sledge J, Gordon S, Knisley M. *Making the shift from financial education to financial capability: Evidence from the financial capability innovation fund.* Center for

Financial Services Innovation, 2011 http://www.cfsinnovation.com/system/files/CFSI_FinCapTrends_Mar2011_final.pdf.

35. CFED 2010, Household financial security framework, http://cfed.org/assets/CFEDHouseholdFramework_4Pager.pdf.

36. Harper A & Rowe M. Financial health and social recovery. *Psychiatric Services*, 2014, 65 (6), 707.

Chapter 8

1. Much of this summary of focus group themes is edited from comments by Matthew Gambino, a psychiatry fellow on the *Citizens Collaborative* team, based on detailed typewritten notes taken during the focus groups. Additional comments from other investigators and me are integrated into the text.

2. Noordsy et al., op cit.

3. My descriptions of the physical characteristics of Bill and Kathy are different than those of the actual interviewees, but I think reflect something of their manner and carriage.

4. See also MacKay, op cit.

5. *Citizens Collaborative* lunch hosts wrote detailed notes, especially for the last three lunch guests. The quotes I give here are close to verbatim for the latter but somewhat less so with the first guest, Rachel. I've tried to take as few liberties as possible with her comments, and "quoted" only those that "read" to me most like speech.

6. See https://www.glide.org/.

7. Weiss, op cit.

8. See also Ponce AN, Lawless M, Rowe M. Homelessness, behavioral health disorders and intimate partner violence: Barriers to services for women. *Community Mental Health Journal*. doi: 10.1007/s10597-014-9712-0. Martha Lawless was the project director of the program I refer to in the text.

9. Salyers MP & Tsemberis S. ACT and recovery: Integrating evidence-based practice and recovery orientation on assertive community treatment teams. *Community Mental Health Journal*, 2007, 43 (6), 619–641.

Chapter 9

1. Tocqueville, op cit.

2. Weber M. *The Protestant ethic and the spirit of capitalism.* T Parsons trans. London: Allen & Unwin, 1976.

3. Weber M. *The theory of social and economic organization.* AM Henderson & T Parsons, trans. London: Collier Macmillan Publishers, 1947.

4. Schwartz, op cit.

5. Susser E, Valencia E, Conover S, Felix A, Tsai W-Y, Wyatt RJ. Preventing recurrent homelessness among mentally ill men: A "critical time" intervention in the aftermath of discharge from a shelter. *American Journal of Public Health*, 1997, 87, 256–262.

6. Paul Johnston, a sociologist at Yale during the 1990s, is the source of this phrase.

7. Goldman HH & Morrissey JP. The alchemy of mental health policy: homelessness and the fourth cycle of reform. *American Journal of Public Health*, 1985, 75 (7), 727–731. doi: 10.2105/AJPH.75.7.727.

8. Charles Perrow, in his book *Normal accidents: Living with high-risk technologies* (New York: Basic Books, 1984), writes of tightly coupled systems for high-technology, high-risk organizations in which each step in the work process must be closely linked with the previous and following steps for the system to function properly and to avoid a potentially disastrous malfunction. In loosely coupled, generally low-technology systems—academia is a good example—work in different parts of the system need not be closely linked with other parts for the system to fulfill its functions.

9. Mandiberg J. Another way: Enclave communities for people with mental illness. *American Journal of Orthopsychiatry*, 2010, 80 (2), 170–176. doi: 10.1111/j.1939-0025.2010. 01020.x.

10. Mandiberg J. The failure of social inclusion: An alternative approach through community development. *Psychiatric Services*, 2012, 63, 458–460. doi: 10.1176/appi.ps. 201100367.

11. Mandiberg J & Warner R. Sustainable innovations for subsistence marketplaces. *Journal of Business Research*, 2012, 65 (12), 1736–1742.

12. Wichowsky A & Moynihan DP. Measuring how administration shapes citizenship: A policy feedback perspective on performance management. *Public Administration Review*, 2008, September-October, 908–920.

13. Rowe, Kloos, et al., op cit.

14. Colomy P & Brown DJ. Goffman and interactional citizenship. *Sociological Perspectives*, 1996, 39 (3), 371–381.

15. Davidson & Rowe, op cit.

16. Rowe & Baranoski, 2000, op cit.

17. Ewalt JR & Ewalt PL. History of the community psychiatry movement. *American Journal of Psychiatry*, 1969, 126 (1), 43–52.

18. Southwick SM & Charney DS. Resilience: The science of mastering life's greatest challenges. New York: Cambridge University Press, 2012.

BIBLIOGRAPHY

Agranoff R. Human service integration: Past and present challenges in public administration. *Public Administration Review*, 1991, 51, 533–542.

Anderson ES. What is the point of equality? *Ethics*, 1999, 109, 287–337.

Anthony WA. Recovery from mental illness: The guiding vision of mental health service systems in the 1990s. *Psychosocial Rehabilitation Journal*, 1993, 16, 11–23.

Baillargeon J, Binswanger IA, Penn JV, Williams BA, Murray OJ. Psychiatric disorders and repeat incarcerations: The revolving prison door. *American Journal of Psychiatry*, 2009, 166, 103–109.

Baillargeon J, Hoge SK, Penn JV. Addressing the challenge of community reentry among released inmates with serious mental Illness. *American Journal of Community Psychology*, 2010, 46, 361–375.

Barr M. *Financial services for low- and moderate-income households: Detroit area household financial services study*. Ann Arbor: Survey Research Center, University of Michigan, 2006.

Barrett-Leonard GT. Dimensions of therapist response as causal factors in therapeutic change. *Psychological Monographs*, 1962, 76, 1–36.

Baumgartner JN & Herman DB. Community integration of formerly homeless men and women with severe mental illness after hospital discharge. *Psychiatric Services*, 2012, 63 (5), 435–437.

Bellah RN, Madsen R, Sullivan WM, Swidler A, Tipton SM. *Habits of the heart: Individualism and commitment in American life*. Berkeley, CA: University of California Press, 1996.

Bellamy CD, Garvin C, MacFarlane P, Mowbray OP, Mowbray CT, Holter MC. An analysis of groups in consumer-centered programs. *American Journal of Psychiatric Rehabilitation*, 2006, 9 (3), 219–240.

Benedict P, Guy K, Bellamy PD with Rowe M, Baranoski M, Hunter-Gamble C, Herring Y, TwoBears L, Harper A, Crespo M, Antunes K. *Guide to implementing a citizenship project*, New Haveen, Connecticut: Yale Program for Recovery and Community Health, 2014.

Berger PL & Neuhaus RJ. *To empower people: The role of mediating structures in public policy*. Washington, DC: American Enterprise Institute for Public Policy, 1977.

Bolton JM, Robinson J, Sareen J. Self-medication of mood disorders with alcohol and drugs in the National Epidemiologic Survey on Alcohol and Related Conditions. *Journal of Affective Disorders*, 2009, 115 (3), 367–375.

Bourdieu P. Forms of capital. In JG Richardson, ed. *Handbook of theory and research for the sociology of education*. New York: Greenwood Press, 1983, 241–258

Brown S. *Student-teacher interviews*. New Haven, Connecticut: Yale Program for Recovery and Community Health, Unpublished report.

Buckley R & Bigelow DA. The multi-service network: Reaching the underserved multi-problem individual. *Community Mental Health Journal*, 1992, 28, 43–50.

Burke-Miller JK, Swarbrick M, Carter TM, Jonikas JA, Zipple A, Fraser V, Cook JA. Promoting self-determination and financial security through innovative asset building approaches. *Psychiatric Rehabilitation Journal*, 2010, 34 (2), 104–112. doi: 10.2975/34.2.2010.104.112

Burns JK & Esterhuizen T. Poverty, inequality and the treated incidence of first-episode psychosis: An ecology study from south Africa. *Social Psychiatry and Psychiatric Epidemiology*, 2008, 43, 331–335.

Burns T, Catty J, Baker T, Drake RE, Fioritti A, Knapp M, Lauber C, Rössler W, Tomov T, Busschbach JV, White S, Wiersma D. The effectiveness of supported employment for people with severe mental illness: A randomised controlled trial. *Lancet*, 2007, 370 (9593), 1146–1152.

Butterfoss FD, Goodman RM, Wandersman A. Community coalitions for prevention and health promotion. *Health Education Research*, 1993, 8 (3), 315–330, 315.

Callahan S, Mayer N, Palmer K, Ferlazzo L. Rowing the boat with two oars. *NFG Reports*, 1998, 3 (5), 3.

Carpenter-Song E. Anthropological perspectives on money management: Considerations for the design and implementation of interventions for substance abuse. *The American Journal of Drug and Alcohol Abuse*, 2012, 38, 49–54. doi:10.3109/00952990.2011. 643980

Cast AD & Burke PJ. A theory of self-esteem. *Social Forces*, 2002, 80 (3), 1041–1068.

CFED 2010. *Household financial security framework*, http://cfed.org/assets/CFEDHouse holdFramework_4Pager.pdf.

Chafetz L. Why clinicians distance themselves from the homeless mentally ill. In RH Lamb, LL Bachrach & FI Kass, eds. *Treating the homeless mentally ill: A report of the task force on the homeless mentally ill*. Washington, DC: American Psychiatric Association, 1992, 95–107.

Chiricos T, Barrick K, Bales W, Bontrager S. The labeling of convicted felons and its consequences for recidivism. *Criminology*, 2007, 45 (3), 547–581. doi: 10.1111/j.1745-9125. 2007.00089.x

Christens BD. Toward relational empowerment. *American Journal of Community Psychology*, 2012, 50 (1–2), 114–128. doi: 10.1007/s10464-011-9483-5

Clayton A, O'Connell M, Bellamy C, Benedict P, Rowe M. The citizenship project, part II: Impact of a citizenship intervention on clinical and community outcomes for persons with mental illness and criminal justice charges. *American Journal of Community Psychology*, 2012, 45 (2). doi: 10.1007/s10464-012-9549-z

Cohen NL & Marcos LR. Outreach intervention models for the homeless mentally ill. In RH Lamb, LL Bachrach & FI Kass, eds. *Treating the homeless mentally ill: A report on the task force on the homeless mentally ill*. Washington, DC: American Psychiatric Association, 1992, 141–157.

Cohen NL & Tsemberis S. Emergency psychiatric interventions on the street. *New Directions for Mental Health Services*, 1991, 52, 3–16.

Cohen P & Cohen J. The clinician's illusion. *Archives of General Psychiatry*, 1984, 41 (12), 1178–1182. doi: 10.1001/archpsyc.1984.01790230064010

Coleman JS. *Foundations of social theory*. Cambridge, MA: Belknap, 1990.

Colomy P & Brown DJ. Goffman and interactional citizenship. *Sociological Perspectives*, 1996, 39 (3), 371–381.

Concept System Software, Version 4.0. Ithaca, NY: Concept Systems, Inc., 2007.

Connors GJ, Tonigan JS, Miller WR. A longitudinal model of intake symptomatology, AA participation and outcome: Retrospective study of the project MATCH outpatient and aftercare samples. *Journal of Studies on Alcohol*, 2001, 62, 817–825.

Cook JA & Mueser K. Economic security: An essential component of recovery. *Psychiatric Rehabilitation Journal*, 2013, 36 (1), 1–3. doi: 10.1037/h0094739

Copeland ME. What is wellness recovery action plan® (WRAP®)? http://www.mental-healthrecovery.com/wrap. Accessed on January 5, 2014.

Davidson L. *Living outside mental illness: Qualitative studies of recovery in schizophrenia*. New York: New York University Press, 2005.

Davidson L, Chinman M, Sells D, Rowe M. Peer support among adults with serious mental illness: A report from the field. *Schizophrenia Bulletin*, 2006, 32 (3), 443–450.

Davidson L, Mezzina R, Rowe M, Thompson K. "A life in the community": Italian mental health reform and recovery. *Journal of Mental Health*, 2010, 19 (5), 436–443.

Davidson L & Roe D. Recovery from versus recovery in serious mental illness: One strategy for lessening confusion plaguing recovery. *Journal of Mental Health*, 2007, 16 (4), 459–470. doi: 10.1080/09n638230701482394

Davidson L & Rowe M. *Peer support within criminal justice settings: The role of forensic peer specialists*. National GAINS Center, 2007.

Davidson L, Stayner DA, Nickou C, Styron TH, Rowe M, Chinman MJ. "Simply to be let in": Inclusion as a basis for recovery from mental illness. *Psychiatric Rehabilitation Journal*, 2001, 24, 375–388.

Davidson L, Tondora J, O'Connell M, Lawless M, Rowe M. *Transforming mental health care: A practical guide to recovery-oriented practice*. New York: Oxford University Press, 2008.

Davidson ML. *Multidimensional scaling*. New York: Wiley, 1983.

Department of Justice. Mental health problems of prison and jail inmates. *Bureau of Justice Statistics Special Report*. 2006, NCJ 213600.

American Psychiatric Association. *Diagnostic and statistical manual of mental disorders* (4th ed., Text Revision). Washington, DC: Author, 2000.

Duffy S. The citizenship theory of social justice: exploring the meaning of personalisation for social workers. *Journal of Social Work Practice: Psychotherapeutic Approaches in Health, Welfare, and the Community*, 2010, 24 (3), 253–267. doi: 10.1080/02650533.2010.500118

Durkheim É. *Division of labor in society*. G Simpson, trans. London: Collier Macmillan, 1933.

Edgley A, Stickley T, Wright N, Repper J. The politics of recovery in mental health: A left libertarian policy analysis. *Social Theory & Health*, 2012, 10 (2), 121–140. doi: 10.1057/sth.2012.1

Elbogen E, Bradford D, Swartz M. A recovery-oriented money management intervention. *Psychiatric Services*, 2013, 64 (1), 99.

Elbogen E, Tiegreen J, Vaughan C, Bradford DW. Money management, mental health, and psychiatric disability: A recovery-oriented model for improving financial skills. *Psychiatric Rehabilitation Journal*, 2011, 34 (3), 223–231.

El-Mallakh P. Doing my best: Poverty and self-care among individuals with schizophrenia and diabetes mellitus. *Archives of Psychiatric Nursing*, 2007, 21 (1), 49–60

Erikson K. *A new species of trouble: Explorations in disaster, trauma, and community.* New York: Norton, 1994.

Erikson K. *Everything in its path: Destruction of community in the Buffalo Creek Flood.* New York: Simon and Schuster, 1976.

Everitt B. *Cluster analysis, 2nd ed.* New York: Halsted, 1980.

Ewalt JR & Ewalt PL. History of the community psychiatry movement. *American Journal of Psychiatry*, 1969, 126 (1), 43–52.

Farmer P. Investigating the root causes of the global health crisis: Paul Farmer on TED book *The Upstream Doctors.* http://blog.ted.com/2013/06/05/investigating -the-root-causes-of-the-global-health-crisis-paul-farmer-on-the-upstream-doctors/.

FDIC 2012. National survey of unbanked and underbanked households. https://www.fdic. gov/householdsurvey/2012_unbankedreport.pdf.

Fine M, Torre ME, Boudin K, Bowen I, Judith C, Hylton D, Martinez M, Rivera M, Roberts RA, Smart P, Upegui D. Participatory action research: from within and beyond prison bars. In Camic J, Rhodes JE, Yardley L, eds. *Qualitative research in psychology: Expanding perspectives in methodology and design.* Washington, DC: American Psychological Association, 2003, 173–198.

Fisk D, Rowe M, Brooks R, Gildersleeve D. Integrating consumer staff into a homeless outreach project: Critical issues and strategies. *Psychiatric Rehabilitation Journal*, 2000, 23 (3), 244–252.

Flores PJ. *Group therapy with addicted populations: An integration of twelve-step and psychodynamic theory, 2nd ed.* New York: The Haworth Press, 1997.

Fram DH. Group methods in the treatment of substance abusers. *Psychiatric Annals*, 1990, 20 (7), 385–388.

Francisco VT, Paine AL, Fawcett SB. A methodology for monitoring and evaluating community health coalitions, *Health Education Research*, 1993, 8, 403–416.

Freedman DA. *Statistical models: Theory and practice.* Cambridge, UK: Cambridge University Press, 2003.

Gambino MJ. *Mental health and ideals of citizenship: Patient care at St. Elizabeth's Hospital in Washington, D.C., 1903–1962.* Urbana, IL: University of Illinois, 2011.

Garvin CD. A task-centered group approach to work with the chronically mentally ill. *Social Work with Groups*, 1992, 15 (2/3), 67–80.

Garvin CD. *Contemporary group work.* Boston: Allyn and Bacon, 1997.

Geronimus AT. The weathering hypothesis and the health of African-American women and infants: Evidence and speculations. *Ethnicity & Disease*, 1992, 2 (3), 207–221.

Giddens A. *Modernity and self-identity: Self and society in the late modern age.* Stanford, CA: Stanford University Press, 1991.

Goffman, E. *Asylums: Essays on the social situation of mental patients and other inmates.* New York: Anchor Books, 1961.

Goffman E. *Strategic interaction.* Philadelphia: University of Pennsylvania Press, 1969.

Goldman HH & Morrissey JP. The alchemy of mental health policy: Homelessness and the fourth cycle of reform. *American Journal of Public Health*, 1985, 75 (7), 727–731. doi: 10.2105/AJPH.75.7.727

Gutierrez LM. Beyond coping: an empowerment perspective on stressful life events. *Journal of Sociology and Social Welfare*, 1994, 21 (3), 201–219.

Habermas J. *Legitimation crisis*. T McCarthy, trans. Boston: Beacon Press, 1973.

Hall S & Cheston R. Mental health and identity: The evaluation of a drop-in centre. *Journal of Community and Applied Social Psychology*, 2002, 12 (1), 30–43.

Hannum R, Myers-Parelli A, Schoenfeld P, Cameron C, Campbell H, Chrismer L. Promoting social integration among people with psychiatric disabilities. *Innovations & Research*, 1994, 3, 17–23.

Harper A. *Improving the financial health of Connecticut Mental Health Center (CMHC) clients*. Consultancy report for the CMHC Foundation, 2012.

Harper A, Clayton A, Foss-Kelly L, Bailey M, Sernyak M, Rowe M. Financial health and mental health: Making the connections. 2014.

Harper A & Rowe M. Financial health and social recovery. *Psychiatric Services*, 2014, 65 (6), 707.

Hartwell S. Triple stigma: Persons with mental illnesses and substances abuse problems in the criminal justice system. *Criminal Justice Policy Review*, 2004, 15, 84–99.

Heater D. *A brief history of citizenship*. New York: New York University Press, 2004.

Hocking RR. The analysis and selection of variables in linear regression. *Biometrics*, 1976, 32.

Hoffman RE. A social deafferentation hypothesis for induction of active schizophrenia. *Schizophrenia Bulletin*, 2007, 33 (5), 1066–1070. doi: 10.1093/schbul/sbm079

Hogan D & Owen D. Social capital, active citizenship and political equality in Australia. In I. Winter, ed., *Social capital and public policy in Australia*. Melbourne: Australian Institute of Family Studies, 2000, 74–103.

Hoge SK. Providing transition and outpatient services to the mentally ill released from correctional institutions. In R. B. Greifinger, ed. *Public health behind bars: From prisons to communities*. New York: Springer, 2007, 461–477.

Honneth A. *The struggle for recognition: The moral grammar of social conflict*. J Anderson, trans. Cambridge, MA: MIT Press, 1995.

Hopper K. Redistribution and its discontents: On the prospects of committed work in public mental health and like settings. *Human Organization*, 2006, 65 (2), 218–226.

Hopper K. Reframing early psychiatric crises: A capabilities-informed approach. *Journal of Human Development, Disability, and Social Change*, 2009, 20 (2), 23–29.

Hopper K. Rethinking social recovery in schizophrenia: What a capabilities approach might offer. *Social Science & Medicine*, 2007, 65, 868–879.

Hopper K. The counter-reformation that failed? A commentary on the mixed legacy of supportive housing. *Psychiatric Services*, 2012, 63 (5), 461–463.

Hopper K & Baumohl J. Held in abeyance: Rethinking homelessness and advocacy. *American Behavioral Scientist*, 1994, 37 (4), 522–552. doi: 10.1177/0002764294037004007

Hopper K, Jost J, Hay T, Welber S, Haugland G. Homelessness, severe mental illness and the institutional circuit. *Psychiatric Services*, 1997, 48 (5), 659–665.

https://www.glide.org/.

http://sakisan.hubpages.com/hub/What-is-K2-drug-Answered.

http://www.participatorybudgeting.org/who-we-are/mission-approach/.

http://www.photovoice.org/about/.

http://www.prainc.com/soar/cms-assets/documents/74697-776854.homelessness-defs081512.pdf.

http://store.samhsa.gov/shin/content/SMA04-3870/SMA04-3870.pdf.

http://homeless.samhsa.gov/ResourceFiles/0abwdb1u.pdf.

http://www.socialresearchmethods.net/kb/convdisc.php.

Hudson C. Socioeconomic status and mental illness: Tests of the social causation and selection hypotheses. *American Journal of Orthopsychiatry*, 2005, 75 (1), 3–18.

Humphreys K. Professional interventions that facilitate 12-step self-help group involvement. *Alcohol Research and Health*, 1999, 23, 93–98.

Humphreys K, Moos RH, Cohen C. Social and community resources and long-term recovery from treated and untreated alcoholism. *Journal of Studies on Alcohol*, 1997, 58 (3), 231–239.

Jacobs J. *The death and life of great American cities*. New York: Vintage Books, 1961.

Jacobson N. *Dignity and health*. Nashville: Vanderbilt University Press, 2012.

Janoski T. *Citizenship and civil society: A framework of rights and obligations in liberal, traditional, and social democratic regimes*. Cambridge, MA: Cambridge University Press, 1998.

Jenkins R, Bhugra D, Bebbington P, Brugha T, Farrell M, Coid J, Fryers T, Weich S, Singleton N, Meltzer H. Debt, income and mental disorder in the general population. *Psychological Medicine*, 2008, 38, 1485–1493.

Johnson SL, Sandrow D, Myer B, Winters R, Miller I, Solomon D, Keitner G. Increase in manic symptoms after life events in goal attainment. *Journal of Abnormal Psychology*, 2000, 109 (4), 721–727.

Johnston K. The messy link between slave owners and modern management. http://hbswk.hbs.edu/item/7182.html.

Kant I. Grounding for the metaphysics of morals. In Michael Morgan, ed. *Classics of moral and political theory*. Indianapolis: Hackett, 1992, 991–1041.

Kelly PD. The power gap: Freedom, power and mental illness. *Social Science & Medicine*, 2006, 63 (8), 2118–2128.

Kessler RC, Berglund P, Demler O, Jin R, Merikangas KR, Walters E. Lifetime prevalence and age-of-onset distributions of DSM-IV disorders in the National Comorbidity Survey Replication. *Archives of General Psychiatry*, 2005, 62, 593–602. doi: 10.1001/archpsyc.62.6.593

Kloos B, Benedict P, TwoBears L, Rowe M. *Citizens process evaluation: Documenting the creation of a community-based organization*. New Haven, CT: Consultation Center, 1999.

Kretzmann & McKnight J. *Building communities from the inside out: A path toward finding and mobilizing a community's assets*. Evanston, IL: Institute for Policy Research, Northwestern University, 1996.

Kurtz LF. *Self-help and support groups: A handbook for practitioners*. Thousand Oaks, CA: Sage, 1997.

Lamb HR & Weinberger L. The shift of psychiatric inpatient care from hospitals to jails and prisons. *Journal of the American Academy of Psychiatry and the Law*, 2005, 33 (4), 529–534.

Lamberti JS, Weisman R, Faden DI. Forensic assertive community treatment: Preventing incarceration of adults with severe mental illness. *Psychiatric Services*, 2004, 55 (11), 1285–1293. doi: 10.1176/appi.ps.55.11.1285

Lehman AF. A quality of life interview for the chronically mentally ill. *Evaluation and Program Planning*, 1988, 11, 51–62.

Lister R. Dialectics of citizenship. *Hypatia*, 1997, 12 (4), 6–26. doi:10.1111/j.1527-2001.1997. tb00296.x

MacBeth G. Collaboration can be elusive: Virginia's experience in developing an inter-agency system of care. *Administration and Policy in Mental Health*, 1993, 20, 259–281.

MacKay K. Compounding conditional citizenship: To what extent does Scottish & English mental health law increase or diminish citizenship? *British Journal of Social Work*, 2011, 41, 931–948. doi: 10.1093/bjsw/bc010

Manchanda R. *The upstream doctors: Medical innovators track sickness to its source*. New York: TED Books, 2013.

Mandiberg J. Another way: Enclave communities for people with mental illness. *American Journal of Orthopsychiatry*, 2010, 80 (2), 170–176. doi: 10.1111/j.1939-0025.2010 .01020.x

Mandiberg J. The failure of social inclusion: An alternative approach through community development. *Psychiatric Services*, 2012, 63, 458–460. doi: 10.1176/appi.ps.201100367

Mandiberg J & Warner R. Sustainable innovations for subsistence marketplaces. *Journal of Business Research*, 2012, 65 (12), 1736–1742.

Marshall TH. *Class, citizenship and social development*. Chicago: University of Chicago Press, 1964.

Maruna S. Reentry as a rite of passage. *Punishment and Society*, 2011, 13, 3–28.

Maruna S & LeBel TP. Welcome home? Examining the "re-entry court" concept from a strengths-based perspective. *Western Criminology Review*, 2003, 4 (2), 91–107.

Mattison A, Benedict P, TwoBears L. *As I sat on the green: Living without a home in New Haven*. New Haven, CT: Citizens Project/Columbus House, 2000.

McKellar J, Stewart E, Humphreys K. Alcoholics Anonymous involvement and positive alcohol-related outcomes: Cause, consequence, or just a correlate? A prospective 2-year study of 2,319 alcohol-dependent men. *Journal of Consulting and Clinical Psychology*, 2003, 71, 302–308.

McKnight JL. Regenerating community. *Social Policy*, 1987, Winter, 54–58.

McMillan D & Chavis D. Sense of community: A definition and theory. *Journal of Community Psychology*, 1986, 14, 6–23.

McNeil DE, Binder RL, Robinson JC. Incarceration associated with homelessness, mental disorder, and co-occurring substance abuse. *Psychiatric Services*, 2005, 56, 840–846.

McKnight JL. Regenerating community. *Social Policy*, 1987, Winter, 54–58.

Meissen G, Powell TJ, Wituk SA, Girrens K, Arteaga S. Attitudes of AA contact persons toward group participation by persons with a mental illness. *Psychiatric Services*, 1999, 50, 1079–1081.

Moos RH & Moos BS. Participation in treatment and alcoholics anonymous: A 16-year follow-up of initially untreated individuals. *Journal of Clinical Psychology*, 2006, 62 (6), 735–750.

Moos RH & Moos BS. Sixteen-year changes and stable remission among treated and untreated individuals with alcohol use disorders. *Drug and Alcohol Dependence*, 2005, 80 (3), 337–347.

Morse GA, Calsyn RJ, Miller J, Rosenberg P, West L, Gilliland J. Outreach to homeless mentally ill people: Conceptual and clinical considerations. *Community Mental Health Journal*, 1996, 32 (3), 261–274.

Mouffe C. *The return of the political.* London: Verso Press, 2005.

Mueser K, Myer PS, Penn DL, Clany R, Clancy DM, Salyers MP. The illness management and recovery program: Rationale, development, and preliminary findings. *Schizophrenia Bulletin Suppl 1,* 2006, 32, S32–S43.

Myers J, Lindenthal J, Pepper M. Life events, social integration and psychiatric symptomology. *Journal of Health and Social Behavior,* 1975, 16 (4), 421–427.

Nisbet RA. *The quest for community: A study in the ethics of order & freedom.* New York: Oxford University Press, 1953.

Noordsy D, Torrey W, Mueser K, Mead S, O'Keefe C, Fox L. Recovery from severe mental illness: An intrapersonal and functional outcome definition. *International Review of Psychiatry,* 2002, 14, 318–326.

O'Connell MJ, Clayton A, Stern E, Bellamy C, Benedict P, Rowe M. Reliability and validity of a newly-developed measure of citizenship among persons with mental illness. 2014.

Ohmer ML. How theory and research inform citizen participation in poor communities: the ecological perspective and theories on self- and collective efficacy and sense of community. *Journal of Human Behavior in the Social Environment,* 2010, 20 (1), 1–19. doi: 10.1080/1091135093126999

Osher FC & Steadman HJ. Adapting evidence-based practices for persons with mental illness involved with the criminal justice system. *Psychiatric Services,* 2007, 58, 1472–1478.

Outhwaite W. *The Habermas reader.* Cambridge, UK: Polity Press, 1996.

Panas L, Yael C, Fournier E, McCarty D. Performance measures for outpatient substance abuse services: Group versus individual therapy. *Journal of Substance Abuse Treatment,* 2003, 25 (4), 271–278.

Perrow C. *Normal accidents: Living with high-risk technologies.* New York: Basic Books, 1984.

Pickett SA, Cook JA, Cohler BJ. Caregiving burden experienced by parents of offspring with severe mental illness: Impact of off-timedness. *Journal of Applied Social Sciences,* 1994, 18, 199–207.

Polcin DL & Zemore S. Psychiatric severity and spirituality, helping, and participation in Alcoholics Anonymous during recovery. *American Journal of Drug and Alcohol Abuse,* 2004, 30 (3), 577–592.

Ponce AN, Clayton A, Noia J, Rowe M, O'Connell MO. Making meaning of citizenship: Mental illness, forensic involvement, and homelessness. *Journal of Forensic Psychology Practice,* 2012, 12 (4), 349–365. doi: 10.1080/15228932.2012.695660

Ponce AN, Lawless M, Rowe M. Homelessness, behavioral health disorders and intimate partner violence: Barriers to services for women. *Community Mental Health Journal.* doi: 10.1007/s10597-014-9712-0

Portes A. Social capital: Its origins and applications in modern sociology. *Annual Review of Sociology* 24, 1998, 1–24.

Portis EB. Citizenship & personal identity. *Polity,* 1986, 18 (3), 457–472.

Randolph F. Improving service systems through systems integration: The ACCESS program. *American Rehabilitation,* 1995, 21, 36–38.

Randolph F, Blasinsky M, Leginski W, Parker LB, Goldman HH. Creating integrated service systems for homeless persons with mental illness: the ACCESS Program. Access to Community Care and Effective Services and Supports. *Psychiatric Services*, 1997, 48 (3), 369–373.

Rans SA & Green M. Project Friendship, Prince George, BC: Bridging the gap. In Rans SA & Mike Green (authors), Kretzmann JP & McKnight JL (co-directors). *Building community connections by engaging the gifts of people on welfare, people with disabilities, people with mental illness, older adults, young people.* Evanston, IL: School of Education and Social Policy, Northwestern University, 2005, 27–40.

Reaching out: A guide for service providers. Washington, DC: Interagency Council on the Homeless, 1991.

Ridgway P. The recovery markers questionnaire. Unpublished.

Roman C & Travis J. *Taking stock: Housing, homelessness, and prisoner reentry.* Washington, DC: Urban Institute, 2004.

Rosen M. The check effect reconsidered. *Addiction*, 2011, 106, 1071–1077.

Rossi PH. *Down and out in America: The origins of homelessness.* Chicago: University of Chicago Press, 1989.

Rowe M. Alternatives to outpatient commitment. *Journal of the American Academy of Psychiatry and the Law*, 2013, 41 (3), 332–336.

Rowe M. *Crossing the border: Encounters between homeless people and outreach workers.* Berkeley, CA: University of California Press, 1999.

Rowe M & Baranoski M. Citizenship, mental illness, and the criminal justice system. *International Journal of Law and Psychiatry*, 34, 2011, 303–308.

Rowe M & Baranoski M. Mental illness, criminality, and citizenship. *Journal of the American Academy of Psychiatry and the Law*, 2000, 28 (3), 262–264.

Rowe M, Bellamy C, Baranoski M, Wieland M, O'Connell M, Benedict P, Davidson, L, Buchanan J, Sells D. Reducing alcohol use, drug use and criminality among persons with severe mental illness. *Psychiatric Services*, 2007, 58 (7), 955–961.

Rowe M, Benedict P, Falzer P. Representation of the governed: Leadership building for people with behavioral health disorders who are homeless or were formerly homeless. *Psychiatric Rehabilitation Journal*, 2003, 26 (3), 240–248.

Rowe M, Benedict P, Sells D, Dinzeo T, Garvin C, Schwab L, Baranoski M, Girard V, Bellamy C. Citizenship, community, and recovery: A group- and peer-based intervention for persons with co-occurring disorders and criminal justice histories. *Journal for Groups in Addiction and Recovery*, 2009, 4 (4), 224–244.

Rowe M, Clayton A, Benedict P, Bellamy C, Antunes K, Miller R, Pelletier J, Stern E, O'Connell MJ. Going to the source: Citzenship outcome measure development. *Psychiatric Services*, 2012, 63, 461–463.

Rowe M, Hoge M, Fisk D. Critical issues in serving people who are homeless and mentally ill. *Administration and Policy in Mental Health*, 1996, 23 (6), 555–565.

Rowe M, Hoge MA, Fisk D. The bright yellow sneakers: A case example of assertive outreach with mentally ill homeless persons. *Continuum: Developments in Ambulatory Health Care*, 1996, 3 (4), 265–269.

Rowe M, Kloos B, Chinman M, Davidson L, Cross AB. Homelessness, mental illness and citizenship. *Social Policy and Administration*, 2001, 35, 14–31.

Rowe M & Pelletier J-F. Citizenship: A response to the marginalization of people with mental illnesses. *Journal of Forensic Psychology Practice*, 2012, 12 (4), 366–381. doi: 10.1080/15228932.2012.697423

Rowe M, Serowik KL, Ablondi K, Wilber C, Rosen MI. Recovery and money management. *Psychiatric Rehabilitation Journal*, 2013, 36 (2), 116–118.

Salyers MP & Tsemberis S. ACT and recovery: Integrating evidence-based practice and recovery orientation on assertive community treatment teams. *Community Mental Health Journal*, 2007, 43 (6), 619–641.

Schur L, Shields T, Kruse D, Schriner K. Enabling democracy: Disability and voter turnout. *Political Research Quarterly*, 2002, 55 (1), 167–190. doi: 10.1177/106591290205500107

Schwartz DB. *Who cares? Rediscovering community*. Boulder, CO: Westview Press, 1999.

Sells D, Black R, Davidson L, Rowe M. Beyond generic support: The incidence and impact of invalidation within peer-based and traditional treatment for clients with severe mental illness. *Psychiatric Services*, 2008, 59 (11), 1322–1327.

Sells D, Davidson L, Jewell C, Falzer P, Rowe M. The treatment relationship in peer-based and regular case management services for clients with severe mental illness. *Psychiatric Services*, 2006, 57 (8), 1179–1184.

Sen A. Well-being, agency and freedom: The Dewey lectures, 1984. *The Journal of Philosophy*, 1985, 82 (4), 169–221.

Servon L. The real reason the poor go without bank accounts. *The Atlantic Cities Place Matters*, 2013. http://www.theatlanticcities.com/jobs-and-economy/2013/09/why-poor-choose-go-without-bank-accounts/6783/.

Silver H & Miller SM. Social exclusion: The European approach to social disadvantage. *Indicators*, 2003, 2 (2), 1–17.

Simmons J, Roberge L, Kendrick BS. The interpersonal relationship in clinical practice: The Barrett-Leonard Inventory as an assessment instrument. *Evaluation and the Health Professions*, 1995, 18, 103–112.

Simon J. *Poor discipline: Parole and the social control of the underclass, 1890–1990*. Chicago: University of Chicago Press, 1993.

Sledge J, Gordon S, Knisley M. *Making the shift from financial education to financial capability: Evidence from the financial capability innovation fund*. Chicago: Center for Financial Services Innovation, 2011 http://www.cfsinnovation.com/system/files/CFSI_FinCapTrends_Mar2011_final.pdf.

Snow DA & Anderson L. Identity work among the homeless. *American Journal of Sociology*, 1987, 97, 1337–1371.

Snow DA, Baker SG, Anderson L, Martin M. The myth of pervasive mental illness among the homeless. *Social Problems*, 33 (5), 407–423.

SPSS, IBM. *SPSS Statistics Version 19.0.0.1*, 2010.

Stanton A & Revenson T. Adjustment to chronic disease: progress and promise in research, In Friedman HS & Silver RC, *Foundations of Health Psychology*. New York: Oxford University Press, 2006.

Stellar JE, Manzo VM, Kraus MW, Keltner D. Class and compassion: Socioeconomic factors predict responses to suffering. *Emotion*, 2012, 12 (3), 449–459. doi: 10.1037/a0026508

Streiner DL. Starting at the beginning: An introduction to coefficient alpha and internal consistency. *Journal of Personality Assessment*, 2003, 80, 99–103.

Stryker S & Burke PJ. The past, present, and future of an identity theory. *Social Psychology Quarterly*, 2000, 63 (4), 284–297.

Substance Abuse and Mental Health Services Administration. *Services integration: A twenty-year perspective*, 1991.

Sue DW, Capodilupo CM, Torino GC, Bucceri JM, Holder AMB, Nadal KL, Esquilin M. Racial microaggressions in everyday life: Implications for clinical practice. *American Psychologist*, 2007, 62 (4), 271–286.

Susser E, Valencia E, Conover S, Felix A, Tsai W-Y, Wyatt RJ. Preventing recurrent homelessness among mentally ill men: A 'critical time' intervention in the aftermath of discharge from a shelter. *American Journal of Public Health*, 1997, 87, 256–262.

Swarbrick M. Asset-building, financial self-management service model: Piecing together consumer financial independence. *Journal of Psychosocial Nursing and Mental Health Services*, 2006, 44 (10), 22–26.

Swayze FV. Clinical case management with the homeless mentally ill. In RH Lamb, LL Bachrach & FI Kass, eds. *Treating the homeless mentally ill: A report of the task force on the homeless mentally ill*. Washington, DC: American Psychiatric Association, 1992, 203–219.

Swidler A. Culture in action: Symbols and strategies. *American Sociological Review*, 1986, 51, 273–286.

Taxman FS & Bouffard JA. Substance abuse counselors' treatment philosophy and the content of treatment services provided to offenders in drug court programs. *Journal of Substance Abuse Treatment*, 2003, 25 (2), 75–84.

Teplin LA: Psychiatric and substance abuse disorders among male urban jail detainees. *American Journal of Public Health*, 1994, 84, 290–293.

The President's New Freedom Commission on Mental Health. Achieving the promise: transforming mental health care in America. Rockville, MD: DHHS Pub. No. SMA-03-3832, 2003.

Thoits PA. Multiple identities: Examining gender and marital status differences in distress. *American Sociological Review*, 1986, 51 (2), 259–272.

Tocqueville AD. *Democracy in America: Volumes I & II*. H Reeve, trans. New York: Alfred E. Knopf, 1953, 1945.

Trochim WM & Kane M. Concept mapping: An introduction to structured conceptualization in health care. *International Journal for Quality in Health Care*, 2005, 17, 187–191.

Tsai J, Mares S, Rosenheck RA. Does housing chronically mentally ill adults lead to social integration? *Psychiatric Services*, 2012, 63 (5), 427–434.

Turner-Crowson J & Wallcraft J. The recovery vision for mental health services and research: A British perspective. *Psychiatric Rehabilitation Journal*, 2002, 25, 245–254.

Uggen C, Manza J, Thompson M. Citizenship, democracy, and the civic reintegration of criminal offenders. *Annals, American Academy of Political and Social Science*, 2006, 281–310.

Vannicelli M. *Removing the roadblocks: Group psychotherapy with substance abusers and family members*. New York: Guilford Press, 1992.

Viswanathan M, Ammerman A, Eng E, Garlehner G, Lohr KN, Griffith D, Rhodes S, Samuel-Hodge C, Maty S, Lux L, Webb L, Sutton SF, Swinson T, Jackman A, Whitener L. *Community-based participatory research: Assessing the evidence*. AHRQ pub no 04-E022-2. Rockville, MD: Agency for Healthcare Research and Quality, 2004.

Voting and Registration in the Election of November 2012—Detailed Tables. United States Census Bureau, 2012. http://www.census.gov/hhes/www/socdemo/voting/publications/p20/2012/tables.html.

Wakefield S & Uggen C. Incarceration and stratification. *Annual Review of Sociology*, 2010, 36, 387–406. doi: 10.1146/annurev.soc.012809.102551

Wallerstein NB & Duran B. Using community-based participatory research to address health disparities. *Health Promotion Practice*, 2006, 7, 312–323.

Wang C & Burris MA. Empowerment through Photo Novella: Portraits of participation. *Health Education & Behavior*, 1994, 21 (2), 171–186. doi:10.1177/109019819402100204

Ware NC, Hopper K, Tugenberg T, Dickey R, Fisher D. A theory of social inclusion as quality of life. *Psychiatric Services*, 2008, 59 (1), 27–33.

Ware NC, Hopper K, Tugenberg T, Dickey B, Fisher D. Connectedness and citizenship: Redefining social integration. *Psychiatric Services*, 2007, 58 (4), 469–474.

Warren, Rose S, Bergunder AF. *The structure of urban reform*. Lexington, MA: Lexington Books, 1974.

Weber M. *The theory of social and economic organization*. AM Henderson & T Parsons, trans. London: Collier Macmillan Publishers, 1947.

Weber M. *The Protestant ethic and the spirit of capitalism*. T Parsons, trans. London: Allen & Unwin, 1976.

Weisser J, Morrow M, James B. *A critical exploration of social integration in the mental health recovery literature*. Vancouver, BC: Centre for the Study of Gender, Social Inequities, and Mental Health (CCSM), http://www.socialinequities.ca/wordpress/wp-content/uploads/2011/02/Recovery-Scoping-Review.Final_.STYLE_.pdf, 2011.

Werbner P & Yuval-Davis N. Women and the new discourse of citizenship. In N Yuval-Davis & P Werbner, eds: *Women, citizenship and difference*. New York: Zed Books, 1999, 1–31.

Whitley R, Strickler D, Drake RE. Recovery center for people with severe mental illness: A survey of programs. *Community Mental Health Journal*, 2012, 48, 547–556.

Wichowsky A & Moynihan DP. Measuring how administration shapes citizenship: A policy feedback perspective on performance management. *Public Administration Review*, 2008, September-October, 908–920.

Wiseman J. *Stations of the lost: The treatment of Skid-Row alcoholics*. Englewood Cliffs, NJ: Prentice-Hall, 1970.

Wolfe T. *The right stuff*. New York: Farrar, Strauss & Giroux, 1979.

Yanos PT, Stefanic A, Tsemberis S. Objective community integration of MH consumers living in supported housing and of others in the community. *Psychiatric Services*, 2012, 63 (5), 438–444.

Yule G. *The study of language, third ed*. Cambridge, UK: Cambridge University Press, 2006.

INDEX

Note: The letters "f" and "n" after a page number indicate a figure or a footnote respectively.

Aaron (disorderly conduct) 37
abstract reflection, capacity for 162
ACCESS (Access to Community Care and
    Effective Services and Supports) 4, 18
    definition of homelessness 7
    outreach team 192
    push for peer support work 43
    seeking solutions system of care 193
accountability, for those who break the law 104
ACT (assertive community treatment) team 187,
    188
action group, developing community connec-
    tions for the *Collaborative*, 139
addiction, money and 154
administrative theory, giving priority to cost
    achievement over citizenship values 198
advisory group, for the collaborative 187
advocacy 167, 173
Affordable Care Act (ACA)
    biggest driver of change, xiv
    creating even greater health disparities 180
    impact of 190
African-American adults, incarceration of 36
African American women, health deteriorating
    in early adulthood 123
age, of *Citizens Project* students, 70
agency freedom 18
Age of Enlightenment 12
Alfredo 52
Alice. *See* Mattison, Alice
alienation, from the domiciled community 10
Allison. *See* Ponce, Allison
Alonso, interest in biking 135–136
Americans with Disabilities Act, class on 41
Anderson; Elizabeth 13–14
Andrea 52, 53, 54
"And with that I pass" closer line 79
Angela 200
Annie. *See* Harper, Annie
Anthony, William 15
anti-recovery (AR), versus pro-recovery (PR)
    16–17
apartments, like sensory deprivation
    chambers 11

appointments, difficulty keeping
    109–110
Aristotle, on citizenship 11
As I Sat on the Green, addressing the objective of
    community education, 23
aspirational nature, of citizenship 205n1
"assaults on dignity," strong theme across focus
    groups 107–108
assertive community treatment (ACT) team
    187, 188
assertiveness class 42
asset building 151
asset limits, imposed by the benefits system 157
"associationalism," 208n23
"associational life," 191, 208n23
"associational world," 191
attention, shifting from recidivism to citizen-
    ship 36
awareness, stumbling into 7

back of the bus syndrome 17
"bad attitudes," 50
Bailey, Peggy 20, 121, 128, 188
bank account, downside of not having 157
Baranoski, Madelon 35, 36, 39, 44, 56
barrier, to voter registration 126
baseline interviews, completed 49
"basic trust," 90
behavioral health problems, Rita's 87
being housed, providing a foundation to achieve
    citizenship 112
being responsible to and for yourself 169, 171
Bellah, Robert 12
Bellamy, Chyrell 95, 119–120, 122–123, 205n1
Benedict, Patty 20, 23, 26, 27, 28, 38, 39, 44,
    45–46, 47, 48, 51, 52, 53, 56, 59, 60, 64–65,
    69, 74, 76, 79, 80, 85, 86, 89, 115, 137, 139,
    169, 179, 201
benefits, fear of losing 157
Bernice 52
Bill 167–170, 202
Billy 137, 139
birth certificate, original 126–127
board and committee training, planning of 26

board members, pleased with experience with the interns 29
Bobby *Citizens Project* student, 78–82, 83
boundary encounters, of Jim and Ed 188
bounded citizenship 11, 193, 194, 195
bounded conditions, working with people living under 149
brewing conflict, knowing when to walk away from 83
bridges, building between community members, people who were homeless, and social service folk 32
Brokeback Mountain, meaning of, 144
Bromage, Billy 128–129, 130, 134
Brown, David 198
Brown, Stacy 48
Bruce, Lucile 119, 126, 130, 200
budgeting, difficulties with 154
budgeting principles 153

capabilities, posing a risk to basic securities 18
capabilities theory 18–19, 197
"care management," xv
"care manager," xv
"carers," need to be on time and stay in place over time 182
caretaker, Kathy as 173
Caring for Self and Others, Domain 3, 103
Carl, in the *Citizens Project*, 58
Carlos 54
"case management," xv
case managers, xv 43–44
Cecilia (check casher) 179, 183–185
change(s)
    Affordable Care Act (ACA) as biggest driver of, xiv
    in *Citizens Project*, 63–70
    gatekeeping organizations resisting 4
    happening at precisely the same time 9
    having jumps and hobblings 81
    in policy 190
    readiness for 79
    as unpleasant and meeting resistance 120
Charles, on Methadone and other medications 54
check-cashing stores, and their staff 183
children, as a big part of Rita's recovery 87
choice
    lack of 165
    latent as well as active 165
Choices, Domain 6, 102
Chomsky, Noam 16
Christ Church community room 39
Christens, Brian 43
Chyrell. *See* Bellamy, Chyrell

citizens 19–23
    standing in relations of equality to each other 13
Citizens Collaborative
    foundational ideas 116–123
    hosting people who might not be supportive of citizenship work 179
    linking two main paths to citizenship 161
    placing members on mental health center's treatment teams 188
    projects and research 123–133
    selecting as a name 119
    suggesting an outline of a model 195
    summing up 185–188
    three principles 185
Citizens Council, member of, 171
citizenship, xiii 96–97
    for all 120
    application of a theoretical framework of, xvi
    for Bobby 80
    buying into the basic principles of 119
    definitions of 14, 39
    developing an individual instrument to measure 95–99
    as an exclusionary as well as inclusionary title 94
    health and socioeconomic disparities and racism in connection with 122–123
    hostile to large segments of humanity 13
    identifying and celebrating from the ground floor up 122
    intending to help individuals 190
    involving rights, privileges and corresponding responsibilities 15
    keys to 13
    as levels of political participation 12
    linking with mental health, xiv
    literature on 11
    naming practices we associate with 122
    need for more empirical data on the elements of 95
    new concept in mental health care 190
    opening up and restricting freedom 13
    positively correlated with trust in government and volunteering 101
    practical and symbolic importance of, xiv
    as a program versus as a community 77–78
    proposing the 5 Rs (rights, responsibilities, roles, resources, and relationships) 193
    roots in outreach work 1–11
    seven cluster concept mapping construct of, 106f
    seven-domain map of 105
    shared understanding of, xv

started on a grand scale on the community-level pathway to citizenship 33
taking to scale (Citizens Collaborative I) 114–133
taking to scale (Citizens Collaborative II) 134–159
taking to scale (Citizens Collaborative III) 160–188
theoretical framework of 94
citizenship and mental health
  current landscape of, 194f
  future model, 196f
  model of 189–199
  premodel of 194–195, 194f
citizenship approach 26
citizenship benefits, entitlement to 104
citizenship-building project 40
citizenship claims, made by and for excluded groups, xiii
Citizenship Council, one-year funding for, 60
citizenship course, in the *Citizens Project*, 47–51
citizenship efforts, initial 193–194
citizenship framework
  as guide for addressing gaps in policy 32
  not assumed to be applicable in other areas, regions, and urban or rural settings 191
  possibilities for 32
  relevance for mental health care, xvi
  resonated with commonly held values 32
  resonating with Norma Ware and colleagues 15
citizenship-informed clinical care 118
citizenship intervention
  helping people attend to long jumps and hobblings of change 81
  linked to clinical care at a mental health center, xv
  plus standard clinical care at the mental health center 60
  students 61
citizenship lunches 141, 178–185
citizenship manual, dilemma of 116
citizenship map, in regard to responsibility 107
citizenship measure
  capturing elements of citizenship 102
  items to include in 98
  scores on positively associated with scores on quality of life 101
citizenship model 164, 198–199
citizenship-oriented care 117
  bringing into individual treatment 186
  centered in individual treatment teams 160
  under "citizenship-oriented systems of care," 189
  developing, xiii 116

dilemma suggested by 116
focus groups 161–166
integrated with the clinical work of teams 188
most formidable barrier to 175
notion of, xv 40
pilot projects 187
reflected in the mental health system of care 196
working principles for 160
citizenship-oriented planning processes 199
citizenship-oriented systems of care, toward a model of 192–199
citizenship-oriented work, happening "undercover," 122
citizenship program, starting 38
citizenship projects, varying with local constraints and opportunities 33
citizenship rights 12, 15
citizenship scores 100–101
citizenship statements 97
citizenship themes, dialectical pairs of 14
citizenship theory, of social justice 13
Citizens Project
  about citizenship, not about being antitreatment 40
  activities with 173
  aims of 19
  assessing students' progress toward full community membership 99
  becoming a small supportive community 71
  as being a "refuge," 92
  changes 63–70
  combining social activist elements with appeals to democratic ideals 34
  as a community-level intervention 39
  continued for more than a decade 63
  contradiction at the heart 77
  creating 36–45
  distinct from other group-based interventions 39
  evaluation of 31–34
  forcing into the strictures of a manual 123
  four-month intervention 40
  from four to six months 63–64
  giving a test run at a community-level approach 194
  going back to help people build on what they've got started 86
  having elements of both social activism and democratic ideals 193
  having one foot in the mental health system of care and the other in a mainstream world 195
  manual 116, 123–125, 185
  member of 171

Citizens Project (*Cont.*)
  mentors 44
  model not being locked into 185
  modified as it became a mini-community 194
  naming of 19
  nearly all-male domain 115
  Ned talking about 202
  negotiated its contradictions by being an
    enduring community 116
  not reporting on participant's status 40
  as one source of information and example 160
  ongoing 63–93
  peer work on 43
  porous nature of 195
  as a refuge or sanctuary 90
  as a replacement family 85
  representing 80
  straddling the margins and mainstreams of
    society 195
  student characteristics 69–70
  students excluded from full participation 195
  took up the second, individual-level approach
    194
  touched on the 5 Rs 34
  trial run at a community-level approach 34
civic-collective participation 14
civic consciousness, form of 129
civic education activities, associated with voting
  127
civic reintegration 36
"civic republican" model of citizenship 12
civil and legal rights 12
Civil Rights, Domain 4, 102
class instructors, for the Leadership Project 27
class rules, developing a set of 27
class topics, relationship with the main R
  addressed 124–125
Clayton, Ashley 122, 130, 179
"client," used instead of "patient", xv
clients
  identifying 205n2
  interest in voting and helping others get reg-
    istered 129
  interviewing those making citizenship progress
    166
  interviews with 167–173
  potential for harming themselves or others 164
  structure of services for working against rep-
    resentation 26
  working diligently to manage money 159
clinical care, incorporating discussion of financial matters into 150
clinical treatment, defined as addressing mental
  health symptoms, xiv
clinicians

"already doing," 122
  contributed to redefining criminals as mental
    patients 38
  encouraging to consider citizenship-oriented
    goals with clients 122
  interviewing those supporting clients' citizen-
    ship goals 166
  interviews with 167, 173–178
  viewing clients as people needing constant
    monitoring 121
clinicians and clinical teams, introduction of any
  new project or new mandate to 121
"clinician's illusion," falling prey to a variety
  of 78
Cole, Robert 118
Colomy, Paul 198
Columbus House 19–20, 27, 38
comfort zone, as a difficulty for many clients 174
"committed work," 137
communicative action, theory of 75
communities
  getting people engaged in 138
  introducing to each other 23
  of rather than in 188
  welcoming people in from its margins 19
community
  building 130–133, 178
  including animals and nature 172
  including sub-communities 55
  as morally neutral 187
  power of coming from people "having equal
    standing," 145
  providing a place to be in 105
  sense of connection with 93
  strong sense of 71
community action group
  community focus groups 187
  conducted a series of focus groups 141
  served as a think tank 139
community banks, offering low- or no-fee
  accounts 158
community barriers, types of 50
community-based participatory research (CBPR)
  95–96
community-based resources, understanding students' knowledge of 48
"community coalition," 21
"community connections," 134
community connections, contacts, and resources,
  linked directly to clinical teams 186
Community Council 19, 20, 21
community inclusion 114, 146
"community integration." *See* citizenship
community-level citizenship projects, ideas about
  future 32

community-level interventions, xvi
community members, most dependable 21
community recognition, of the previously
    excluded group's legitimacy 14
community release efforts, expanded 199
community resources and opportunities, building
    strong connections to 160
Community Soup Kitchen 39
community support systems 193
community valued role projects 43
"community within a community," 180
concept-mapping research design 95
concept-mapping sessions, treated as separate
    sub studies 96
concept-mapping software 97
concern, over risk to clients 165
"conditional citizenship," 117
confidentiality rule, in "What's Up?," 66–67
connectedness and social inclusion, importance
    of 162
Connecticut Department of Mental Health and
    Addiction Services (DMHAS) 38, 116, 187
Connecticut Mental Health Center, xiii
connection, geography of 142
conservator or representative payee mechanisms
    156
consistency, of care 182
"consolation community," 172
constituency groups, recruiting representatives
    from 20
consumer society, members of 154
Continuum of Care Committee, establishment
    of 25
"Continuum of Care" plan, localities to develop
    25
convergent validity 100
Copeland, Mary Ellen 42
core recovery themes 149
co-researcher team (CRT), recruiting an
    eight-member 96
core themes, of the *Citizenship Project*, 70–78
council members, trying to recruit strong 22
couples, in current relationship not allowed to
    join subsequent cohorts 52
course, of the *Citizens Project*, 41–43
"creaming," 30
criminal charges, changed criteria to 70
criminal histories, people with 36
criminal justice focus group 103
criminal justice system
    classes on 41
    keep clear of in the future 49
    link with citizenship and mental illness
    198
criminal record, having 50

critical mass, helping to make activities and com-
    munity building happen 145
"cultural competence," lesson in 25
cultural miscommunication, Lezley's caution
    against 137
culture as a "toolkit," 71
culture of citizenship 115
Cunningham, Alison 21
"customer satisfaction," promoting to replace a
    "last resort for the poor" reputation 118

Daniel (poet) 56
Dansinghani, Mary 123
Dante, wanted to join a running group 136
David, in the *Citizens Project*, 59
Davidson, Larry 15, 144
"deals," clients' vulnerability to 153
death, preparations for 104
deinstitutionalization 4, 15
democratic citizenship 13
dendrogram, arranging statistically significant
    clusters 98
Denise, as peer mentor 57
Denise (widow) 23
deprivation, fueling spending sprees 177
de Tocqueville, Alexis 12
developmental model, Marshall's 12
developmental phase 112
dignity, assaults on 107–108
disabilities, people with 13, 125–126
discriminant validity 100
discrimination
    against people with mental illnesses 102
    by potential employers' or property owners
    162
disincentives, to working 157–158
"diversity," 78
DMHAS. *See* Connecticut Department of
    Mental Health and Addiction Services
    (DMHAS)
domain map 105–106
door, opening into a new life 83
Double Trouble in Recovery (DTR) 68
Downtown Evening Soup Kitchen 5
drugs, street culture of 46
drug use, decreased exacerbating symptoms 61
Duffy, Simon 13
Durkheim, Emile 12E
Ed, stock trader 136–137, 138, 200–201
Edgley, Alison 16
education, importance of students understand-
    ing of the training material 28
effective citizenship, enhancing 13
electronic clearinghouse, creating a shared
    139

Ellen, focus group attendee 141–142, 145, 146–147
empathy
  for the struggles of others 112
  teaching a class on 55
employment and housing, focus group issues 111–112
end-of-course interviews, not conducted 48
engagement, ACA advancing the notion of, xiv
enjoying time, spent with others 73
entitlement programs, class on 42
entry, involving inclusion in the decision-making process 149
Erikson, Kai 1, 7
"essential client," 20
ethnicity, of *Citizens Project* students, 69
European Union nations, social inclusion among 17
European view, of poverty 17
evaluation, with participant observation 21
everyone, citizenship directed toward 120
everyone speaks rule, in "What's Up?," 67
exit, plan for "release" or staged release 149

face-to-face meetings, supporting students in 44
"failing," as a catalyst growth, or community building 55
"Fake it 'til you make it," 169
"fallacy of comparison," 68
family, as important to John 85
family members, as primary relationships 171
family reunions, desired by John 85
Farmer, Paul 122
FBI 200–201
federal prisons, inmates in 35
feedback, characteristics of 68
Feeling Good with the Blues seminar, 57
felony conviction, stigma accompanying 108
female clients, drawing from a much larger group 69
finances, control of as an intolerable constraint 156
"financial capability," 150, 151
financial health 148, 187
  citizenship and 158–159
  growing field of 151
  research and scholarly literature on 150
financial services, using formal 156–157
financial tools and services, in the New Haven area 151
finishing, something of value to the person 72
Fisk, Deborah (Debbie) 43, 56, 200
5 Rs (rights, responsibilities, roles, resources, and relationships) 193
  asking people about 86

centrality of 119–120
of citizenship 41, 47
of citizenship in Ned's words 203
Citizens touched on, 34
connection to 14
in definition of citizenship 39
having to stick people deep 169
linking to distinct program components in the *Citizens Project*, 94
"flourishing," 203
focus, on simply keeping clients alive 175
focus groups 96–97
  with clients who reported having money problems 151
  with clinicians and direct care staff on finances of clients 151–152
  connecting clients of the mental health center outside the mental health center 141
  treated separate as separate sub studies 96
focus group transcripts 102–105
focusing on yourself rule, in "What's Up?," 67
focus on feedback, keeping on the person who just spoke 68
food pantries, depending on 153
food stamps 6, 153
forensic assertive community treatment (FACT) 38
"forensic peer staff," in prerelease and re-entry programs 198
"forensic peer work," 44
formal citizenship 12
forward movement diminished 115
freedom, to keep one's private life private 143
"free" job training problems, betrayed by 109
"functionings," people's 18
funding cuts, cynicism about 181

Gambino, Matthew 13, 219n1
gap, between citizenship theory and practice 94
gatekeeping organizations 4
"gateway act," 126
geese, community of 93
gender, of *Citizens Project* students, 69
"generalizability," of the citizenship framework 191
geography, standing in the way of connection 142
giving back 107, 112
Glide, "spiritual movement," 180
God
  gave Rita kids 87
  showing the way 83
Goffman, Erving 13, 198
Goldman, Howard 193
"go to the source," 95

Government and Infrastructure, Domain 2, 102
graduation, from the *Citizens Project*, 44–45, 58
group, fostering a strong and supportive 41
group-based intervention, choosing 39
group component, of the *Citizens Project*, 40–41
group identity, encouragement of 30
group rules and norms, students developing 41
group treatment experience 110
guide, compared to a manual 123–124
Gutierrez, Lorraine 29–30
Guy, Kimberly 119, 123

Habermas, Jurgen 75
Harp, Toni 82, 128
Harper, Annie 83, 149–150, 159, 183
health, taking care of 169
health care, changing in the United States, xiv
healthy alternatives, class on 42
help, isn't always helpful 109
helping others 92–93, 107
Herring, Yolanda 119
hierarchical cluster analysis, performing 98
hierarchy, differentiating the need for 197
"higher power" language 73
HIV/AIDS prevention class 42
home care 181–183
homeless community, isolation from peers in 10
homeless encounters, involving instrumental
    elements 5
homelessness
    definitions of 7
    depending on how you define it 200
    link between instrumental and affective ele-
        ments of exiting 111
    looking more like home than an apartment 10
    otherness to the experience of 1
    oversimplification of 192
    required less responsibility 107
    satisfaction of being able to survive it 6
homeless outreach 3, 193
homeless people
    attuned to in-the-moment meanings 112
    idea of a book written by 22–24
Homeless Survivors group 168
home visits, to patients 177
Honneth, Alex 14, 73, 119
Hopper, Kim 16, 105, 137
"housed community," sympathetic hearing from
    94
"housed person," identity of being a 6
housing
    barriers to 111
    community inclusion classes and 42
    employment programs and 112
    worries associated with 6

Housing and Urban Development programs,
    funding approach for 25
humans, suffering 92
hybrid community system 197
hybrid status, leap to 196

ideal-future model 196
identity theory 15
identity transactions, understanding 7
"identity work," 30
Illness Management and Recovery (IMR) 38,
    114
impulse spending, avoiding 153
inadequate income. *See also* poverty, resulting in
    a struggle to meet basic needs, 150
inclusion
    based on a disability paradigm 17
    beginning with respect and belonging 120
    dilemma of 148
    European policies to promote 17–18
    importance of 147
income and goods, not adequate measures of
    "well-being," 18
individual efforts, encouragement of 30
individuality, outward expressions of 105
individual rights and freedom, paired 14
individuals, supporting the citizenship of 33
individual snapshots, of students 58
individual therapy 164
individual valued role projects 56
informal economy, opportunities in 153
institutionalized clients 182
integrated mental health system of care 196, 197
integrated systems of care, ideal of 192
interaction, shared values in 72–73
interactional rights and obligations, study of
    198
interaction order, microanalysis of 198
Interagency Council on Homelessness 18
interests, helping people identify 135
interests in common, importance of having
    143–144
internal consistency 100
internships
    beginning before the end of the class period 30
    for graduates 28
    sponsoring 27
interventions
    expanded from four to six months 64
    freestanding helping two dozen or so people
        a year 95
    for individuals 94
    with Jennie 21
    length of 63
    as a mini-community theme 71–72

interventions (*Cont.*)
  proposal to develop and evaluate financial services and supports 159
  in systems of care and local communities 190
interviews
  with clients 167–173
  with clinicians 173–178
  results of 101–102
  with students 48
  with students of *Citizens Project*, 78–93
intimate partner violence, in some clients' lives 182
intimate relationships class 42
invitation 142–143
involuntary interventions, attention to entry, process, and exit in regard to 149
iterative learning-and-action process 189

Jacobs, Jane 143, 172
jail diversion 35, 37
jail diversion clients 70
jail diversion response 38
jail time, substituting for mental health care 38
James, focus group attendee 141, 143, 147
Janoski, Thomas 12, 15
Jennie (poet) 21
Jessica 52, 54
Jill (arrested for recycling) 37
Jim
  citizenship foundation story of 124
  getting in touch with 200–201
  story of 43
Jobs, Steve 185
jobs and education classes 42
jobs project, networking and planning for 24–25
Joe, community for valued role project 55
John *Citizens Project* student, 80, 83–85
Jonathan 53
Joseph
  fascinated with idea of stock trading 136–137
  ready to make the next contact 138
judges, using incarceration to contain and ensure treatment for defendants 35

K2, smoking 93
Kant, Immanuel 73
Kathy
  client interview 167, 170–173
  handling finances 155–156
Kelvin (self-destructive) 23
kindness, small acts of 171
knowledge, created in collaboration 95–96

latent citizenship 90
Latin Chiefs 78–79

Laub, Dori 8
Laura, focus group attendee 141, 143–145, 147
Lawless, Martha 182
leadership, initial classes on 27
Leadership Project
  considering funding needed for ongoing support 31
  creation of 25
  major shortcoming of 29
  not measuring changes in levels of stress 30
  recruiting students for 27
  as a start 33
learning, giving people a place for 203
legal aspect, of citizenship 94
legal critique, of citizenship, xiii
legal issues class 41
legal rights, included right to fair treatment 103
Legal Rights, Domain 5, 102
Lehman's Quality of Life Scale, 100
letter writing, to persons helping in their recovery and community living 55
Lezley. *See* TwoBears, Lezley
"liberal state" model, of citizenship 12
life, building a new 85
life changes, socially positive associated with anxiety and agitation 61
life changing experience, natural to divide life into a before and after 81
life disruptions, categories broadly defined 99
life "disruption" theory 95
life interruptions, removing them from mainstream for long periods of time 109
"life in the community"
  ideal of 117
  for people with mental illness 190
  relationship and connectedness strongest elements of 173
  supporting 132
lifeworld, penetrating the system 191
linear regression models, determining total amount of variance 101
listening first, and then giving feedback 68
Lister, Ruth 13
"literal" homelessness 7
Liz, psychologist in training 56
local communities, supporting clients' place and participation in 117
local mental health authorities (LMHAs) 192
love of dogs, connecting Kathy with people 172
lower income people, showing greater concern and compassion for the suffering of others 112
Lucile 128
luxury, desire for 155, 184

Mackay, Kathryn 117
Madelon. *See* Baranoski, Madelon
mainstream society, with associational life and
systems of health and social care 195
mainstream status, with citizenship rights and
obligations 14
Mandiberg, Jim 197
manual
after 12 years 185
development for the *Citizens Project*, 123–125
writing a detailed for the *Citizens Project*, 116
Manuel 53
"maps" or visual representations, of data collected 95
Marc, interest in kayaking 136
marginalization, accepting or applying for goods
and services bringing to light 6
marginalized status and membership with
restricted rights and obligations 14
margins of society, occupants of 195
Maria. *See* O'Connell, Maria
Marshall, Thomas 12
Maruna, Shadd 205n1
Masterson, Sheila 21
master status 13
material means, people needing 14
Mattison, Alice 23, 53
Mattison, Edward 21
McKnight, John 134
McMahon, Linda 127
measure of citizenship, 12-item version of 161
measure validation, as process as much as product 100
medical care, access to 103
Melissa, visiting nurse 179, 181
Melville Charitable Trust 19, 22
men, outnumbering women in *Citizens Project*,
69
mental health, citizenship and 14–19
mental health agency, accepting responsibility
for providing treatment 35
mental health care
increased access to, xiv
as multifaceted work 177
not providing clients with an entrée to a full
membership and participation in the community 15
mental health center
as a community 138, 172
people arriving at in crisis 175
providing leadership, clinical care, and case
management 4–5
reasons for bringing citizenship into 118
mental health community, difficulty breaking
out of 174

mental health outreach, to people who are
homeless, xiii
mental health reform, recurring historical cycles
of 199
mental health stigma, as preventing finding work
50
mental health symptoms, helping people manage
their 38
mental health system
clients too comfortable in 163
not supporting social inclusion of its clients
197
mental health systems of care
forms of 192
limits of all 193
occupying a marginal space in society 195
mental illnesses
of *Citizens Project* students, 69–70
energy required to deal with people with 147
few people with dangerous or violent 146
hearing from people with on citizenship ideas
and aspiration 95
only one aspect of a person's life 16
people with 36, 146
mental or physical health, making it difficult to
follow through with connections 137
"mental patient," taking on the title of 5
mentorship, relational process of 43
"microaggressions," conference devoted in part
to 123
micro-interactional level, in communities and
associational life 198
Miller, Rebecca 139
"model," 191
Model Cities programs, in the 1960s 4
"model" figure 191
model of citizenship and mental health, making
certain assumptions 190
modern business management techniques, pioneered by slave owners in the 1800s 122
money
it's all about 185
logistics of managing 156
paid to attend *Citizens Project*, 74
triggering impulses 154
money management, usually involving coercion
148
moral code, strong 90
moral failures, of Nicholas' parents 91
Morris, Christa 201, 204
Morrissey, Joseph 193
Mouffe, Chantal 14
Moynihan, Donald 198
multidimensional scaling analysis 97–98
Murphy, Chris 127

mutual disconnection, among neighbors and community members 143
mutual group support, creating right conditions for developing 30

names, changing in this book for people 205n2
Nancy (brush with the law) 55
Nathan 201–202
natural associations 198
"naturally occurring" communities 186
Ned 45–47, 201–204
negative personal attitudes, changing 49
negativity, sense of 46
neighborhood, residents' identification with their 140
neighborhood leaders, "giving back" to 140
New Haven community, social and economic borders of 5
New Haven outreach team 4
"new homelessness," of the late 1970s and early 1980s 3
"new person," emerged from thousands of years 72
Nicholas *Citizens Project* student, 89–93
Nisbet, Robert 72
"no cross-talking" rule, in "What's Up?," 67–68
Noordsy, Douglas 148–149
"Now what?" question 77

O'Connell, Maria 95, 105
"off-timedness" theory 95
Ohmer, Mary 140
Oliver, wanted to join a book club 135
Olsen, Steve 135, 139
"ontological security," 90
"other side of the coin" connection 100
out-of-the-mainstream location, in poor sections of town 5
Outreach, doing its work "Outside Society" in the ideal-future model 196
outreach teams
  limitations of 9
  price of accepting services from 6
  tied to local mental health system of care 192
outreach work 192–193, 194–195, 194f
  citizenship roots in 1–11
  by Jim 1–3
  not the answer to community inclusion 9
outreach workers
  ability to support a life in the community 10
  bringing a wide range of services 192
  connecting with Jim 3
  growing awareness of the limit of their help 11
  helping people remain in housing 11
  leaving their offices for the streets 3–4

social encounters with people who were homeless 5
  trying to keep the focus on what they can do 11
"Outside Society," heading 194, 194f
"overqualification," as a code term 111
overqualified people, competing for the same low-wage jobs 111
ownership, importance of 104

pardons process 123
parents, sins of, imparting a special hurt 91
participation
  elements of 14
  rights 12
participatory budgeting (PB), as a democratic process 130
Participatory Budgeting Project 130
partisanship, avoiding appearance of 127
paternalism, toward interns 30
pathways, for achieving citizenship 193
patient advocacy class 41
Patty. *See* Benedict, Patty
Paul, focus group attendee 141, 142, 145, 146, 147–148
payees, reliable hard to find 150
Pedersen, Kyle 118, 149–150
Peer Engagement Specialist Project 43
peer mentor component
  of *Citizens Project*, 75
  growing pains 58
peer mentors
  backgrounds of 56
  hiring, training, and work of 125
peer mentor support, increased 60
peer mentor work 44
peers
  coming in many forms 184
  as staff in mental health care 43
peer specialists, motivating people unengaged in treatment 43
peer staff, valuable resource for one-to-one counseling with clients 158
peer-staffed recovery centers, freestanding 118
peer-to-peer work, in self-help groups 43
peer workers, making contact with and persuading people "unengaged" in care to accept it 3
Peggy. *See* Bailey, Peggy
people, bringing together 146
People's Center 20
people with disabilities 13, 125–126
personal agency, exercise of 19
personal barriers, types of 50
personal capacities, central to achievement of social inclusion 17

personalities, shifting 53
personality mismatches, of peer mentors and students 58
"personalization," by "users" 13
personal readiness, allowing for 80
Personal Responsibilities: Domain 1, 102
personal responsibility and empowerment, classes in 42
personal stories, having to tell over and over again 108
persons with mental illness, self-sustaining social and economic enclaves of 197
person-to-person connection, tension with bureaucratic distinctions of "helper" and "the one helped," xv
person-to-person work, with people who are socially excluded 137
Peter, ham radio interest 52, 135
photo I.D. cards, clients not having 126
place, possibilities of 76–77
planning efforts, key themes from 119–123
pluralistic democracy, attention to marginalized groups 14
poetry reading, for people with traumatic brain injuries 56
Police Academy Presentation 52–53
police-in-training, explaining homelessness to 52
policy changes, impact on the development of citizenship-oriented system of care 190
political rights 12
politics 12
Ponce, Allison 105, 120, 121–122, 205n1
Portis, Edward 104
post-graduation support, after the *Citizens Project*, 59–60
poverty
    coping strategies 153–154
    intensity of 152–153
    interconnection with mental illness 150
    lack of upward mobility and 70
    US view of 17
"power-based" model 33
powerlessness
    to achieve future goals 109
    of clinical staff 176
    sense of 183
practice and evaluation, stages of, xiii
predictors, examining 101
pre-existing conditions, disallowing for denying coverage, xiv
"premodel" figure 191, 194, 194f
prerelease citizenship programs 199
present, staying in 88
price, of a loss of privacy or of anonymity 5
problems, posed by clinicians 166

process, including training in handling of finances 149
"process logs," weekly 21–22
"program citizenship," 116, 117, 118
Program for Recovery and Community Health (PRCH), peer staff member in 68
Project Connect, community connections and citizenship-oriented care, 134–141
Project Friendship, in Prince George, British Columbia, 134
pro-recovery (PR), versus anti-recovery (AR) 16–17
psychiatry's role, via mental institutions 13
public mental health institutions, providing a bare bones social world 117
public speaking 47, 71–72
public speaking classes 28, 42, 64
public speech, giving a successful 65

"qualitative" research, in context of larger "quantitative" studies 148
"quality of life crimes," 61

R. *See also* 5 Rs (rights, responsibilities, roles, resources, and relationships)
    of legal, civil, and social rights 119
    of relationship 115
race, in relation to citizenship 122
race and ethnicity, of *Citizens Project* students, 69
Rachel, primary care physician 179–180
racism and racial profiling 102
radical individualism, American culture of 12–13
randomized controlled trial (RCT)
    of the *Citizens Project*, 60–62
    of peer specialists 43
rapid-fire exchanges, on the street leading to devastating outcomes 68
"rationalization of the world," 191
readiness, for change 79
"real community," definition of 143
recipient-doer dilemma, in mental health field 18
recognition
    concept of 119
    involving immediate mutual acknowledgement 73
recovery 15–17
Recovery Markers Questionnaire-Revised, 100
recovery movement, top-down 121
recovery-oriented care 117, 118
    lesson from 120–122
recovery-related interventions 118
relationship-building class 42
relationships
    classes 42

relationships (*Cont.*)
  delaying new social networks and social
    "moments," 11
  developing and maintaining a variety of 69
  with fellow students and with fellow board
    members 34
  as first-named R 179
religion and spirituality 73–74
religion rights, in a mental health facility 170
religious beliefs and spirituality, connecting with
  74
rescue animals, house full of 172
research, qualitative and quantitative 217n12
resources
  5 Rs tied up with 180
  links among 177
  at the mental health center 176
  offered by clinicians 166
  represented modestly work experience 34
  sharing information on community 69
respect, being treated with 173
"respect" R, needed for the other Rs to work
  119–120
responsibilities
  classes on 41
  of John 84
  roles defined by 180
responsibility
  biggest to myself 169, 171
  of giving back and helping others 104
  meaning different things in different contexts
    107
  meaning reaching out to those in similar cir-
    cumstances 84
  practicing 69
  required people to accept 34
  taking 86
results, of interviews 101–102
reverse encroachment 191
"reverse" questions, about the meaning of each
  of 5 Rs 129
Reyes, Tomas 126, 128
rights
  applying to a broader range of issues 104
  classes on the criminal justice system 41
  if arrested 50
  as members of a voluntary community 69
  of people to be represented 34
  in relation citizenship 82
risk, kinds and levels of 143
risk assessment, vicious circle of 164–165
Rita *Citizens Project* student, 85–89
rites of passage 44, 76, 205n1
Robert, peer mentor 46, 57
rocking, back and forth in staff meetings 56

Roe, David 15
role model, for the next generation 103–104
role model, mentor, or messenger, saying something at the right time 168
roles
  being a board member 34
  defined by responsibilities 180
  examining 69
roles and resources, five classes grouped under 42
rolling enrollment, undermining the logical flow
  of classes 115
Ron (breach of the peace) 37
Ron (peer outreach worker) 43
Rosen, Marc 148
Rosenthal, Caitlin 122
Rs. *See also* 5 Rs (rights, responsibilities, roles,
  resources, and relationships), overlap
  among, 41
Russian roulette, playing 89

sabotaging success, class on 41
safe haven *Citizens Project* as, 81–82
safety, as a prominent theme 163
Salvation Army shelter, not qualifying as an
  emergency shelter 213n53
SAMHSA. *See* Substance Abuse and Mental
  Health Services Administration (SAMHSA)
Sandra, wanted to join a needlepoint group 135
Sandy, in the *Citizens Project*, 58–59
San Francisco, characteristics of 180
savings, concept of 176
schizophrenia, recovery from 15
school, Rita going back to 87–88
Schwartz, David 191
"screening off," constant influx of data in
  modern life 90
secondary institutions, as buffers between
  the individual and the state 12
second chance 79, 162
self-advocacy 173
self-defeating attitudes, students bringing with
  them 88
self-esteem, not achieved in isolation 14
self-help groups, strengths and drawbacks of 42
self-inventory, of one's personal citizenship 120
"self-medication" theory 61
self-respect, cannot be achieved in isolation 14
Sells, David 43
Sen, Amartya 18
"sense of belonging." *See* citizenship
The Sense of Community Index II, 100
Sernyak, Michael 126, 130, 197
service obligations, to the state 12
service providers, used to running programs 32
seven-cluster domain "solution," 98

shadow citizenship, homelessness conferring 11
sharing value 73
Shelter Plus 86
Silver, Hilary 17
skill and citizenship building, as a theme 71–72
small community, feel and character of 78
social and economic rights, to health care, education, and welfare 12
social and political theory, citizenship in 12
social beings, people as 104
Social Capital Scale, 100
social capital theory, focus on developing personal networks 15
social commitment, as a universal quality in human affairs 104
social connectedness 15, 162
social connection and community, high standards for 143
social inclusion 17–18, 198. *See also* citizenship
social integration 110
social isolation, as a trigger for psychosis 9
social justice theory, paying little attention to needs of people with disabilities 13
socially positive life changes, associated with anxiety and agitation 61
'socially solvent,' 180
social networks, involving strategic help 138
social policies, impact of 198
social recovery 15–16, 149, 197
social service organizations, taking advantage 109
social service programs, ill treatment of clients by staff members of 108
social service providers, contacts with 31
social work, building on a grand tradition 199
social zones, taking first step outside 138
socioeconomic subcommunities, offering promise 197
something to do, keeping you going 73
specialized interests, connecting people with 136
specificity, of capabilities theory 19
"speech community," 75
speeches
    emphasis on 64
    powerful impact on students 65
speech rules, agreed-upon 75
Spell, Stacy 141
spending sprees 178
Spiritual Roundtable 123
SPSS statistical software, analyzing data from 110 interviews 100–102
SSI (Supplemental Security Income) 18
SSI disability income, accepting 6
stability, assumed 190
Stacy 48, 49, 50, 52

stand-alone citizenship intervention, continuing to exist 196
stardom, pressures of 85
state, giving legal sanction to citizenship norms 12
state mental health authority 192
statements, sorting and rating of 97
state prisons, inmates in 35
statistical analysis 97–99
statistical validation study 100–102
"staying in school," importance of 51
Staying in School projects 51–52
St. Elizabeth, as a fieldwork site for theory, 13 ?
Stollar, Jennifer 112
stigma
    associated with incarceration, homelessness, and mental illness 109
    attached to homelessness 6
    attached to mental illness 162
    available everywhere 180
    as a barrier 174
    of having a felony conviction 108
    mental health 50
"street speech," with its different considerations 76
stress and anger management classes 42
structured support, needed beyond the *Citizens Project*, 78
struggles, ongoing 59
students
    in citizenship intervention 61
    designing individual and group projects 43
    interviews conducted with students of *Citizens Project*, 78–93
    receiving individual and group "wraparound" peer mentor support 40
    value of being 72
study participants, including people with life disruptions 96
sub-communities 55
sub-groups, marginalized even within already-marginalized communities 180
Substance Abuse and Mental Health Services Administration (SAMHSA) 4
    ACCESS program 193
    definition of homelessness 7
    push for peer support work 43
substance abuse disorders, co-occurring existing 36
substance use, of *Citizens Project* students, 69–70
substantive citizenship 12
Sue, Derald 123
Supplemental Security Income (SSI) 6, 18
supported employment 38

survey instrument, measuring individual achievement of citizenship, xvi
Suzanne, psychiatrist 174, 176–178
Swidler, Ann 71
system encroachment, on the various forms of associational life 191
system integration theory 4, 181
"systems," 191
systems integration 4, 192

Ted 145, 146
Thanksgiving dinner, as a valued role project 55
themes
    from citizenship-oriented care focus groups 161–166
    of the *Citizenship Project*, 70–78
    core recovery 149
    dialectical pairs of citizenship 14
    from focus groups on finances 152
    from planning efforts 119–123
    skill and citizenship building 71–72
    time pervasive in focus groups 109–111
Theresa, patient 181–183
tightly coupled systems 220n8
Tim, as peer mentor 56–57
time
    as a pervasive theme of focus groups 109–111
    spending so much surviving 73
Tocquevillian-Durkheimian tradition 14–15
Tom, guide for all things homeless 72–73
tool-kit idea, as exemplified in classes 71
"total institutions," 13
"tough love," working when coming from peers 44
tragedies, endured by Peggy 20
transition, to a focus on action and tangible projects 186
"transitional" housing 7
treatment plan, concept of recovery-oriented, person-centered 175
"treatment system and community living" character, of public mental health 190
treatment team, focus group with 165
trust relationships, development of in the group 65
2012 Voter Registration Campaign 126–128
TwoBears, Lezley 10–11, 20, 21, 22, 23, 24–25, 33, 38, 45, 52, 66, 86, 114–115, 137

Uggen, Christopher 36
"underclass" status 14
underworld, of non-regulated relationships and care in mental health organizations and systems 191–192

undocumented Latino immigrants, providing care to, xiv
"unfunded mandate," not being an 121
US Army Special Forces, dream of joining 91
utility bills 153–154

validation 99, 100
validation studies 99–113
valued role, being a student as 72
valued role projects 47
    as most challenging part of the citizenship intervention 51–56
    as new territory 66
    process and elements of creating and delivering 125
values, different in a community with different characteristics 180
variance 101
veterans, excluded from the measure development process 99
violence, need for protection from it 103
visual means, representing what we mean by citizenship and the 5 Rs 119
voter registration 125–130
    as challenge for mental health centers 129
    infrastructure development 128–130
    linked with *Collaborative*'s work, 185, 186
voting, as a right for people with mental illnesses 126
Voting Rights Act of 1993, 125

Ware, Norma 15, 105
War on Poverty programs 192
"war stories" glamorizing addiction, banned 67
"way station" metaphor 72
"weak ties," benefits of 143
"weathering hypothesis," 122
Weber, Max 191
Weingarten, Richard 21
Weiss, Janet 181
welfare agencies, encouraging dependency 117
"welfare dependents," 117
"wellbeing deprivation," 19
"wellbeing freedom," 18
Wellness Recovery Action Plan* 42
Wendy, clinician 174–176
Werbner, Pnina 13
West River Neighborhood Association 140, 187
"What comes next?," 59
"What's Up?"
    compared to other self-help groups 68
    evolved to become a core component of the *Citizens Project*, 65–69
    occupying the center of the project 115
    origins of 66

"What's Up?" (*Cont.*)
  rules structuring 66–69
  speech in 75
"what's up?" discussion, starting citizenship
    meetings 47
Whitley, Rob 118
Wichowsky, Amber 198
Williamson, Bridgett 139
Wiseman, Jacqueline 116–117
work
  competition for 111
  disincentives to 157–158
  importance of 164
  issue of looking for 110
  raising sense of self worth 174

work groups, addressing overarching mission
    123
working hypotheses, for *Citizens*, 22
workplace, being discriminated against
    108–109
world, being able to be out in 203
World Stewardship, as most possible to achieve
    107
World Stewardship, Domain 7, 103

Yale Art Gallery 119
Yale Center for British Art 119
Yale Institution for Social and Policy Studies
    60
Yuval-Davis, Nira 13